Healthy Calendar
Diabetic Cooking

Lara Rondinelli, RD, LDN, CDE and
Chef Jennifer Bucko

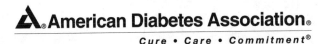

American Diabetes Association

Cure • Care • Commitment®

Director, Book Publishing, John Fedor; *Associate Director, Consumer Books,* Sherrye Landrum; *Editor,* Laurie Guffey; *Associate Director, Book Production,* Peggy M. Rote; *Composition,* Circle Graphics; *Cover Design,* Kathy Tresnak, Koncept, Inc.; *Interior photographs: Photographer,* John Burwell, Burwell & Burwell Photography; *Set Stylist,* Claudia Burwell; *Food Stylist,* Lisa Cherkasky; *Printer,* Port City Press, Inc.

Printed in the United States of America
1 3 5 7 9 10 8 6 4 2

The suggestions and information contained in this publication are generally consistent with the *Clinical Practice Recommendations* and other policies of the American Diabetes Association, but they do not represent the policy or position of the Association or any of its boards or committees. Reasonable steps have been taken to ensure the accuracy of the information presented. However, the American Diabetes Association cannot ensure the safety or efficacy of any product or service described in this publication. Individuals are advised to consult a physician or other appropriate health care professional before undertaking any diet or exercise program or taking any medication referred to in this publication. Professionals must use and apply their own professional judgment, experience, and training and should not rely solely on the information contained in this publication before prescribing any diet, exercise, or medication. The American Diabetes Association—its officers, directors, employees, volunteers, and members—assumes no responsibility or liability for personal or other injury, loss, or damage that may result from the suggestions or information in this publication.

⊚ The paper in this publication meets the requirements of the ANSI Standard Z39.48-1992 (permanence of paper).

ADA titles may be purchased for business or promotional use or for special sales. To purchase this book in large quantities, or for custom editions of this book with your logo, contact Lee Romano Sequeira, Special Sales & Promotions, at the address below, or at LRomano@ diabetes.org or 703-299-2046.

American Diabetes Association
1701 North Beauregard Street
Alexandria, Virginia 22311

Library of Congress Cataloging-in-Publication Data
Bucko, Jennifer, 1974–
    Healthy calendar diabetic cooking / Jennifer Bucko, Lara Rondinelli.
        p. cm.
    Includes index.
    ISBN 1-58040-160-0 (pbk. : alk. paper)
        1. Diabetes—Diet therapy—Recipes. 2. Menus. I. Rondinelli, Lara M. 1974– II. Title.

RC662.B82 2004
641.5′6314—dc22   2004057548

❖ Contents ❖

❖ Acknowledgments ❖

This book surely would not have been possible had it not been for my co-author and lifelong best friend, Lara Rondinelli. Lara, your knowledge and experience made this book what it is and continuously inspire me to be healthy; and your unconditional friendship inspires me to be a better person. This book started as a dream and became our reality, and I wouldn't want to share this experience with anyone else. Thanks for always being there for me and for being such a great best friend. What would I do without you?

I want to thank my family of amazing chefs, especially my mom, Judy Bucko, for constantly inspiring me to follow my dreams, do what I love, and make a killer pot of soup. Mom, you are the reason I'm the woman I am today. To my entire family: Jill, Rob, Kate, and Erin Kilhefner; Jane, Mike, Gabrielle, and Camille DiMartin; Jackie, Patrick, Penny, and Ella Burke; and Jim, Paula, and Lily Bucko, thank you for your constant support, your outstanding recipe ideas, your feedback, and your senses of humor . . . all of which I couldn't have survived this project without. And to my dad, Jack Bucko, who would have loved this book. Dad, I wish you could have been here to see and experience all of this.

To all of our friends who acted as our official taste-testers at our Cookbook Taste Testing Parties: you guys made this project even more fun than it already was. Thanks for all of the great bottles of wine. Thank you to Chris Janos, who tasted our very first dish and to Elizabeth Mills for some great recipe ideas. To Draga and Rodney Beckner, Jenny and Josh Jacobs, and Jenny and Dan Jaworski, thanks for always being there for us and letting us try out our recipes on you.

To all my friends from NFA, especially Larry Dyekman, Laura Oatney, Mary Alice Patton, Deborah and Mark Loehrke, Heather Cook, Audrey West, and Julie Sick, thanks for being such outstanding cheerleaders through culinary school and this project. Thank you to my culinary school instructors at the Cooking and Hospitality Institute of Chicago for inspiring me to do great things and to my co-chefs-in-training for the laughs, support, and inspiration, especially Lisa Larson, Theresa Gaither, Rhonda Kottke, Todd Ronna, Greg Barwick, and Greg Kolacinski, the original CHIC crew.

Thank you to everyone at the American Diabetes Association, especially John Fedor, Director of Book Publishing, for your support, belief in us, and words of wisdom. Thank you to our outstanding ADA editor, Laurie Guffey, for your talent, expertise, and optimism about this book, and to Madelyn Wheeler, for your unbelievable dedication in completing the nutrition analysis of the recipes. Thank you for making our dream come true.

Finally, I would like to thank Jilly. If our paths hadn't crossed, this book may never have happened.

— Jennifer Bucko

I would like to thank my parents for supporting me throughout all the stages in my life this far and for raising me to pursue my dreams. This book was a dream that became a reality with the help of many people!

Thank you to my coauthor and best friend of 18 years, Jennifer Bucko, for making this project fun, as well as offering your creative expertise in cooking and journalism. I learned so much from you, and I couldn't have done this book with anyone else. I would like to thank my sister, Jennifer Sebring, for trying so many of the recipes on her family, along with providing much feedback and enthusiasm for this book. Also, thank you to my mother, Jane Rondinelli, and my sister, Kari Mender, and other family members who gave us their delicious recipes to recreate.

The making of this cookbook created great memories that I will cherish forever, and I thank everyone involved. Thank you to the many wonderful people in my life who shared in my excitement and this experience. Thank you for your support, feedback, marketing, and attendance at our cookbook taste-testing events.

This book wouldn't have been possible without the efforts of many people at the American Diabetes Association. A very big thanks goes to John Fedor, Director of Book Publishing, for seeing the potential and for believing in our idea and us at the earliest stage. You were a key factor in making this book a reality, and I thank you. Thank you to our wonderful ADA editor, Laurie Guffey, for your expertise and dedication to this project, and Madelyn Wheeler for your diligent completion of the nutrition analysis of the recipes—you both were a joy to work with.

Finally, thank you to all my patients with diabetes who gave me the idea to write this book. I hope this makes your life with diabetes a little easier and healthier.

— Lara Rondinelli, RD, LDN, CDE

January

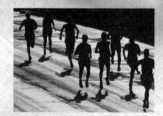

Put those New Year's resolutions to good work! You don't have to become a marathon runner—just get a little exercise each day. You don't have to change everything about how you eat all at once— just make some small changes now. Start with some of this month's recipes!

A Fresh Start

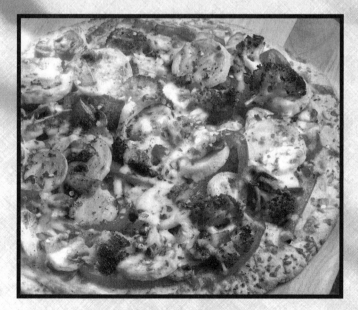

Veggie Pizza (page 48)
You can add almost any veggie you like to this healthy, satisfying pizza and it will taste delicious! Have a pizza party and let your guests make their own pizzas.

January ❖ Recipes

RECIPE LIST

DAY 1: Sloppy Joes **4**
Corn Salad **5**

DAY 2: Spinach and Mushroom Pizza **6**

DAY 3: Tangy Apricot-Glazed Pork
Tenderloin **7**
Lucky Black-Eyed Peas **8**

DAY 4: Peanut-Crusted Cod **9**

DAY 5: Tortellini Soup **10**

GROCERY LIST

Fresh Produce
Onions – 2
Garlic – 1 head
Green bell pepper – 3
Red onion – 1
Red bell pepper – 2
Fresh basil – 1 bunch
Spinach – 1 bunch
Mushrooms – 1 pint

Meat/Poultry/Fish
Lean ground beef –
1 pound
Pork tenderloin –
1 pound
Cod filets – 4 (4-ounce)
filets
Lean Italian turkey
sausage – 1 package
(about 4–5 links)

Grains/Bread/Pasta
Whole-wheat hamburger
buns – 6 buns
Prepackaged 12-inch
pizza crust – 1

Dairy and Cheese
Shredded, reduced-fat
mozzarella cheese –
1 bag
9-ounce package three-
cheese tortellini –
1 package
Eggs
Margarine

Canned Goods
and Sauces
8-ounce can tomato
sauce – 1 can
15-ounce can no-salt-
added diced
tomatoes – 2 cans
Light sugar-free apricot
preserves – 1 jar
15.5-ounce can black-
eyed peas – 2 cans
14.5-ounce can fat-free,
reduced-sodium
chicken broth – 3 cans

Frozen Foods
Corn – 1 bag

Staples/Seasonings/
Baking Needs
Salt/ground black pepper
Cooking spray
Yellow mustard
Worcestershire sauce
Balsamic vinegar
Olive oil
Dried basil
Dried oregano
Dried sage
Dried thyme
Crushed red pepper
flakes
All-purpose flour
Cayenne pepper
Apple cider vinegar

Miscellaneous
Red wine
Unsalted peanuts –
small jar

Sloppy Joes

1 pound lean ground beef
1/2 cup diced onions
2 garlic cloves, minced
8-ounce can tomato sauce
1/2 cup water
1 cup diced tomatoes (fresh or canned; if canned, drain juice)
1 tablespoon yellow mustard
2 tablespoons Worcestershire sauce
1/4 teaspoon salt (optional)
1/2 teaspoon ground black pepper
6 whole-wheat hamburger buns

1. In a large skillet, cook ground beef over medium-high heat for approximately 5 minutes. Drain fat.

2. Add onions and cook 3 minutes or until onions begin to turn clear. Add garlic and cook 1 more minute.

3. Add remaining ingredients except buns and simmer for 10 minutes.

4. Serve on whole-wheat buns.

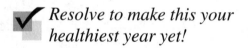

Resolve to make this your healthiest year yet!

Exchanges
1 1/2 Starch	2 Vegetable
2 Lean Meat	1/2 Fat

Calories 293
  Calories from Fat 78
Total Fat . . . . 9 g
  Saturated Fat . . . . 3 g
Cholesterol . . . . 46 mg
Sodium . . . . 691 mg
Total Carbohydrate . . . . . . 33 g
  Dietary Fiber . . . . 3 g
  Sugars . . . . 10 g
Protein . . . . 20 g

Dietitian's Tip: To reduce this recipe's fat content even further, use lean ground turkey instead of beef.

Corn Salad

2 cups frozen corn
1 cup finely diced green bell pepper
1 cup finely diced red bell pepper
1/2 cup finely diced red onion
1/2 teaspoon chopped fresh basil
1/4 cup balsamic vinegar
2 teaspoons olive oil
1/2 teaspoon salt
1/4 teaspoon ground black pepper

1. Place frozen corn in a colander and run under cold water for about 5 minutes to thaw.

2. In a medium bowl, toss together corn, green and red pepper, red onion, and basil.

3. In a small bowl, whisk together remaining ingredients and pour over salad. Toss to coat.

Exchanges

1 Starch

Calories 71
  Calories from Fat 14
Total Fat . . . . 2 g
  Saturated Fat . . . . 0 g
Cholesterol . . . . 0 mg
Sodium . . . . 170 mg
Total Carbohydrate . . . . . . 15 g
  Dietary Fiber . . . . 2 g
  Sugars . . . . 4 g
Protein . . . . 2 g

Chef's Tip: Place a wet paper towel under your cutting board to anchor it while you are dicing vegetables.

Spinach and Mushroom Pizza

4 cups fresh spinach, washed, stemmed, and coarsely chopped

2 cups sliced mushrooms

1 1/2 tablespoons olive oil, divided

1/2 teaspoon salt (optional)

1/2 teaspoon ground black pepper

1/2 tablespoon dried basil

1/2 tablespoon dried oregano

1 12-inch prepackaged pizza crust

3 garlic cloves, minced

1/2 cup shredded, part-skim mozzarella cheese

1. Preheat oven to 375 degrees. In a medium nonstick skillet, sauté spinach and mushrooms in 1/2 tablespoon olive oil. Add salt, pepper, basil, and oregano. Sauté until all the moisture is evaporated (about 10 minutes).

2. Rub pizza crust with 1 tablespoon olive oil. Sprinkle minced garlic on top. Spread the spinach and mushroom mixture evenly over the pizza crust.

3. Sprinkle the cheese on top and bake for 15 minutes or until cheese is bubbly and lightly browned.

Exchanges

3 Starch	1 1/2 Fat
1 Medium-Fat Meat	

Calories	380
Calories from Fat	129
Total Fat	14 g
Saturated Fat	3 g
Cholesterol	8 mg
Sodium	686 mg
Total Carbohydrate	47 g
Dietary Fiber	3 g
Sugars	3 g
Protein	16 g

Dietitian's Tip: Serve this pizza with a fresh green salad.

Tangy Apricot-Glazed Pork Tenderloin

Makes: 4 servings   *Serving Size: 1/4 recipe*   *Prep Time: 5 minutes*

1 pound pork tenderloin
1/2 cup light sugar-free apricot preserves
1/4 cup apple cider vinegar
1/2 tablespoon dried sage
1/2 tablespoon dried basil
1/2 tablespoon dried thyme
2 garlic cloves, minced
1/2 teaspoon salt
1/2 teaspoon ground black pepper

1. Preheat oven to 350 degrees. Trim tenderloin of all visible fat. Set aside.

2. In small saucepan, combine preserves, vinegar, herbs, and garlic over medium heat. Simmer for 3 minutes to make a glaze.

3. Season all sides of the tenderloin with salt and pepper. Place tenderloin in a shallow baking dish.

4. Coat tenderloin with apricot glaze and bake for 30 minutes or until pork is done.

Exchanges

3 Very Lean Meat
1/2 Carbohydrate

Calories 161
  Calories from Fat 38
Total Fat . . . . 4 g
  Saturated Fat . . . . 1 g
Cholesterol . . . . 65 mg
Sodium . . . . 338 mg
Total Carbohydrate . . . . 7 g
  Dietary Fiber . . . . 0 g
  Sugars . . . . 1 g
Protein . . . . 24 g

Chef's Tip: The tenderloin is a lean cut of any meat. Typically, round or loin cuts are leaner meats.

Lucky Black-Eyed Peas

2 tablespoons olive oil

1 green bell pepper, cut into 1-inch strips

2 garlic cloves, minced

2 15.5-ounce cans black-eyed peas, rinsed and drained

1/2 teaspoon crushed red pepper flakes

1. Add oil to a large nonstick skillet over medium-high heat. Add green pepper and sauté for approximately 10 minutes. Add garlic and sauté 30 seconds.

2. Add black-eyed peas and red pepper flakes and sauté 5–10 more minutes.

Exchanges

1 Starch	1/2 Fat
1 Very Lean Meat	

Calories 140
 Calories from Fat 39
Total Fat . . . . 4 g
 Saturated Fat . . . . 1 g
Cholesterol . . . . 0 mg
Sodium . . . . 138 mg
Total Carbohydrate . . . . . . 19 g
 Dietary Fiber . . . . 6 g
 Sugars . . . . 4 g
Protein . . . . 7 g

Dietitian's Tip: Black-eyed peas are high in fiber: 6 grams per 1/2 cup. A high-fiber food contains 5 grams dietary fiber or more per serving.

Peanut-Crusted Cod

Makes: 4 servings   *Serving Size: 1 filet*   *Prep Time: 5 minutes*

1/2 cup all-purpose flour
1/4 teaspoon cayenne pepper
1/2 cup chopped unsalted peanuts
4 4-ounce cod filets
1/2 teaspoon salt
1/4 teaspoon ground black pepper
2 egg whites, lightly beaten
   Cooking spray
1 teaspoon margarine

1. In a small bowl, combine flour and cayenne pepper. Spread flour mixture on a plate. Spread peanuts on a separate plate.

2. Season filets with salt and pepper on both sides. Dredge one filet through flour and shake off excess. Dip floured filet into egg whites. Press one side of the filet into chopped peanuts.

3. Coat a large nonstick skillet with cooking spray. Melt margarine over medium heat. Place filets peanut side down in skillet and cook for about 3 minutes on each side.

Exchanges

3 Lean Meat   1 Carbohydrate

Calories 234
  Calories from Fat 76
Total Fat . . . . 8 g
  Saturated Fat . . . . 2 g
Cholesterol . . . . 50 mg
Sodium . . . . 399 mg
Total Carbohydrate . . . . . . 12 g
  Dietary Fiber . . . . 1 g
  Sugars. . . . . 1 g
Protein . . . . 27 g

Chef's Tip: You can use tilapia, orange roughy, or perch instead of cod in this recipe.

Tortellini Soup

Makes: 7 servings *Serving Size: 1 cup* *Prep Time: 10 minutes*

Cooking spray
2 cups reduced-fat or lean Italian turkey sausage, crumbled
1/2 cup finely diced onion
1/4 cup red wine
1/2 tablespoon dried basil
1/2 tablespoon dried oregano
1 15-ounce can no-salt-added diced tomatoes with juice
3 14.5-ounce cans fat-free, reduced-sodium chicken broth
2 1/2 cups uncooked three-cheese tortellini
1/2 teaspoon ground black pepper

1. Coat a large soup pot with cooking spray. Add sausage and onion and cook over medium-high heat for 7 minutes or until sausage begins to brown.

2. Add wine to deglaze pan. Cook for 2 minutes or until wine is almost completely evaporated.

3. Add basil and oregano and cook for 1 more minute. Add tomatoes and broth. Bring to a boil, then reduce heat and simmer for 5 minutes.

4. Add tortellini and pepper. Cook for another 10 minutes.

✔ *January is National Volunteer Blood Donor Month . . . donate blood today!*

Exchanges

1 Starch	1 Vegetable
2 Lean Meat	

Calories 216
Calories from Fat 63
Total Fat . . . . 7 g
Saturated Fat . . . . 2 g
Cholesterol . . . . 43 mg
Sodium . . . . 858 mg
Total Carbohydrate . . . . . . 23 g
Dietary Fiber . . . . 2 g
Sugars . . . . 5 g
Protein . . . . 16 g

Chef's Tip: If you don't want to use wine in this recipe, you can substitute 1 tablespoon red wine vinegar or balsamic vinegar.

RECIPE LIST

DAY 1: Blackened Catfish **12**

DAY 2: Turkey Chili **13**

DAY 3: Chili Mac **14**

DAY 4: Pecan Chicken **15**
Spaghetti Squash **16**

DAY 5: Hearty Lentil Soup **17**
Cucumber Onion Salad **18**

GROCERY LIST

Fresh Produce
Green bell pepper – 1
Onions – 3
Spaghetti squash –
1 medium
Celery – 1 bag
Carrots – small bag
Fresh dill – 1 bunch
Cucumbers – 2 large

Meat/Poultry/Fish
Catfish filets – 4
(4-ounce) filets
Lean ground turkey –
1 1/4 pounds
Boneless, skinless
chicken breasts – 4
(4-ounce) breasts
Lean smoked precooked
turkey sausage (kiel-
basa) – 14 ounces

Grains/Bread/Pasta
Elbow macaroni – 1 box
Cornflakes – 1 small box

Dairy and Cheese
Eggs
Grated Parmesan cheese
Plain, fat-free yogurt –
8 ounces
Light sour cream – small
container

Canned Goods and Sauces
14.5-ounce can no-salt-
added diced
tomatoes – 4 cans
15.5-ounce can kidney
beans – 2 cans
14.5-ounce can fat-free,
reduced-sodium
chicken broth – 1 can

Staples/Seasonings/ Baking Needs
Salt/ground black pepper
Cooking spray
Paprika
Cayenne pepper
Chili powder
Cumin
Garlic salt
Onion salt
All-purpose flour
Olive oil
Bay leaf
White wine vinegar
Sugar substitute

Miscellaneous
1.25-ounce chili season-
ing packet – 1 packet
Pecans, chopped – small
bag
Dried lentils – 1 bag

Blackened Catfish

2 tablespoons paprika
1 teaspoon cayenne pepper
1 tablespoon chili powder
1 teaspoon cumin
1/2 teaspoon salt
1/2 teaspoon ground black pepper
4 4-ounce catfish filets
   Cooking spray

1. In a small bowl, combine the first six ingredients and stir well.

2. Rub one side of each filet well with spice mixture.

3. Coat a large nonstick skillet with cooking spray. Over medium-high heat, place each filet spice side down and cook for 3 minutes on each side or until fish is done.

Exchanges
3 Lean Meat

Calories 164
   Calories from Fat 79
Total Fat . . . . 9 g
   Saturated Fat . . . . 2 g
Cholesterol . . . . 65 mg
Sodium . . . . 239 mg
Total Carbohydrate . . . . 2 g
   Dietary Fiber . . . . 1 g
   Sugars . . . . 1 g
Protein . . . . 19 g

Chef's Tip: If you prefer this dish less spicy, reduce the cayenne pepper to 1/2–3/4 teaspoon. Couscous and broccoli make excellent side dishes for this entrée.

Turkey Chili

Makes: 9 servings   *Serving Size: 1 cup*   *Prep Time: 15 minutes*

1 1/4 pounds lean ground turkey
       Cooking spray
   1   green bell pepper, finely
       diced
   1   small onion, finely diced
   2   14.5-ounce cans no-salt-
       added diced tomatoes
   2   15.5-ounce cans kidney
       beans, undrained
   1   1.25-ounce chili seasoning
       packet

1. In a large soup pot, cook turkey over medium-high heat until brown. Remove turkey from pot and drain fat.

2. Spray pot with cooking spray and sauté green pepper and onion for 3–4 minutes.

3. Add cooked turkey back to pot with the remaining ingredients. Bring to a boil, cover, and simmer 10 minutes. Reserve 4 cups chili for Chili Mac recipe (see page 14).

Exchanges

1 Starch   1 Vegetable
2 Lean Meat

Calories 226
  Calories from Fat 61
Total Fat . . . . 7 g
  Saturated Fat . . . . 2 g
Cholesterol . . . . 47 mg
Sodium . . . . 557 mg
Total Carbohydrate . . . . . . 23 g
  Dietary Fiber . . . . 6 g
  Sugars . . . . 6 g
Protein . . . . 19 g

Dietitian's Tip: This recipe not only tastes good, but has great nutritional value as well. The meat and beans provide iron, and the vitamin C in the tomatoes helps your body absorb the iron.

Chili Mac

Makes: 4 servings   *Serving Size: 1 cup chili and*   *Prep Time: 10 minutes*
                            3/4 cup cooked pasta

4 cups Turkey Chili, heated
(see recipe, page 13)

3 cups cooked elbow macaroni
(about 1 1/2 cups uncooked
macaroni)

Mix pasta and Turkey Chili and serve.

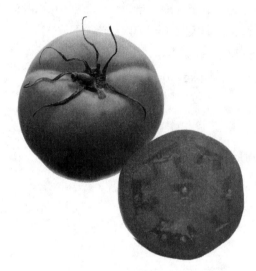

Exchanges

3 Starch   1 Vegetable
2 Lean Meat

Calories 374
   Calories from Fat 67
Total Fat . . . . 7 g
   Saturated Fat . . . . 2 g
Cholesterol . . . . 47 mg
Sodium . . . . 558 mg
Total Carbohydrate . . . . . . 53 g
   Dietary Fiber . . . . 8 g
   Sugars . . . . 8 g
Protein . . . . 24 g

Dietitian's Tip: To boost the
fiber in this recipe, try whole-
wheat pasta, found in many grocery and health food stores.

Pecan Chicken

Makes: 4 servings   *Serving Size: 1 chicken breast*   *Prep Time: 10 minutes*

Cooking spray
1 cup cornflake crumbs
1/2 cup chopped pecans
1/2 teaspoon garlic salt
1/2 teaspoon onion salt
1 egg
2 egg whites
2 tablespoons all-purpose flour
4 4-ounce boneless, skinless chicken breasts

1. Preheat oven to 350 degrees. Coat a shallow baking pan with cooking spray.

2. In a medium bowl, combine cornflake crumbs, pecans, garlic salt, and onion salt. In a separate bowl, lightly beat egg and egg whites. Put the flour in a third bowl.

3. Dip each chicken breast in the flour, then the egg mixture, then in the cornflake and pecan mixture. Coat each side of the chicken breast.

4. Place chicken breasts in the baking pan. Spray chicken lightly with cooking spray and bake 30–35 minutes or until chicken juices run clear.

Exchanges

1 Starch	4 Lean Meat

Calories	312
Calories from Fat	112
Total Fat	12 g
Saturated Fat	2 g
Cholesterol	122 mg
Sodium	519 mg
Total Carbohydrate	18 g
Dietary Fiber	2 g
Sugars	2 g
Protein	31 g

Dietitian's Tip: Pecans are high in fat, so this recipe only uses a small amount . . . but a small amount provides big flavor!

Spaghetti Squash

Makes: 5 servings   *Serving Size: 1/2 cup*   *Prep Time: 45 minutes*

1 medium spaghetti squash
  Cooking spray
1 teaspoon olive oil
2 tablespoons grated Parmesan
  cheese
1/4 teaspoon salt
1/4 teaspoon ground black pepper

1. Preheat oven to 400 degrees. Cut ends off squash and then cut squash in half lengthwise. Scoop out seeds and wash and dry both sides.

2. Coat a large metal or glass baking dish with cooking spray. Place squash halves face down on baking dish and spray the skins lightly with cooking spray.

3. Bake for 40 minutes.

4. Remove squash meat from rind with fork and place in a medium bowl. Discard rind. Drizzle oil over squash, sprinkle with Parmesan cheese, salt, and pepper, and stir.

Exchanges

1 Starch	1/2 Fat

Calories 92	
Calories from Fat 22	
Total Fat . . . . 2 g	
Saturated Fat . . . . 1 g	
Cholesterol . . . . 3 mg	
Sodium . . . . 211 mg	
Total Carbohydrate . . . . . . 16 g	
Dietary Fiber . . . . 3 g	
Sugars . . . . 5 g	
Protein . . . . 3 g	

Chef's Tip: If you've never tried this mild-flavored squash before, you're in for a fun treat!

Hearty Lentil Soup

Makes: 9 servings   *Serving Size: 1 cup*   *Prep Time: 20 minutes*

Cooking spray

14 ounces lean smoked pre-cooked turkey sausage (Kielbasa), sliced

1 cup diced celery

1 medium onion, diced

1 carrot, diced

3 cups water

1 14.5-ounce can fat-free, reduced-sodium chicken broth

2 14.5-ounce cans no-salt-added diced tomatoes

1 cup dried lentils

1/2 teaspoon salt (optional)

1 teaspoon ground black pepper

1 bay leaf

1. Coat a large soup pot with cooking spray. Over medium-high heat, sauté sausage until lightly brown. Remove from pan.

2. Add celery, onion, and carrots to pot and sauté over medium-high heat for approximately 4 minutes.

3. Add the sausage and all remaining ingredients. Bring to a boil; reduce heat and simmer for 1 hour.

4. Remove bay leaf and serve.

Exchanges

1 Starch   1 Vegetable
1 Lean Meat

Calories 168
   Calories from Fat 39
Total Fat . . . . 4 g
   Saturated Fat . . . . 1 g
Cholesterol . . . . 28 mg
Sodium . . . . 825 mg
Total Carbohydrate . . . . . . 20 g
   Dietary Fiber . . . . 7 g
   Sugars . . . . 7 g
Protein . . . . 13 g

Dietitian's Tip: Lentils, along with all legumes, contain both carbohydrate and protein and are an excellent source of fiber.

Cucumber Onion Salad

Makes: 5 servings   *Serving Size: 1/5 recipe*   *Prep Time: 5 minutes*

1/2 cup plain, fat-free yogurt
1/4 cup light sour cream
1 tablespoon minced fresh dill
1/2 teaspoon garlic salt
1 1/2 tablespoons white wine vinegar
1/4 teaspoon ground black pepper
1 packet sugar substitute
2 large cucumbers, peeled and thinly sliced
1 medium onion, thinly sliced

1. In a medium bowl, whisk together all ingredients except cucumber and onion.

2. Add cucumber and onion and toss to coat well. Serve chilled.

✔ *January is National Eye Care Month. Take care of your eyes with annual exams by an ophthalmologist.*

Exchanges

2 Vegetable

Calories 55
Calories from Fat 11
Total Fat . . . . 1 g
Saturated Fat . . . . 1 g
Cholesterol . . . . 5 mg
Sodium . . . . 160 mg
Total Carbohydrate . . . . 9 g
Dietary Fiber . . . . 1 g
Sugars . . . . 7 g
Protein . . . . 3 g

Chef's Tip: Dill has a distinctive flavor that may be too strong for some people. If you don't care for dill, just leave it out.

RECIPE LIST

DAY 1: Turkey and Wild Rice Soup **20**

Spinach Salad with Mushrooms **21**

DAY 2: Sweet and Sour Pork **22**

DAY 3: Chicken Breasts with
Raspberry Balsamic Glaze **23**

Candied Walnut Salad **24**

DAY 4: Creamy Macaroni and Cheese **25**

DAY 5: Stuffed Peppers **26**

GROCERY LIST

Fresh Produce
Carrots – 1 small bag
Onions – 2
Celery – 1 bunch
Mushrooms – 1 pint
Garlic – 1 head
10-ounce bag baby
spinach – 1 bag
Mixed field greens –
4 cups
Green bell pepper – 7

Meat/Poultry/Fish
Roasted turkey breast –
12–14 ounces
Boneless, center-cut
pork chops – 1 pound
Boneless, skinless
chicken breasts – 4
(4-ounce) breasts
Lean ground beef –
1 pound

Grains/Bread/Pasta
Wild and long grain
rice – 1 box or bag
Elbow macaroni – 1 box
Instant brown rice –
1 box or bag

Dairy and Cheese
Margarine
Light Ranch dressing –
1 bottle
Fat-free milk
Shredded, reduced-fat
cheddar cheese –
1 bag

Canned Goods and Sauces
14.5-ounce can no-salt-
added diced
tomatoes – 2 cans
14.5-ounce can fat-free,
reduced-sodium
chicken broth – 4 cans
Pineapple chunks (in
juice) – 1 can
Light sugar-free seedless
raspberry preserves –
1 jar
Sweet-and-sour sauce –
small bottle
Dijon mustard – small
bottle

Staples/Seasonings/Baking Needs
Salt/ground black pepper
Cooking spray
All-purpose flour
Dried thyme
Bay leaf
Evaporated fat-free milk
Olive oil
Canola oil
Balsamic vinegar
Red wine vinegar
Brown sugar
Hot pepper sauce

Miscellaneous
Sunflower seeds –
small bag
Walnuts – small bag

Turkey and Wild Rice Soup

Makes: 7 servings *Serving Size: 1 cup* *Prep Time: 15 minutes*

2 teaspoons margarine
1 cup finely diced carrot
1 cup finely diced onion
1/2 cup finely diced celery
1 cup sliced mushrooms
1 garlic clove, minced
2 tablespoons all-purpose flour
3 14.5-ounce cans fat-free, reduced-sodium chicken broth
1/4 teaspoon dried thyme
1 bay leaf
2 cups roasted turkey breast, chopped
1 cup uncooked wild and long-grain rice
1/2 cup evaporated fat-free milk
1/4 teaspoon salt (optional)
1/4 teaspoon ground black pepper

1. Heat margarine in a large soup pot over medium-high heat. Add carrots, onion, celery, and mushrooms and sauté until beginning to brown. Add garlic and sauté for 1 more minute.

2. Add flour, stirring constantly, and cook for 1 minute. Add chicken broth and stir (make sure to scrape the brown bits on the bottom of pan).

3. Add thyme, bay leaf, turkey, and rice; bring to a boil.

4. Reduce heat to a simmer; cover and cook for 25 minutes. Add evaporated milk; bring to a boil for 1 minute. Add salt and pepper. Remove bay leaf before serving.

Exchanges

1 Starch   1 Vegetable
2 Very Lean Meat

Calories	175
Calories from Fat	15
Total Fat	2 g
Saturated Fat	0 g
Cholesterol	33 mg
Sodium	678 mg
Total Carbohydrate	21 g
Dietary Fiber	2 g
Sugars	5 g
Protein	18 g

Chef's Tip: Save yourself some prep time and buy presliced mushrooms.

Spinach Salad with Mushrooms

Makes: 4 servings   *Serving Size: 1 1/2 cups*   *Prep Time: 5 minutes*

1 10-ounce bag baby spinach
1 cup sliced mushrooms
1/4 cup sunflower seeds
1/3 cup light Ranch dressing

1. In a large salad bowl, toss spinach and mushrooms together.

2. Sprinkle sunflower seeds over the top and drizzle with dressing. Toss well to coat.

Exchanges

1 Vegetable   2 Fat

Calories 121
  Calories from Fat 81
Total Fat . . . . 9 g
  Saturated Fat . . . . 1 g
Cholesterol . . . . 0 mg
Sodium . . . . 244 mg
Total Carbohydrate . . . . . . 7 g
  Dietary Fiber . . . . 3 g
  Sugars . . . . 1 g
Protein . . . . 5 g

Chef's Tip: Bagged spinach will save you time in this recipe.

Sweet and Sour Pork

Makes: 4 servings   *Serving Size: 1/4 recipe*   *Prep Time: 10 minutes*

6 tablespoons jarred sweet-and-sour sauce

3/4 cup fat-free, reduced-sodium chicken broth

1 pound boneless center-cut pork chops, cubed

1 teaspoon ground black pepper

1 tablespoon olive oil, divided

1 green bell pepper, diced

1 cup pineapple chunks packed in juice, drained

1. Mix sweet and sour sauce with chicken broth and set aside.

2. Sprinkle pork with pepper. In a large nonstick skillet or wok, sauté pork cubes in 1/2 tablespoon olive oil over medium-high heat until cooked through and beginning to brown. Set the cooked pork aside in a bowl.

3. In the same pan, sauté green peppers in 1/2 tablespoon olive oil for 2 minutes. Add the pork and pineapple to the peppers. Pour sauce over pork mixture and simmer for 5 minutes. Serve over rice.

Exchanges

3 Lean Meat   1 Carbohydrate
1/2 Fat

Calories 269
  Calories from Fat 96
Total Fat . . . . 11 g
  Saturated Fat . . . . 3 g
Cholesterol . . . . 72 mg
Sodium . . . . 292 mg
Total Carbohydrate . . . . . . 17 g
  Dietary Fiber . . . . 1 g
  Sugars . . . . 13 g
Protein . . . . 26 g

Chef's Tip: You can ask your butcher to cube the pork for you, saving yourself a step in this recipe.

Chicken Breasts with Raspberry Balsamic Glaze

Makes: 4 servings   *Serving Size: 1 chicken breast*   *Prep Time: 10 minutes*

- **1** teaspoon canola oil
- **2** garlic cloves, minced
- **1/2** cup light sugar-free seedless raspberry preserves
- **1/4** cup balsamic vinegar
- **1/4** teaspoon ground black pepper
- **4** 4-ounce boneless, skinless chicken breasts
  Cooking spray

1. Preheat oven to 350 degrees. In a small saucepan, heat oil, add garlic, and sauté for 30 seconds over medium-high heat.

2. Add raspberry preserves, balsamic vinegar, and pepper and bring to a low boil; simmer 3 minutes or until mixture gets a glaze-like consistency.

3. Reserve half of glaze and set aside. Brush chicken breasts on both sides with remaining glaze.

4. Coat a baking dish with cooking spray. Place chicken breasts in dish and bake 30 minutes. Pour remaining glaze over chicken breasts.

Exchanges

3 Very Lean Meat	1/2 Fat
1/2 Carbohydrate	

Calories	176
Calories from Fat	36
Total Fat	4 g
Saturated Fat	1 g
Cholesterol	68 mg
Sodium	60 mg
Total Carbohydrate	9 g
Dietary Fiber	0 g
Sugars	2 g
Protein	25 g

Chef's Tip: Your guests will ask for the recipe for this quick and tasty dish.

Candied Walnut Salad

Makes: 4 servings   *Serving Size: 1/4 recipe*   *Prep Time: 15 minutes*

2 tablespoons red wine vinegar
1 tablespoon olive oil
1 teaspoon Dijon mustard
1 tablespoon margarine
2 tablespoons brown sugar
1/4 cup chopped walnuts
4 cups mixed field greens
1/2 cup shredded carrots

1. Preheat oven to 350 degrees. In a small bowl, whisk together vinegar, oil, and mustard; set aside.

2. In a small bowl, combine margarine and brown sugar. Microwave on high for 30 seconds to melt margarine, then stir well. Toss walnuts with margarine and sugar and spread on a small baking sheet. Bake for 15–20 minutes or until beginning to brown.

3. In a large salad bowl, toss remaining salad ingredients with the candied nuts. Drizzle dressing over salad and toss to coat.

Exchanges
1 Vegetable   1/2 Carbohydrate
2 Fat

Calories	142
Calories from Fat	97
Total Fat	11 g
Saturated Fat	1 g
Cholesterol	0 mg
Sodium	79 mg
Total Carbohydrate	11 g
Dietary Fiber	1 g
Sugars	9 g
Protein	2 g

Chef's Tip: Sweet, crunchy walnuts add great texture to this dish.

Creamy Macaroni and Cheese

Makes: 6 servings   *Serving Size: 1/2 cup*   *Prep Time: 25 minutes*

8 ounces uncooked elbow macaroni
2 teaspoons margarine
2 tablespoons all-purpose flour
1 1/2 cups fat-free milk
1 1/4 cups shredded, reduced-fat cheddar cheese (reserve 2 tablespoons)
1/2 teaspoon salt
1/2 teaspoon ground black pepper
1/4 teaspoon hot pepper sauce
Cooking spray

1. Preheat oven to 350 degrees. Cook macaroni according to directions on box, omitting salt. Drain.

2. In a small nonstick skillet, heat margarine over medium heat. Stir in flour and cook for 4–5 minutes to create a roux.

3. In a small saucepan, add milk and bring to a boil; whisk in roux. Reduce to a simmer for 7 minutes.

4. Add cheese (except reserved 2 tablespoons) to pan and whisk while simmering 2 more minutes. Add salt, pepper, and hot pepper sauce.

5. In a large bowl, combine noodles and cheese sauce and mix well.

6. Coat an 8-inch glass baking dish with cooking spray. Spread macaroni mixture in dish. Sprinkle remaining cheese over the top.

7. Bake for 15 minutes.

Exchanges

2 Starch   1 Medium-Fat Meat

Calories	250
Calories from Fat	62
Total Fat	7 g
Saturated Fat	3 g
Cholesterol	18 mg
Sodium	444 mg
Total Carbohydrate	34 g
Dietary Fiber	1 g
Sugars	4 g
Protein	13 g

Dietitian's Tip: Enjoy this great low-fat, guilt-free version of a traditional favorite.

Stuffed Peppers

Makes: 6 servings   *Serving Size: 1 stuffed pepper*   *Prep Time: 20 minutes*

2/3 cup uncooked instant brown rice
6 medium green bell peppers
1 pound lean ground beef
1 small onion, chopped
2 14.5-ounce cans no-salt-added diced tomatoes
2 garlic cloves, minced
1/4 teaspoon ground black pepper

1. Preheat oven to 350 degrees. Cook rice according to package directions, omitting salt.

2. Fill a large saucepan with water and bring to a boil. Cut the tops off the green peppers and remove the seeds and membranes. Place the peppers in the boiling water and boil for 5 minutes. Remove and drain.

3. In a large skillet, brown ground beef and onion. Drain fat.

4. Add the brown rice and diced tomatoes to the skillet with ground beef and mix well. Add garlic and black pepper.

5. Place peppers right side up in a large baking dish. Fill peppers with beef and rice mixture. Bake, covered, for 30 minutes.

Exchanges

1/2 Starch	4 Vegetable
2 Lean Meat	

Calories 236
  Calories from Fat 64
Total Fat . . . . 7 g
  Saturated Fat . . . . 2 g
Cholesterol . . . . 46 mg
Sodium . . . . 107 mg
Total Carbohydrate . . . . . . 27 g
  Dietary Fiber . . . . 6 g
  Sugars . . . . 9 g
Protein . . . . 18 g

Chef's Tip: Using instant brown rice is a great way to get this dinner on the table fast. You can always use instant rice as a time-saver in any recipe.

RECIPE LIST

GROCERY LIST

Fresh Produce
Onions – 2
Lettuce – 1 head
Tomato – 1 large
Garlic – 1 head
Fresh oregano – 1 bunch
Asparagus –
1 1/2 pounds
Fresh parsley – 1 bunch
Bananas – 4–5

Meat/Poultry/Fish
Cooked ham steak –
12–14 ounces
90% lean ground beef –
1 pound
Tuna steaks – 4
(4-ounce) steaks
Lean ground turkey –
1 pound

Grains/Bread/Pasta
Flour or corn tortillas – 8

Medium shell pasta –
1 box
No-boil lasagna noodles –
1 box
Old-fashioned oats –
small container

Dairy and Cheese
Eggs
Shredded, reduced-fat
cheddar cheese – 1 bag
Shredded, part-skim
mozzarella cheese –
1 bag
Grated Parmesan cheese
Fat-free ricotta cheese –
15 ounces
Low-fat buttermilk –
small container

Canned Goods
and Sauces
14.5-ounce can fat-free,
reduced-sodium
chicken broth – 2 cans
16-ounce can Great
Northern beans –
2 cans
8-ounce can creamed
corn – 1 can
14.5-ounce can no-salt-
added diced
tomatoes – 1 can
26-ounce jar marinara
pasta sauce – 2 jars

Frozen Foods
9-ounce package
chopped spinach –
1 package

Staples/Seasonings/
Baking Needs
Salt/ground black
pepper
Cooking spray
Bay leaf
Cumin
Chili powder
Cayenne pepper
Onion salt
Olive oil
Canola oil
All-purpose flour
Sugar
Baking powder
Baking soda
Sugar substitute
Mini semi-sweet choco-
late chips – small bag

Miscellaneous
8.5-ounce box corn
muffin mix – 1 box
Kalamata olives –
1 small jar

Ham and White Bean Soup

Makes: 6 servings   *Serving Size: 1 cup*   *Prep Time: 12 minutes*

Cooking spray
1 medium onion, finely diced
1/2 cup chopped cooked ham
2 14.5-ounce cans fat-free,
reduced-sodium chicken broth
2 16-ounce cans Great Northern
beans, rinsed and drained
1/2 teaspoon ground black pepper
1 bay leaf

1. Spray a large soup pot with cooking spray. Add onion and sauté with chopped ham 2 minutes over medium-high heat. Add all remaining ingredients and bring to a boil.

2. Reduce heat and simmer 15 minutes. Remove bay leaf before serving.

Exchanges
1 1/2 Starch   1 Very Lean Meat

Calories 151
  Calories from Fat 10
Total Fat . . . . 1 g
  Saturated Fat . . . . 0 g
Cholesterol . . . . 7 mg
Sodium . . . . 653 mg
Total Carbohydrate . . . . . . 23 g
  Dietary Fiber . . . . 7 g
  Sugars . . . . 4 g
Protein . . . . 13 g

Dietitian's Tip: Rinsing canned beans helps remove some of the sodium.

Quick Creamy Cornbread

Makes: 8 servings   *Serving Size: 1 slice*   *Prep Time: 5 minutes*

1 8.5-ounce box corn muffin mix
1 egg
1 8-ounce can creamed corn
  Cooking spray

1. Preheat oven to 400 degrees. In a medium mixing bowl, combine corn muffin mix, egg, and creamed corn.

2. Pour batter into an 8 × 8-inch baking pan coated with cooking spray. Bake 20–25 minutes.

3. Cool. Cut into 8 slices.

Exchanges
1 1/2 Starch

Calories 115
  Calories from Fat 26
Total Fat . . . . 3 g
  Saturated Fat . . . . 1 g
Cholesterol . . . . 27 mg
Sodium . . . . 339 mg
Total Carbohydrate . . . . . . 26 g
  Dietary Fiber . . . . 1 g
  Sugars . . . . 8 g
Protein . . . . 3 g

Chef's Tip: Cornbread can't get much easier than this. The creamed corn adds a unique touch.

Quick Tacos

1 pound 90% lean ground beef
2/3 cup water
1 teaspoon cumin
1 tablespoon chili powder
1/4 teaspoon cayenne pepper
1 teaspoon onion salt
8 6-inch flour or corn tortillas
1/2 cup shredded, reduced-fat
   cheddar cheese
1 cup shredded lettuce
1 large tomato, diced
   Hot pepper sauce (optional)

1. Brown beef in a large nonstick skillet over medium-high heat until thoroughly cooked and no longer pink. Drain fat.

2. Add water, cumin, chili powder, cayenne pepper, and onion salt and simmer 2–4 minutes.

3. Warm tortillas. Fill each tortilla with 1/4 cup taco meat, 2 tablespoons cheese, lettuce, tomato, and hot pepper sauce.

Exchanges

1 Starch	1 Vegetable
1 Lean Meat	1 Fat

Calories. 211
  Calories from Fat. 77
Total Fat . . . . 9 g
  Saturated Fat . . . . 3 g
Cholesterol . . . . 39 mg
Sodium . . . . 410 mg
Total Carbohydrate. . . . . . 19 g
  Dietary Fiber . . . . 2 g
  Sugars. . . . . 2 g
Protein. . . . . 16 g

Dietitian's Tip: If you need to watch your sodium intake, use onion powder instead of onion salt.

Spinach Pasta Shells

Makes: 5 servings   *Serving Size: 1 cup*   *Prep Time: 20 minutes*

5 ounces uncooked medium shell pasta (about 2 cups)
9 ounces frozen, chopped spinach
2 tablespoons olive oil, divided
4 garlic cloves, minced
1/4 cup grated Parmesan cheese

1. Cook pasta according to package directions, omitting salt. While pasta is cooking, defrost spinach in microwave. Squeeze all liquid from spinach.

2. In a medium nonstick skillet, sauté spinach in 1 tablespoon olive oil over medium-high heat for approximately 5 minutes. Add garlic and Parmesan cheese; sauté 1 minute.

3. Drain pasta. Add spinach mixture and 1 tablespoon olive oil to pasta and toss.

Exchanges

1 1/2 Starch	1 1/2 Fat

Calories 191	
Calories from Fat 69	
Total Fat . . . . 8 g	
Saturated Fat . . . . 2 g	
Cholesterol . . . . 6 mg	
Sodium . . . . 139 mg	
Total Carbohydrate . . . . . . 24 g	
Dietary Fiber . . . . 2 g	
Sugars . . . . 2 g	
Protein . . . . 8 g	

Dietitian's Tip: Olive oil is a great source of monounsaturated fat and is good for you (in the right portion sizes!).

Tuna with Tomatoes and Olives

Makes: 4 servings   *Serving Size: 1 tuna steak*   *Prep Time: 10 minutes*

Cooking spray
4 4-ounce tuna steaks
1 teaspoon olive oil
1 large onion, thinly sliced (about 1 1/2 cups)
1 14.5-ounce can no-salt-added diced tomatoes with juice
1/2 cup Kalamata olives, pitted and chopped
2 tablespoons chopped fresh oregano (or 1 tablespoon dried oregano)
1 packet sugar substitute
1/4 teaspoon ground black pepper

1. Coat a large sauté pan with cooking spray. Over medium-high heat, sear tuna on each side about 2 minutes. Remove from pan.

2. Add olive oil to pan. Add onion and cook for about 5 minutes or until beginning to brown. Reduce heat to low. Add tomatoes, olives, and oregano and simmer for another 3 minutes. Mix in sugar substitute and black pepper.

3. Add tuna back to mixture, cover, and cook 3 more minutes.

Exchanges

3 Lean Meat	2 Vegetable

Calories 231
  Calories from Fat 77
Total Fat . . . . 9 g
  Saturated Fat . . . . 0 g
Cholesterol . . . . 42 mg
Sodium . . . . 220 mg
Total Carbohydrate . . . . . . 12 g
  Dietary Fiber . . . . 4 g
  Sugars . . . . 7 g
Protein . . . . 27 g

Dietitian's Tip: Tuna is a great source of omega-3 fatty acids, which have been found to protect against heart disease.

Roasted Asparagus

Makes: 6 servings   *Serving Size: 1/6 recipe*   *Prep Time: 5 minutes*

1 1/2 pounds fresh asparagus
     Cooking spray
1 tablespoon olive oil
1/4 cup grated Parmesan cheese

1. Preheat oven to 450 degrees. Wash asparagus and cut off ends. Coat a baking dish with cooking spray.

2. Place asparagus in baking dish, drizzle with olive oil, and sprinkle with Parmesan cheese.

3. Bake 15 minutes.

Exchanges

1 Vegetable	1 Fat

Calories 53
   Calories from Fat 35
Total Fat . . . . 4 g
   Saturated Fat . . . . 1 g
Cholesterol . . . . 5 mg
Sodium . . . . 91 mg
Total Carbohydrate . . . . 2 g
   Dietary Fiber . . . . 1 g
   Sugars . . . . 1 g
Protein . . . . 3 g

Dietitian's Tip: Parmesan cheese can add a lot of flavor to many foods without adding too much fat.

Turkey Lasagna

Makes: 10 servings   *Serving Size: 1/10 recipe*   *Prep Time: 15 minutes*

Cooking spray
1 pound lean ground turkey
2 26-ounce jars marinara pasta sauce
1 cup shredded, part-skim mozzarella cheese, divided
15 ounces fat-free ricotta cheese
1/4 cup grated Parmesan cheese
1 egg, slightly beaten
1/4 cup chopped fresh parsley
12 no-boil lasagna noodles

1. Preheat oven to 350 degrees. Coat a 13 × 9 × 2-inch glass baking dish with cooking spray.

2. In a large saucepan, cook turkey over medium-high heat until brown. Drain fat. Lower heat to medium and add pasta sauce. Cook for 5 minutes.

3. In a medium bowl, mix together 1/2 cup mozzarella, ricotta, Parmesan, egg, and parsley.

4. Spread 1 cup pasta sauce on bottom of baking dish. Arrange noodles side by side on top of sauce, over-lapping slightly. Spread 1/4 cup cheese mixture on top of noodles.

5. Repeat layering with pasta sauce, noodles, and cheese mixture 2 more times.

6. Top with remaining 3 noodles and 1 cup sauce. Cover lasagna with foil and bake 25 minutes. Uncover; top with remaining mozzarella cheese and bake additional 25 minutes or until cheese is light golden brown.

Exchanges

1 Starch	3 Vegetable
2 Lean Meat	1/2 Fat

Calories 293
  Calories from Fat 76
Total Fat . . . . 8 g
  Saturated Fat . . . . 3 g
Cholesterol . . . . 97 mg
Sodium . . . . 609 mg
Total Carbohydrate . . . . . . 30 g
  Dietary Fiber . . . . 4 g
  Sugars . . . . 11 g
Protein . . . . 26 g

Chef's Tip: If you haven't used ground turkey before, you will be amazed how great it tastes in this recipe.

Banana Chocolate Chip Bread

Makes: 16 servings   *Serving Size: 1 slice*   *Prep Time: 15 minutes*

Cooking spray
1 1/2 cups very ripe bananas, mashed (about 4 bananas)
2 tablespoons canola oil
1/4 cup low-fat buttermilk
4 egg whites
1 1/2 cups all-purpose flour
1/2 cup old-fashioned oats
1/2 cup sugar
2 teaspoons baking powder
1 teaspoon baking soda
1/2 teaspoon salt
1/3 cup mini semi-sweet chocolate chips (reserve 1 tablespoon)

1. Preheat oven to 350 degrees. Lightly spray an 8 × 4-inch loaf pan with cooking spray.

2. In a medium bowl, combine bananas, oil, buttermilk, and egg whites; mix well. Set aside.

3. In a large bowl, combine flour, oats, sugar, baking powder, baking soda, and salt.

4. Make a well in the center of the dry ingredients. Add banana mixture to dry ingredients all at once and mix well.

5. Stir in 1/3 cup chocolate chips to batter. Pour batter into loaf pan. Sprinkle 1 tablespoon chocolate chips on top of batter.

6. Bake 50–60 minutes or until toothpick inserted in center comes out clean.

Exchanges
1/2 Fat   1 1/2 Carbohydrate

Calories 133
Calories from Fat 29
Total Fat . . . . 3 g
Saturated Fat . . . . 1 g
Cholesterol . . . . 0 mg
Sodium . . . . 215 mg
Total Carbohydrate . . . . . . 24 g
Dietary Fiber . . . . 1 g
Sugars . . . . 12 g
Protein . . . . 3 g

Dietitian's Tip: You'll love this low-fat chocolate version of banana bread.

February

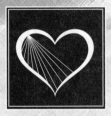

Did you know that diabetes and heart disease are linked? There is a lot you can do to reduce your risk, starting with how you eat. Try more chicken and fish, whole grains, fresh fruits, and crunchy vegetables—and get some exercise, too!

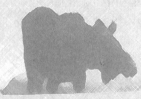

American Heart Month

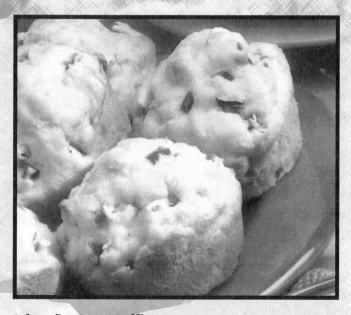

Jalapeño Corn Muffins (page 54)
These light and scrumptious muffins are terrific with
chili or hearty stews. Or make them for Sunday brunch
and serve them in a pretty basket.

February ❖ Recipes

February ❖ Week 1

GROCERY LIST

Fresh Produce
Russet potatoes – 6
Yellow onion – 1
Avocado – 1
Lettuce – 1 head
Tomatoes – 3
Cucumber – 1
Carrots – small bag
Green bell pepper – 1
Red bell pepper – 2
Broccoli – 1–2 heads
Yellow squash – 2
Celery – 1 bag
Scallions – 1 bunch

Meat/Poultry/Fish
Beef tenderloin steaks –
4 (4-ounce) steaks
Thinly sliced, smoked
deli turkey –
12 ounces
Boneless, skinless
chicken breasts –
2 pounds
Tuna steaks – 4
(5-ounce) steaks

Grains/Bread/Pasta
10-inch flour tortillas – 4
Rotini pasta – 1 box
Penne pasta – 1 box

Dairy and Cheese
Fat-free half-and-half –
1 pint
Shredded, reduced-fat
cheddar cheese –
1 bag
Plain, fat-free yogurt –
8 ounces
Grated Parmesan cheese

Canned Goods and Sauces
Fat-free Italian
dressing – 1 bottle
14-ounce can no-salt-
added diced
tomatoes – 1 can
16-ounce can water
chestnuts – 1 can
14.5-ounce can bean
sprouts – 1 can
14.5-ounce can fat-free,
reduced-sodium
chicken broth – 1 can
Lite soy sauce – 1 bottle

Frozen Foods
Peas – 1 bag

Staples/Seasonings/ Baking Needs
Salt/ground black pepper
Cooking spray
Chili powder
Red wine vinegar
Olive oil
Dried basil
Dried oregano
Cornstarch
Balsamic vinegar
Honey

Miscellaneous
White wine

39

Beef Tenderloin

Makes: 4 servings   *Serving Size: 1 steak*   *Prep Time: 5 minutes*

4 4-ounce beef tenderloin steaks
1/2 teaspoon salt
1 teaspoon ground black pepper
Cooking spray

1. Preheat oven to 400 degrees. Trim visible fat from sides of meat. Season both sides of meat with salt and pepper.

2. Coat a large sauté pan with cooking spray. Over high heat, sear meat on both sides about 1 minute. Place steaks in baking pan.

3. Bake in oven for 15 minutes. Turn once halfway through baking.

 National Women's Heart Health Day is February 1. Do the right thing for your heart by eating right and getting plenty of exercise.

Exchanges
3 Lean Meat

Calories 151
    Calories from Fat 63
Total Fat . . . . 7 g
    Saturated Fat . . . . 3 g
Cholesterol . . . . 60 mg
Sodium . . . . 336 mg
Total Carbohydrate . . . . 0 g
    Dietary Fiber . . . . 0 g
    Sugars. . . . . 0 g
Protein. . . . . 20 g

Chef's Tip: After you remove the steaks from the oven, let them sit for 5 minutes before you cut them. This will allow the juices to redistribute themselves, providing maximum flavor!

Scalloped Potatoes

Makes: 6 servings   *Serving Size: 2/3 cup*   *Prep Time: 15 minutes*

6 medium russet potatoes
1 medium yellow onion, cut into thin strips
  Cooking spray
1/4 teaspoon salt
1/4 teaspoon ground black pepper
1 cup fat-free half-and-half
1/2 cup shredded, reduced-fat, sharp cheddar cheese, divided

1. Preheat oven to 400 degrees. Peel potatoes and slice into thin rounds.

2. Coat a large nonstick skillet with cooking spray and sauté onions and potatoes over medium-high heat until the onions turn clear.

3. Spray a pie pan or 8-inch round cake pan with cooking spray.

4. Place a thick layer (about half) of the potatoes and onions in the bottom of pan.

5. Add salt and pepper to half-and-half. Pour 1/2 cup of the half-and half over the potatoes. Sprinkle 1/4 cup of the cheese on top.

6. Add the remaining potatoes and pour 1/2 cup half-and-half over the potatoes and top with remaining cheese.

7. Bake for 40 minutes or until potatoes are soft.

Exchanges

2 Starch

Calories	160
Calories from Fat	24
Total Fat	3 g
Saturated Fat	1 g
Cholesterol	9 mg
Sodium	243 mg
Total Carbohydrate	30 g
Dietary Fiber	3 g
Sugars	6 g
Protein	6 g

Dietitian's Tip: Try fat-free half-and-half in any recipe where you want creaminess without added fat.

Turkey and Avocado Wraps

Makes: 4 servings   *Serving Size: 1 wrap*   *Prep Time: 25 minutes*

1/2 avocado
3 tablespoons plain, fat-free yogurt
1/4 teaspoon chili powder
2 cups chopped lettuce
2 small tomatoes, seeded and finely diced
2 tablespoons fat-free Italian dressing
4 10-inch flour tortillas
12 ounces thinly-sliced, smoked deli turkey
1 cucumber, thinly sliced

1. In a small bowl, mash the avocado with a fork. Add yogurt and chili powder to avocado and mix well.

2. In a medium bowl, toss lettuce and tomato with Italian dressing.

3. Spread 1 1/2 tablespoons of avocado mixture on tortilla. Add 3 ounces turkey, 1/4 lettuce and tomato mixture, and 5 slices cucumber to tortilla.

4. Fold in the left and right side of the tortilla until the edges are about 1 inch apart and then roll from the top down. Repeat this process for remaining 3 wraps.

Exchanges

3 Starch	1 Vegetable
2 Very Lean Meat	1 Fat

Calories 380
Calories from Fat 81
Total Fat . . . . 9 g
Saturated Fat . . . . 2 g
Cholesterol . . . . 30 mg
Sodium . . . . 1258 mg
Total Carbohydrate . . . . . . 48 g
Dietary Fiber . . . . 5 g
Sugars . . . . 7 g
Protein . . . . 26 g

Dietitian's Tip: Avocados are a good source of potassium, a mineral that helps the body's fluids stay in balance.

Confetti Pasta Salad

Makes: 6 servings   *Serving Size: 1 cup*   *Prep Time: 20 minutes*

DRESSING

1/4 cup red wine vinegar

  2 teaspoons olive oil

1/4 teaspoon dried basil

1/4 teaspoon salt

1/4 teaspoon ground black pepper

SALAD

  5 ounces uncooked rotini pasta
(about 2 cups)

  1 cup fresh or frozen peas

  1 cup finely diced carrot

  1 green bell pepper, finely diced

  1 tomato, seeded and finely
diced

1. In a small bowl, whisk together all the dressing ingredients; set aside.

2. Cook pasta according to package directions, omitting salt. Drain pasta in colander and run under cold water for a few minutes to cool.

3. In a medium bowl, toss together pasta, peas, carrots, peppers, and tomatoes.

4. Drizzle dressing over the salad and toss again to coat.

Exchanges

1 1/2 Starch	1 Vegetable

Calories 150
  Calories from Fat 20
Total Fat . . . . 2 g
  Saturated Fat . . . . 0 g
Cholesterol . . . . 0 mg
Sodium . . . . 140 mg
Total Carbohydrate . . . . . . 28 g
  Dietary Fiber . . . . 3 g
  Sugars . . . . 5 g
Protein . . . . 5 g

Dietitian's Tip: Most green, deep yellow, and orange vegetables are great sources of vitamin A, important for healthy skin and eyes.

Penne with Chicken and Vegetables

Makes: 6 servings   Serving Size: about 2 cups   Prep Time: 15 minutes

9 ounces uncooked penne pasta
  Cooking spray
1 pound boneless, skinless chicken breasts, cut into 1-inch strips
1 tablespoon olive oil
2 cups broccoli florets
2 medium red bell peppers, sliced into thin strips
2 medium yellow squash, sliced
1 14-ounce can no-salt-added diced tomatoes, juice drained
1/4 cup white wine
1/2 teaspoon dried basil
1/2 teaspoon dried oregano
1/4 teaspoon salt
1/4 teaspoon ground black pepper
1/4 cup grated Parmesan cheese

1. Cook pasta according to package directions, omitting salt.

2. Coat a large nonstick skillet with cooking spray. Over medium-high heat, cook chicken strips for approximately 3–5 minutes or until done. Remove from pan and set aside.

3. Add olive oil to pan. Sauté broccoli, red peppers, and squash 3–4 minutes. Add tomatoes, wine, herbs, salt, and pepper. Cook for 5–7 more minutes.

4. Toss chicken and vegetable mixture with drained, cooked penne pasta. Sprinkle with Parmesan cheese.

Exchanges

2 Starch	2 Vegetable
2 Lean Meat	

Calories 333
  Calories from Fat 61
Total Fat . . . . 7 g
  Saturated Fat . . . . 2 g
Cholesterol . . . . 51 mg
Sodium . . . . 250 mg
Total Carbohydrate . . . . . . 40 g
  Dietary Fiber . . . . 5 g
  Sugars . . . . 6 g
Protein . . . . 28 g

Dietitian's Tip: This tasty meal provides protein, carbohydrate, and veggies, all in one dish.

44   WEEK 1 ❖ DAY 3 ❖ FEBRUARY

Cantonese Chicken

Makes: 4 servings   *Serving Size: 1/4 recipe*   *Prep Time: 15 minutes*

Cooking spray
1 pound boneless, skinless chicken breasts, cut into 1-inch cubes
1 cup chopped celery
1 cup sliced, drained water chestnuts
1 14.5-ounce can bean sprouts, rinsed and drained
1 14.5-ounce can fat-free, reduced-sodium chicken broth
2 tablespoons lite soy sauce
1 1/2 tablespoons cornstarch
1/2 teaspoon salt (optional)
1/4 teaspoon ground black pepper

1. Coat a large nonstick skillet with cooking spray. Over medium-high heat, cook chicken for 6 minutes or until chicken is cooked through. Remove chicken from pan.

2. Add celery, water chestnuts, and bean sprouts; stir-fry for about 3 minutes.

3. In a medium bowl, whisk broth, soy sauce, and cornstarch together. Add broth mixture to pan. Bring to a boil; reduce heat and simmer for 5 minutes. Add salt and pepper. Add chicken back to pan and heat through.

4. Serve over Chinese noodles or rice.

Exchanges

3 Very Lean Meat	1/2 Fat
2 Vegetable	

Calories 186
  Calories from Fat 27
Total Fat . . . . 3 g
  Saturated Fat . . . . 1 g
Cholesterol . . . . 68 mg
Sodium . . . . 657 mg
Total Carbohydrate . . . . . . 10 g
  Dietary Fiber . . . . 2 g
  Sugars . . . . 2 g
Protein . . . . 28 g

Chef's Tip: Using a wok for this recipe helps the veggies cook evenly without getting mushy. If you don't have a wok, use a large skillet.

Tuna Steaks with Balsamic Glaze

Makes: 4 servings   *Serving Size: 1 tuna steak*   *Prep Time: 5 minutes*

Cooking spray
4 5-ounce tuna steaks
1/2 teaspoon salt
1/4 teaspoon ground black pepper
3/4 cup balsamic vinegar
1 tablespoon honey
2 scallions, sliced diagonally

1. Coat a large nonstick skillet with cooking spray. Season each side of tuna steaks with salt and pepper. Place tuna steaks in pan and cook over medium-high heat for about 3–4 minutes on each side. Remove from heat.

2. In a small saucepan, combine balsamic vinegar and honey over medium heat. Bring to a low boil and cook until liquid is reduced by half (about 10 minutes). Stir frequently.

3. Spoon balsamic mixture over tuna steaks and top with scallions.

Exchanges
4 Very Lean Meat   1 Carbohydrate
1/2 Fat

Calories 244
Calories from Fat 61
Total Fat . . . . .7 g
Saturated Fat . . . . .0 g
Cholesterol . . . . 53 mg
Sodium . . . . 345 mg
Total Carbohydrate . . . . . . 14 g
Dietary Fiber . . . . .0 g
Sugars. . . . . 11 g
Protein. . . . . 32 g

Dietitian's Tip: This recipe proves fish is easy to cook! You don't want to miss out on the benefits of all those heart-healthy omega-3 fatty acids.

RECIPE LIST

GROCERY LIST

Fresh Produce
Broccoli – 1 head
Yellow squash – 1
Mushrooms – 1 pint
Red bell peppers – 2
Garlic – 1 head
Green bell peppers – 4
Onions – 3
Cabbage – 1 small head
Jalapeño pepper – 1

Meat/Poultry/Fish
Flank steak – 2/3 pound
Oysters, shucked –
1 pound
Bone-in center-cut pork
chops – 4 (5-ounce)
chops
Lean smoked turkey
sausage – 14 ounces

Grains/Bread/Pasta
Prepackaged 12-inch
pizza crust – 1
Bread crumbs –
1 container
Linguine – 1 box
6-inch flour or corn
tortillas – 8
Brown rice – 1 bag

Dairy and Cheese
Shredded, part-skim
mozzarella cheese –
1 bag
Margarine
Fat-free half-and-half –
1 pint
Fresh Parmesan cheese –
1 wedge
Eggs
Low-fat buttermilk –
small container

Shredded, reduced-fat
cheddar cheese –
1 bag

Canned Goods and Sauces
Dijon mustard – 1 bottle
16-ounce can kidney
beans – 2 cans

Frozen Foods
10-ounce box spinach –
1 box

Staples/Seasonings/ Baking Needs
Salt/ground black pepper
Cooking spray
Olive oil
Crushed red pepper
flakes
Canola oil
Chili powder
Cayenne pepper
Cumin
All-purpose flour
Worcestershire sauce
Cornmeal
Baking powder
Honey

Miscellaneous
White wine

Veggie Pizza

Makes: 4 servings   *Serving Size: 2 slices*   *Prep Time: 20 minutes*

1 teaspoon olive oil

1 cup broccoli florets

1 yellow squash, sliced (about 1 cup)

1 cup sliced mushrooms

1 red bell pepper, sliced into thin strips

2 garlic cloves, minced

1 12-inch prepackaged pizza crust

1/2 cup shredded, part-skim mozzarella cheese

1/4 teaspoon ground black pepper

1/4 teaspoon crushed red pepper flakes

1. Preheat oven to 450 degrees. Add olive oil to a large nonstick skillet over medium heat. Add broccoli, squash, mushrooms, and red bell pepper; sauté for 3 minutes. Add garlic and sauté 30 more seconds.

2. Place pizza crust on a baking sheet. Spread the veggie mixture evenly over the pizza. Sprinkle with cheese, black pepper, and red pepper flakes.

3. Bake pizza in oven for 20 minutes or until the cheese begins to lightly brown.

Exchanges

3 Starch	1 Vegetable
1 Lean Meat	1 Fat

Calories 353
  Calories from Fat 96
Total Fat . . . . 11 g
  Saturated Fat . . . . 3 g
Cholesterol . . . . 8 mg
Sodium . . . . 632 mg
Total Carbohydrate . . . . . . 50 g
  Dietary Fiber . . . . 3 g
  Sugars . . . . 5 g
Protein . . . . 15 g

See photo insert.

Dietitian's Tip: Eating pizza can be a great way to sneak more vegetables into your meal plan.

Beef Fajitas

Makes: 4 servings   *Serving Size: 2 fajitas*   *Prep Time: 15 minutes*

Cooking spray

2/3 pound flank steak, cut against the grain into 2-inch strips

1 teaspoon canola oil

2 green bell peppers, sliced into thin strips

1 medium onion, sliced into thin strips

1/4 cup water

1/2 tablespoon chili powder

1/4 teaspoon cayenne pepper

1/4 teaspoon cumin

1/2 teaspoon salt

1/2 teaspoon ground black pepper

8 6-inch flour or corn tortillas

1. Coat a large nonstick skillet with cooking spray. Cook beef over medium-high heat for about 3 minutes. Remove from pan and set aside.

2. Add oil to the pan and heat. Add green pepper and onion; cook for about 7 minutes or until beginning to brown. Add meat and any juices back to pan and cook another 2 minutes.

3. Add water and spices, including salt and pepper. Bring to a boil; reduce heat, and simmer until water evaporates. Serve with tortillas.

Exchanges

2 Starch	2 Vegetable
2 Lean Meat	1 Fat

Calories 350
  Calories from Fat 101
Total Fat . . . . 11 g
  Saturated Fat . . . . 4 g
Cholesterol . . . . 36 mg
Sodium . . . . 635 mg
Total Carbohydrate . . . . . . 41 g
  Dietary Fiber . . . . 4 g
  Sugars . . . . 5 g
Protein . . . . 21 g

Chef's Tip: To cut against the grain means to slice the meat in the opposite direction of the lines—the grain—in the meat.

Oysters Rockefeller

Makes: 2 servings   *Serving Size: about 6 oysters*   *Prep Time: 15 minutes*

Cooking spray

1 tablespoon margarine

2 tablespoons all-purpose flour

1 cup fat-free half-and-half

1/4 teaspoon salt (optional)

1/4 teaspoon ground black pepper

1/4 cup chopped, frozen spinach, thawed and drained

1/4 cup bread crumbs

3 tablespoons grated fresh Parmesan cheese

1 pound fresh oysters, shucked and with juice

2 tablespoons white wine

1. Preheat oven to 350 degrees. Coat an 8-inch pie or cake pan with cooking spray; set aside.

2. In a small nonstick skillet, melt margarine over medium heat. Add flour to margarine, stirring constantly. Cook for 2–3 minutes to make a roux.

3. In a small saucepan, bring half-and-half to a low boil over medium-high heat. Add roux, salt, and pepper to half-and-half while whisking. Boil for 2 minutes; stir in spinach and cook 2 more minutes.

4. In a small bowl, combine bread crumbs and Parmesan cheese; set aside.

5. Line the bottom of the pie or cake pan with the oysters and their juice. Sprinkle wine over the oysters. Pour spinach and sauce mixture over the oysters and sprinkle bread crumb mixture over the top.

6. Bake for 20 minutes or until oysters are done.

Exchanges

1 Lean Meat   2 1/2 Carbohydrate
1 1/2 Fat

Calories	298
Calories from Fat	101
Total Fat	11 g
Saturated Fat	3 g
Cholesterol	34 mg
Sodium	569 mg
Total Carbohydrate	34 g
Dietary Fiber	1 g
Sugars	7 g
Protein	13 g

Chef's Tip: You can buy oysters already shucked in the fresh seafood department. You can also find frozen shucked oysters in the frozen food section.

Honey-Mustard Pork Chops

Makes: 4 servings   *Serving Size: 1 pork chop*   *Prep Time: 10 minutes*

1/2 cup Dijon mustard
  2 tablespoons honey
1/2 teaspoon salt
1/2 teaspoon ground black pepper
  4 5-ounce bone-in, center-cut
    pork chops
    Cooking spray

1. Preheat oven to 400 degrees. In a small bowl, combine Dijon mustard, honey, salt, and pepper.

2. Place pork chops in a baking dish coated with cooking spray. Pour mustard mixture over pork chops and spread to coat.

3. Bake pork chops in oven 30 minutes or until done.

✔ *Keep your hearty healthy this month with low-fat, high-fiber foods and plenty of vegetables!*

Exchanges

3 Lean Meat   1 Carbohydrate

Calories 202
  Calories from Fat 64
Total Fat . . . . 7 g
  Saturated Fat . . . . 2 g
Cholesterol . . . . 59 mg
Sodium . . . . 765 mg
Total Carbohydrate . . . . . . 12 g
  Dietary Fiber . . . . 0 g
  Sugars . . . . 12 g
Protein . . . . 24 g

Dietitian's Tip: Mustard, a free food in the exchange system, adds great flavor without extra fat or calories.

Pasta Cabbage Stir-Fry

Makes: 10 servings   *Serving Size: 1/2 cup*   *Prep Time: 25 minutes*

8 ounces uncooked linguine
1/2 tablespoon olive oil
1 small onion, thinly sliced
4 cups shredded cabbage
1/4 teaspoon salt
1/4 teaspoon ground black pepper

1. Cook pasta according to package directions, omitting salt; drain.

2. Add oil to a large nonstick skillet over medium-high heat. Add onion to pan and cook for 3–5 minutes or until translucent.

3. Add cabbage to pan and stir-fry for 10 minutes or until cabbage is softened and beginning to brown. Add salt and pepper.

4. Add cooked pasta to pan and toss with cabbage mixture; sauté 3 more minutes.

Exchanges

1 Starch	1 Vegetable

Calories	101
Calories from Fat	11
Total Fat	1 g
Saturated Fat	0 g
Cholesterol	0 mg
Sodium	64 mg
Total Carbohydrate	19 g
Dietary Fiber	2 g
Sugars	2 g
Protein	3 g

Chef's Tip: If you don't cook cabbage very often, you might want to reconsider. Stir-frying cabbage with pasta and onions makes a great accompaniment to grilled or broiled meat.

Red Beans and Rice

Makes: 6 servings   *Serving Size: about 1 cup*   *Prep Time: 15 minutes*

Cooking spray

14 ounces lean smoked turkey sausage, sliced

1 medium onion, chopped

1 medium green bell pepper, chopped

1 garlic clove, minced

2 16-ounce cans kidney beans, undrained

1 teaspoon ground black pepper

1/4–1/2 teaspoon cayenne pepper

1 tablespoon Worcestershire sauce

2 cups water

1 cup uncooked brown rice

1. In a large saucepan coated with cooking spray, sauté sausage for 5 minutes over medium-high heat. Add onion and green pepper and sauté another 5 minutes. Add garlic and sauté 30 seconds.

2. Stir in beans, pepper, cayenne pepper, Worcestershire sauce, and water over medium-high heat.

3. Bring to a boil; reduce heat and simmer, uncovered, 25 minutes.

4. Add brown rice, cover, and simmer another 35 minutes.

Exchanges

3 1/2 Starch   1 Medium-Fat Meat

Calories 362
  Calories from Fat 66
Total Fat . . . . 7 g
  Saturated Fat . . . . 2 g
Cholesterol . . . . 42 mg
Sodium . . . . 1553 mg
Total Carbohydrate . . . . . . 53 g
  Dietary Fiber . . . . 7 g
  Sugars. . . . . 9 g
Protein . . . . 20 g

Dietitian's Tip: If you're vegetarian, try this recipe without the sausage.

Jalapeño Corn Muffins

Makes: 12 muffins *Serving Size: 1 muffin* *Prep Time: 13 minutes*

1 1/4 cups all-purpose flour
 3/4 cup cornmeal
   2 teaspoons baking powder
 1/2 teaspoon salt
   2 eggs
   1 cup low-fat buttermilk
   1 tablespoon canola oil
   1 jalapeño pepper, minced
   1 red bell pepper, minced
   1 green bell pepper, minced
 1/2 cup shredded, reduced-fat cheddar cheese

1. Preheat oven to 400 degrees. In a large mixing bowl, sift together flour, cornmeal, baking powder, and salt. Set aside.

2. In a medium mixing bowl, whisk eggs. Add buttermilk and oil; mix well.

3. Add jalapeño pepper, red pepper, green pepper, and cheese to dry ingredients and toss well to coat. Make a well in the center of the dry ingredients.

4. Pour wet ingredients into the well and gently combine just until dry ingredients are moistened. Batter will be thick and lumpy.

5. Spray a muffin pan or line with paper muffin cups. Fill muffin cups 2/3 full. Bake for 25 minutes or until golden brown.

Exchanges

1 1/2 Starch	1/2 Fat

Calories 132
 Calories from Fat 31
Total Fat . . . . 3 g
 Saturated Fat . . . . 1 g
Cholesterol . . . . 40 mg
Sodium . . . . 231 mg
Total Carbohydrate . . . . . . 20 g
 Dietary Fiber . . . . 2 g
 Sugars . . . . 2 g
Protein . . . . 5 g

See photo insert.

Chef's Tip: These muffins are perfect for the holiday season because the bits of red and green pepper make them look very festive.

February ❖ Week 3

RECIPE LIST

DAY 1: Lemon Herb Tilapia with
Zucchini **56**

DAY 2: Broiled BBQ Chicken **57**
Sugar Snap Peas **58**

DAY 3: Salsa Turkey Meat Loaf **59**

DAY 4: Marinated Flank Steak **60**
Garlic and Herb-Mashed
Parsnips **61**

DAY 5: Jerk Chicken **62**

GROCERY LIST

Fresh Produce
Lemon – 1
Garlic – 2 heads
Zucchini – 2
Sugar snap peas –
3 cups
Onion – 1
Limes – 5
Cilantro – 1 bunch
Parsnips – 8 medium
Fresh parsley –
1 bunch
Fresh tarragon – 1 bunch
Shallots – 1–2
Habanero pepper – 1

Meat/Poultry/Fish
Tilapia – 4
(4-ounce) filets
Bone-in chicken breasts –
4 breast halves
Boneless, skinless
chicken breasts – 4
(4-ounce) breasts
Lean ground turkey –
1 pound
Flank steak – 1 pound

Grains/Bread/Pasta
Bread crumbs –
1 container

Dairy and Cheese
Margarine
Eggs
Fat-free milk

Canned Goods and Sauces
15-ounce can tomato
sauce –1
Barbecue sauce –
1 bottle
Lite soy sauce – 1 bottle
Salsa – 1 jar

Staples/Seasonings/ Baking Needs
Salt/ground black pepper
Cooking spray
Dried basil
Dried tarragon
Dried oregano
Dried thyme
Olive oil
Sugar
Ground cinnamon
Allspice
Dry mustard
Dried thyme
Cumin

Miscellaneous
Sesame seeds

55

Lemon Herb Tilapia with Zucchini

Makes: 4 servings   *Serving Size: 1 tilapia filet*   *Prep Time: 25 minutes*
and 1/2 cup zucchini

1/2 cup lemon juice
  3 garlic cloves, minced
  1 teaspoon dried basil
  1 teaspoon dried tarragon
  1 teaspoon dried oregano
  1 teaspoon dried thyme
  4 4-ounce tilapia filets
  2 small zucchini, thinly sliced
    lengthwise
  1 tablespoon margarine
1/4 teaspoon salt
1/4 teaspoon ground black pepper

1. Preheat oven to 400 degrees. Combine lemon juice, garlic, and herbs in a medium bowl. Add fish, cover, and marinate in the refrigerator for 15 minutes.

2. Remove fish from marinade (reserve the marinade). Spray a 12 × 12-inch sheet of aluminum foil with cooking spray.

3. Place 2 filets of fish on the sheet of aluminum foil. Top with half of zucchini. Repeat layering with another layer of fish, then remaining zucchini.

4. Sprinkle chunks of margarine over the top of fish and drizzle 1/4 cup of the marinade over the top. Sprinkle with salt and pepper.

5. Bring foil sides up on both sides and seal. Place on baking sheet and bake in oven for 20 minutes.

Exchanges

3 Very Lean Meat	1/2 Fat
1 Vegetable	

Calories	155
Calories from Fat	50
Total Fat	6 g
Saturated Fat	2 g
Cholesterol	76 mg
Sodium	217 mg
Total Carbohydrate	5 g
Dietary Fiber	1 g
Sugars	2 g
Protein	23 g

Chef's Tip: Cooking with aluminum foil (packet cooking) is a quick, easy, and low-fat method.

Broiled BBQ Chicken

Makes: 4 servings   Serving Size: 1 chicken breast half   Prep Time: 5 minutes

4 chicken breast halves, bone in, skin removed

1/2 teaspoon ground black pepper

1 cup bottled barbecue sauce (reserve 1/4 cup)

1. Preheat oven broiler. Season all sides of each chicken breast with black pepper. Place chicken breast side down in broiler for 10 minutes. Turn chicken over and coat well with 3/4 cup of sauce. Broil for 5 more minutes.

2. Remove chicken from broiler and coat with remaining 1/4 cup of sauce.

 Make the Link! between taking care of your diabetes and keeping your heart healthy . . . ask the American Diabetes Association how today.

Exchanges

4 Very Lean Meat   1/2 Fat
1/2 Carbohydrate

Calories 198
Calories from Fat 39
Total Fat . . . . 4 g
Saturated Fat . . . . 1 g
Cholesterol . . . . 77 mg
Sodium . . . . 577 mg
Total Carbohydrate . . . . . . 8 g
Dietary Fiber . . . . 1 g
Sugars . . . . 7 g
Protein . . . . 29 g

Chef's Tip: This barbecued chicken couldn't be easier—try it outside on the grill in the summer, too!

Sugar Snap Peas

Makes: 6 servings   *Serving Size: 1/2 cup*   *Prep Time: 1 minute*

1/2 teaspoon olive oil

3 cups whole sugar snap peas, washed and dried

1 teaspoon sesame seeds

1 teaspoon lite soy sauce

1. Add oil to a medium nonstick skillet over medium-high heat. Add peas and stir-fry for 2 minutes. Sprinkle with sesame seeds and stir-fry for 2 more minutes.

2. Drizzle peas with soy sauce and stir-fry for 1 more minute.

Exchanges

1 Vegetable

Calories	27
Calories from Fat	6
Total Fat	1 g
Saturated Fat	0 g
Cholesterol	0 mg
Sodium	39 mg
Total Carbohydrate	4 g
Dietary Fiber	1 g
Sugars	2 g
Protein	1 g

Chef's Tip: Sesame seeds provide a lot of flavor—and toasting them enhances that flavor even more.

Salsa Turkey Meat Loaf

Makes: 6 servings   *Serving Size: 1/6 recipe*   *Prep Time: 10 minutes*

Cooking spray
1 pound lean ground turkey
1 egg
1/2 cup bread crumbs
1 finely diced onion
1 garlic clove, minced
3/4 cup salsa, divided

1. Preheat oven to 400 degrees. Coat a 5 × 9-inch loaf pan with cooking spray. In a large mixing bowl, combine turkey, egg, bread crumbs, onion, garlic, and 1/2 cup salsa. Mix thoroughly.

2. Place turkey mixture in loaf pan and spread evenly. Top with remaining 1/4 cup salsa. Bake for 50–60 minutes.

Exchanges

2 Medium-Fat Meat
1/2 Carbohydrate

Calories	185
Calories from Fat	78
Total Fat	9 g
Saturated Fat	3 g
Cholesterol	99 mg
Sodium	265 mg
Total Carbohydrate	10 g
Dietary Fiber	1 g
Sugars	3 g
Protein	17 g

Chef's Tip: Who said meat loaf has to be boring? Serve this zesty dish with Smashed Potatoes (see recipe, page 167).

Marinated Flank Steak

Makes: 4 servings   *Serving Size: 1 steak*   *Prep Time: 20 minutes*

4 limes, juiced (about 1/2 cup lime juice)
1/2 cup whole cilantro leaves
2 garlic cloves, sliced
1 pound flank steak, cut into 4 4-ounce steaks
1/2 teaspoon salt
1/2 teaspoon ground black pepper

1. Prepare an indoor or outdoor grill.

2. Combine lime juice, cilantro, and garlic in a large bowl. Add steaks and marinate for 15 minutes in the refrigerator.

3. Remove steaks from marinade. Season meat on both sides with salt and pepper. Grill over medium-high heat for 5–7 minutes on each side.

4. Slice thinly against the grain to serve.

Exchanges
3 Lean Meat

Calories 172
Calories from Fat 73
Total Fat . . . . 8 g
Saturated Fat . . . . 4 g
Cholesterol . . . . 54 mg
Sodium . . . . 360 mg
Total Carbohydrate . . . . 2 g
Dietary Fiber . . . . 0 g
Sugars . . . . 1 g
Protein . . . . 22 g

Dietitian's Tip: The bold flavors of cilantro, lime juice, and garlic make a great-tasting dish without added fat.

Garlic and Herb-Mashed Parsnips

Makes: 4 servings   *Serving Size: 1/2 cup*   *Prep Time: 15 minutes*

8 medium parsnips, peeled and cubed

4 whole garlic cloves, peeled

3 tablespoons fat-free milk

1 teaspoon chopped fresh parsley

1 teaspoon chopped fresh tarragon

1/2 teaspoon salt

1/4 teaspoon ground black pepper

1. Fill a large saucepan 2/3 full with water and bring to a boil. Add parsnips and garlic cloves. Boil for 10–15 minutes or until parsnips are soft. Drain.

2. In a medium bowl, add all ingredients and, with an electric mixer or a whisk, beat until puréed.

✔ *February is Black History Month. Learn more about a famous black American today!*

Exchanges

2 Starch

Calories 138
 Calories from Fat 4
Total Fat . . . . 0 g
 Saturated Fat . . . . 0 g
Cholesterol . . . . 0 mg
Sodium . . . . 314 mg
Total Carbohydrate . . . . . . 33 g
 Dietary Fiber . . . . 7 g
 Sugars . . . . 7 g
Protein . . . . 3 g

Chef's Tip: If you don't like the flavor of tarragon, try basil in this recipe instead.

Jerk Chicken

Makes: 4 servings   *Serving Size: 1 chicken breast*   *Prep Time: 15 minutes*

2 teaspoons olive oil
2 tablespoons shallots, minced
2 garlic cloves, minced
1 habanero pepper, seeded and minced
1 15-ounce can tomato sauce
2 tablespoons fresh lime juice
2 tablespoons lite soy sauce
1 teaspoon sugar
1/2 teaspoon ground cinnamon
1/2 tablespoon allspice
1/2 tablespoon dry mustard
1 teaspoon dried thyme
1 teaspoon cumin
1/2 teaspoon ground black pepper
Cooking spray
4 4-ounce boneless, skinless chicken breasts

1. Preheat oven to 375 degrees. In a medium saucepan, heat oil over medium-high heat. Add shallots and garlic. Sauté until the shallots are translucent. Add habanero pepper and sauté 1 more minute.

2. Add the remaining ingredients except cooking spray and chicken. Bring to a boil. Reduce heat and simmer for 5 minutes. Place mixture in a blender (or use an immersion blender in the pan) and purée until smooth.

3. Coat a medium glass or metal baking dish with cooking spray. Place chicken breasts in dish. Pour sauce over the top of chicken. Bake for 30 minutes or until chicken is done.

Exchanges

3 Very Lean Meat   1 Fat
1 Carbohydrate

Calories 213
  Calories from Fat 53
Total Fat . . . . 6 g
  Saturated Fat . . . . 1 g
Cholesterol . . . . 68 mg
Sodium . . . . 1009 mg
Total Carbohydrate . . . . . . 13 g
  Dietary Fiber . . . . 2 g
  Sugars . . . . 8 g
Protein . . . . 28 g

Chef's Tip: You should wear plastic or rubber gloves when dealing with hot peppers to prevent any irritation to your eyes or skin.

February ❖ Week 4

GROCERY LIST

Fresh Produce
Onions – 4
Celery – 1 bag
Carrots – 1 bag
Russet potatoes –
  7 medium
Green bell pepper – 2
Zucchini – 2
Mushrooms – 1 pint
Lemon – 2
Fresh parsley – 1 bunch
Idaho potatoes –
  6 medium
Garlic – 1 head
Romaine lettuce –
  12 ounces
Pears – 2 medium

Meat/Poultry/Fish
Lean smoked turkey
  sausage – 1 package
Lean ground turkey –
  1 pound
Bone-in chicken breasts –
  3 breast halves

Grains/Bread/Pasta
Rotini pasta – 1 box
Saltine crackers – small
  box
Old fashioned oats –
  small container
Whole-wheat hamburger
  buns – 6 buns

Dairy and Cheese
Fat-free milk
Grated Parmesan cheese
Eggs
Margarine
Goat cheese –
  1 1/2 ounces

Canned Goods and Sauces
14.5-ounce can fat-free,
  reduced-sodium
  chicken broth – 4 cans
15-ounce can tomato
  sauce – 1 can
14.5-ounce can no-salt-
  added diced
  tomatoes – 1 can
14.75-ounce can
  salmon – 1 can
Dijon mustard – 1 bottle
Fat-free Italian
  dressing – 1 bottle

Frozen Foods
Peas – small bag
8-ounce container
  fat-free whipped
  topping – 1 container

Staples/Seasonings/ Baking Needs
Salt/ground black pepper
Cooking spray
All-purpose flour
Dried sage
Bay leaf
Olive oil
Canola oil
Dried basil
Dried parsley
Dried minced onion
Garlic salt
Cayenne pepper
Chili powder
Cumin
Dried oregano
Dried rosemary
Prepackaged 9-inch pie
  crust – 1 crust
1.4-ounce sugar-free, fat-
  free chocolate pudding
  mix – 2 packages

Miscellaneous
White wine
Almonds – 2 ounces
Mini semi-sweet choco-
  late chips – small bag
Orange juice

Sausage and Potato Soup

Makes: 8 servings   *Serving Size: about 1 cup*   *Prep Time: 20 minutes*

Cooking spray
2 cups lean smoked turkey
    sausage, sliced
1 1/2 cups diced onion
1/2 cup diced celery
1/2 cup diced carrot
2 tablespoons all-purpose flour
3 14.5-ounce cans fat-free,
    reduced-sodium chicken
    broth
4 medium russet potatoes,
    peeled and diced
1/2 teaspoon dried sage
1/2 teaspoon ground black
    pepper
1 bay leaf
1 cup fat-free milk

1. Coat a large soup pot with cooking spray. Cook sausage for 2 minutes. Add onion, celery, and carrots and cook another 5–7 minutes or until beginning to brown.

2. Add flour, stirring well. Cook for 2 minutes. Add broth, potatoes, sage, black pepper, and bay leaf. Bring to a boil, scraping brown bits at the bottom of the pan. Reduce heat and simmer until potatoes are done (about 20 minutes).

3. Add milk and simmer 2 more minutes; do not boil. Remove bay leaf before serving.

February is the focus month of Project Power in African-American churches. Find out more today at your local church.

Exchanges

1 Starch	1 Vegetable
1 Lean Meat	

Calories 151
 Calories from Fat 29
Total Fat . . . . 3 g
 Saturated Fat . . . . 1 g
Cholesterol . . . . 23 mg
Sodium . . . . 922 mg
Total Carbohydrate . . . . . . 21 g
 Dietary Fiber . . . . 2 g
 Sugars . . . . 6 g
Protein . . . . 9 g

Chef's Tip: There's nothing better than homemade soup on a cold winter night!

Ratatouille with Rotini

Makes: 6 servings　　　　*Serving Size: 1 1/2 cups*　　　　*Prep Time: 15 minutes*

8 ounces uncooked rotini pasta
1 tablespoon olive oil
1 medium onion, finely chopped
1 1/2 cups green bell pepper, cut into thin strips
2 medium zucchini, thinly sliced
1 1/2 cups sliced mushrooms
4 garlic cloves, minced
1 15-ounce can tomato sauce
1 14.5-ounce can no-salt-added diced tomatoes
1 teaspoon dried basil
1/2 teaspoon ground black pepper
3 tablespoons grated Parmesan cheese

1. Cook pasta according to package directions, omitting salt; drain.

2. Heat oil in a large nonstick skillet or wok. Over medium-high heat, sauté onion and green pepper until onion is clear. Add zucchini and mushrooms and sauté about 5 more minutes.

3. Add garlic, tomato sauce, and diced tomatoes. Stir in basil and black pepper.

4. Reduce heat and bring to a low boil for 25 minutes. Combine ratatouille with cooked rotini pasta. Sprinkle with Parmesan cheese.

Exchanges

2 Starch　　　　　　　　1/2 Fat
3 Vegetable

Calories 244	
Calories from Fat 41	
Total Fat . . . . 5 g	
Saturated Fat . . . . 1 g	
Cholesterol . . . . 4 mg	
Sodium . . . . 538 mg	
Total Carbohydrate . . . . . . 44 g	
Dietary Fiber . . . . 5 g	
Sugars . . . . 11 g	
Protein . . . . 10 g	

Dietitian's Tip: This meatless meal is a great way to add more vegetables to your meal plan.

Salmon Patties with Lemon Sauce

Makes: 4 patties   *Serving Size: 1 patty*   *Prep time: 15 minutes*

SALMON PATTIES

1 14.75-ounce can salmon

1 egg

1/2 teaspoon ground black pepper

1/4 cup crushed saltine crackers

1 tablespoon Dijon mustard

1 tablespoon dried parsley

LEMON SAUCE

Juice of one lemon

2 tablespoons margarine

1 teaspoon chopped fresh parsley

1. In a medium bowl, combine all patty ingredients together. Divide into 4 equal servings. Shape into 1/4-inch-thick patties.

2. Coat a large nonstick skillet with cooking spray. Cook patties over medium heat approximately 5 minutes on each side or until golden brown.

3. To prepare sauce, combine lemon juice, margarine, and parsley in a saucepan and simmer 5 minutes.

4. Serve 2 teaspoons sauce over each salmon patty.

Exchanges

3 Lean Meat   1/2 Carbohydrate

Calories	241
Calories from Fat	125
Total Fat	14 g
Saturated Fat	2 g
Cholesterol	112 mg
Sodium	814 mg
Total Carbohydrate	5 g
Dietary Fiber	0 g
Sugars	1 g
Protein	23 g

Dietitian's Tip: Salmon is another great source of heart-healthy omega-3 fatty acids—and it's easy to make!

Hearty Turkey Burgers

Makes: 6 servings   *Serving Size: 1 burger*   *Prep Time: 10 minutes*

1 pound lean ground turkey
1 egg
3/4 cup old-fashioned oatmeal
1/2 cup minced fresh mushrooms
2 tablespoons dried minced onion
1/2 teaspoon garlic salt
1/2 teaspoon ground black pepper
6 whole-wheat hamburger buns

1. Prepare an indoor or outdoor grill. Combine all ingredients except buns in a bowl. Divide turkey into 6 equal portions, shaping each into a patty 1/2 inch thick.

2. Place patties on grill rack; grill 7 minutes on each side or until done. (Or coat a large nonstick skillet with cooking spray and cook patties over medium heat for 3–4 minutes per side, or until juices run clear).

3. Serve burgers on whole-wheat hamburger buns.

Exchanges

2 Starch	1/2 Fat
2 Lean Meat	

Calories 301
  Calories from Fat 102
Total Fat . . . . 11 g
  Saturated Fat . . . . 3 g
Cholesterol . . . . 92 mg
Sodium . . . . 374 mg
Total Carbohydrate . . . . . . 28 g
  Dietary Fiber . . . . 3 g
  Sugars . . . . 4 g
Protein . . . . 22 g

Dietitian's Tip: Make sure to buy lean ground turkey—some ground turkey contains dark meat and skin and is higher in fat.

Cajun French Fries

Makes: 6 servings　　　*Serving Size: 1/6 recipe*　　　*Prep Time: 10 minutes*

6 medium Idaho potatoes (6 ounces each), peeled and sliced into eighths
1 tablespoon canola oil
1/4 teaspoon cayenne pepper
1 teaspoon chili powder
1/2 teaspoon cumin
1/2 teaspoon salt
1/4 teaspoon ground black pepper
　　Cooking spray

1. Preheat oven to 350 degrees.

2. Combine potatoes and oil in a large bowl and toss well to coat. In a small bowl, combine cayenne pepper, chili powder, cumin, salt, and black pepper. Sprinkle over potatoes and toss well until all potatoes are coated with seasoning.

3. Coat a large baking sheet with cooking spray. Spread potatoes evenly on baking sheet. Bake for 30 minutes or until golden brown and crispy.

Exchanges
1 1/2 Starch

Calories 125
　Calories from Fat 21
Total Fat . . . . 2 g
　Saturated Fat . . . . 0 g
Cholesterol . . . . 0 mg
Sodium . . . . 204 mg
Total Carbohydrate . . . . . . 24 g
　Dietary Fiber . . . . 2 g
　Sugars . . . . 2 g
Protein . . . . 2 g

Dietitian's Tip: Who says you can't eat French fries? These spicy-sweet fries are so crisp and tasty you won't miss the traditional variety.

Chicken Vesuvio

Makes: 3 servings   *Serving Size: 1 chicken breast*   *Prep Time: 25 minutes*
with 6 potato wedges

3 bone-in chicken breast halves, skin on
1/4 cup all-purpose flour
1 tablespoon olive oil
3 medium russet potatoes, each peeled and cut into 6 wedges
3 garlic cloves, minced
14.5-ounce can fat-free, reduced-sodium chicken broth
2 teaspoons lemon juice
1/4 cup white wine
1 teaspoon dried oregano
1 teaspoon dried rosemary
1/2 cup frozen peas
1/2 teaspoon salt (optional)
1/4 teaspoon ground black pepper

1. Preheat oven to 400 degrees. Remove all excess fat from chicken, leaving the skin on. Dredge the skin side of the chicken in flour and set aside.

2. Add oil to a large nonstick skillet over high heat. Place chicken flour side down in skillet to brown (about 5–6 minutes). Remove chicken from pan and set aside.

3. Microwave potato wedges in a medium bowl for 8 minutes on high.

4. In the same skillet, reduce heat to medium and add the garlic for 30 seconds. Add chicken broth, lemon juice, and wine and cook until liquid is reduced by half. Add the herbs and cook for 1 more minute.

5. Place the chicken skin side up in a medium metal baking pan. Add the chicken broth mixture to the pan, making sure to avoid pouring broth over the top of the chicken. (The liquid should not cover the browned skin).

6. Add the potato wedges to the liquid. Bake in oven for 30 minutes.

7. Take out of oven. Remove potatoes and chicken from pan. Sprinkle with salt and pepper. Pour liquid into the skillet and bring to a boil and reduce by half.

8. Add the frozen peas to the liquid and immediately remove from heat.

9. Serve each breast with 6 potato wedges and 1/2 cup of the broth and peas.

Chef's Tip: You can easily double this recipe when company's coming.

Exchanges

3 Starch	1/2 Fat
3 Lean Meat	

Calories 433
  Calories from Fat . . 113
Total Fat . . . . 13 g
  Saturated Fat . . . . 3 g
Cholesterol . . . . 83 mg
Sodium . . . . 434 mg
Total Carbohydrate . . 41 g
  Dietary Fiber . . . . 5 g
  Sugars . . . . 5 g
Protein . . . . 36 g

Pear Salad with Almonds

Makes: 6 servings   *Serving Size: 1 serving*   *Prep Time: 15 minutes*

1/2 cup fat-free Italian dressing
1/2 cup orange juice
12 ounces chopped romaine lettuce
2 ounces sliced almonds, toasted
1 1/2 ounces goat cheese, crumbled
2 medium pears, peeled and diced

1. In a small bowl, whisk together Italian dressing and orange juice; set aside.

2. In a large salad bowl, toss together remaining ingredients.

3. Drizzle dressing over salad and toss again to coat.

✔ *Eating Disorders Awareness Week is the last week of February. If you think someone may be having eating problems, ask her or him if you can help. Eating problems are symptoms of other issues . . . and those issues can be fixed!*

Exchanges

1 Fruit	1 1/2 Fat

Calories 132
  Calories from Fat 60
Total Fat . . . . 7 g
  Saturated Fat . . . . 1 g
Cholesterol . . . . 7 mg
Sodium . . . . 245 mg
Total Carbohydrate . . . . . . 15 g
  Dietary Fiber . . . . 3 g
  Sugars . . . . 10 g
Protein . . . . 5 g

Chef's Tip: To toast almonds, place them in a small nonstick skillet over low heat and toast for about 4 minutes or until they begin to brown.

Chocolate Mousse Pie

Makes: 8 servings   *Serving Size: 1 piece*   *Prep Time: 5 minutes*

1 9-inch prepackaged pie crust
2 1.4-ounce packages sugar-free fat-free chocolate pudding mix
1 2/3 cups fat-free milk
1 8-ounce container fat-free whipped topping, divided
2 tablespoons mini semi-sweet chocolate chips

1. Preheat oven to 400 degrees. Bake pie crust according to package directions. Remove from oven and cool thoroughly.

2. In a medium bowl, whisk pudding mix and milk. Fold half (4 ounces) of whipped topping into pudding mixture and fold until fully blended.

3. Spread pudding mixture into pie crust and top with remaining whipped topping. Sprinkle top with chocolate chips.

Exchanges

1 Fat   2 Carbohydrate

Calories	194
Calories from Fat	54
Total Fat	6 g
Saturated Fat	2 g
Cholesterol	1 mg
Sodium	253 mg
Total Carbohydrate	30 g
Dietary Fiber	2 g
Sugars	7 g
Protein	4 g

Chef's Tip: Your Valentine will never guess how easy this dessert was to make!

March

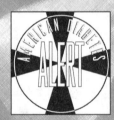

The American Diabetes Alert® is an annual, one-day call-to-action held on the fourth Tuesday of March to help people find out if they are at risk for diabetes. Take the Risk Test at www.diabetes.org and show it to your friends and family.

National Nutrition Month®

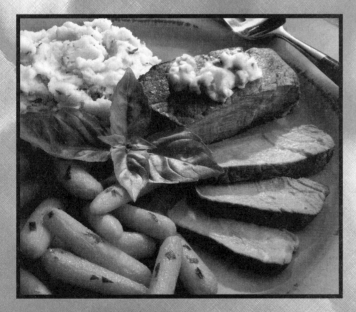

Bleu Cheese–Crusted Steak (page 139)
Basil Mashed Potatoes (page 122)
Honey Tarragon Carrots (page 169)
This meal is fabulous served to dinner guests. It's hearty,
with just the right balance of flavors!

March ❖ Recipes

March ❖ Week 1

DAY 1: Penne with Broccoli
and Herbs **76**

DAY 2: Spice-Rubbed Pork Chops **77**
Roasted Parmesan Zucchini **78**

DAY 3: Turkey Sub Sandwich **79**

DAY 4: Alfredo Orange Roughy and
Rice **80**

DAY 5: Cream of Broccoli Soup **81**
Cheesy Breadsticks **82**

GROCERY LIST

Fresh Produce
Broccoli – 6 heads
Fresh basil – 1 bunch
Fresh Italian (flat-leaf)
parsley – 1 bunch
Garlic – 1 head
Zucchini – 2 large
Lettuce – 1 head
Tomato – 1
Onions – 2 medium

Meat/Poultry/Fish
Bone-in pork chops –
4 (5-ounce) chops
Sliced deli turkey –
12 ounces
Orange roughy filets – 4
(4-ounce) filets

Grains/Bread/Pasta
Penne pasta – 1 box
3-ounce sub rolls – 4
Brown rice – 1 box
or bag

Dairy and Cheese
Fresh Parmesan cheese –
1 wedge
3/4-ounce slices
reduced-fat Swiss
cheese – 4 slices
Fat-free half-and-half –
2 pints
Shredded, reduced-fat
cheddar cheese –
1 bag

Canned Goods and Sauces
14.5-ounce can fat-free,
reduced-sodium
chicken broth – 3 cans
Dijon mustard –
1 container
Light Italian dressing –
1 bottle

Staples/Seasonings/Baking Needs
Salt/ground black pepper
Cooking spray
Dried oregano
Paprika
Cayenne pepper
Chili powder
Garlic salt
Olive oil
Cornstarch
Red wine vinegar

Miscellaneous
White wine
Ready-made refrigerated
breadsticks – 1 can
(12 breadsticks)

Penne with Broccoli and Herbs

Makes: 4 servings   *Serving Size: 1/4 recipe*   *Prep Time: 15 minutes*

2 tablespoons chopped fresh basil

2 tablespoons chopped fresh Italian parsley

1 garlic clove, minced

2 tablespoons olive oil

2 teaspoons red wine vinegar

1/4 teaspoon salt

Dash ground black pepper

8 ounces uncooked penne pasta

2 cups broccoli florets (fresh or frozen)

1. Whisk first seven ingredients together in a small bowl.

2. Cook pasta in a large pot of boiling water until almost tender, about 6 minutes. Add broccoli and cook about 2 more minutes. Drain and transfer to serving bowl.

3. Add dressing and toss well to coat.

Exchanges

2 1/2 Starch	1 Vegetable
1 1/2 Fat	

Calories	284
Calories from Fat	71
Total Fat	8 g
Saturated Fat	1 g
Cholesterol	0 mg
Sodium	160 mg
Total Carbohydrate	45 g
Dietary Fiber	3 g
Sugars	3 g
Protein	8 g

Chef's Tip: You can always add ingredients to your food to enhance the flavor without piling on fat and calories. Shake some crushed red pepper flakes onto this delicious pasta dish, or add extra herbs, such as chopped fresh oregano or chives.

Spice-Rubbed Pork Chops

Makes: 4 servings   *Serving Size: 1 pork chop*   *Prep Time: 5 minutes*

1 tablespoon dried oregano
2 tablespoons paprika
1 teaspoon cayenne pepper
1 teaspoon chili powder
1/2 teaspoon salt
1/2 teaspoon ground black pepper
4 5-ounce, bone-in pork chops
   Cooking spray

1. In a small bowl, combine the first six ingredients and stir well.

2. Rub one side of each pork chop well with spice mixture.

3. Coat a large nonstick skillet with cooking spray. Over medium-high heat, place each chop spice side down and cook for four minutes on each side or until done.

Exchanges
3 Lean Meat

Calories 148
   Calories from Fat 56
Total Fat . . . . 6 g
   Saturated Fat . . . . 2 g
Cholesterol . . . . 59 mg
Sodium . . . . 194 mg
Total Carbohydrate . . . . 2 g
   Dietary Fiber . . . . 1 g
   Sugars . . . . 1 g
Protein . . . . 21 g

Chef's Tip: To make these pork chops even spicier, add 1/2 teaspoon crushed red pepper flakes to the rub.

Roasted Parmesan Zucchini

Makes: 5 servings   *Serving Size: 1/2 cup*   *Prep Time: 5 minutes*

Cooking spray
2 large zucchini, sliced into
  2-inch wedges
2 teaspoons olive oil
1/2 teaspoon garlic salt
3 tablespoons grated Parmesan
  cheese

1. Preheat oven to 450 degrees. Coat a roasting pan with cooking spray.

2. Place zucchini in pan. Drizzle olive oil over zucchini and sprinkle evenly with garlic salt and Parmesan cheese.

3. Roast approximately 20 minutes.

Exchanges
1 Vegetable   1/2 Fat

Calories 52
  Calories from Fat 30
Total Fat . . . . 3 g
  Saturated Fat . . . . 1 g
Cholesterol . . . . 5 mg
Sodium . . . . 208 mg
Total Carbohydrate . . . . 4 g
  Dietary Fiber . . . . 2 g
  Sugars . . . . 2 g
Protein . . . . 3 g

See photo insert.

Chef's Tip: Roasting vegetables enhances their flavor quickly, making it more concentrated and sweet.

Turkey Sub Sandwich

Makes: 4 servings   *Serving Size: 1 sandwich*   *Prep Time: 10 minutes*

- **4** teaspoons Dijon mustard
- **4** 3-ounce sub rolls
- **12** ounces sliced deli turkey
- **4** 3/4-ounce slices reduced-fat Swiss cheese
- **1** cup shredded lettuce
- **1** tomato, thinly sliced
- **1** medium onion, thinly sliced
- **4** tablespoons light Italian dressing

1. Spread 1 teaspoon Dijon mustard on one side of each sub roll. Add 3 ounces turkey, 1 slice cheese, 1/4 cup lettuce, tomato slices, and onion slices to each roll.

2. Repeat for remaining three subs.

3. Drizzle 1 tablespoon dressing on top of lettuce, tomato, and onion on every sandwich.

Exchanges

3 Starch	1 Vegetable
3 Lean Meat	

Calories 408
  Calories from Fat 82
Total Fat . . . . 9 g
  Saturated Fat . . . . 4 g
Cholesterol . . . . 47 mg
Sodium . . . . 1512 mg
Total Carbohydrate . . . . . . 49 g
  Dietary Fiber . . . . 3 g
  Sugars . . . . 9 g
Protein . . . . 33 g

Chef's Tip: Now you can make your own great subs anytime the mood strikes!

Alfredo Orange Roughy and Rice

Makes: 4 servings   *Serving Size: 1 filet and*   *Prep Time: 5 minutes*
                        1/2 cup brown rice

Cooking spray

4 4-ounce orange roughy filets

2 garlic cloves, minced

1/2 cup dry white wine

1 pint fat-free half-and-half

1/2 cup grated fresh Parmesan
    cheese

1/2 teaspoon salt (optional)

1/8 teaspoon ground black pepper

2 cups cooked brown rice

✔ *March is the beginning*
  of SELF *magazine's*
  annual 3-month fitness
  and nutrition challenge!
  Go to www.SELF.com
  for more information.

1. Coat a large sauté pan with cooking spray. Over medium-high heat, sear fish on both sides about 2 minutes.

2. Remove from pan and set aside. Spray pan again with cooking spray; add garlic. Cook for about 30 seconds; do not let it brown.

3. Add wine; cook until liquid evaporates by half. Add half-and-half and Parmesan cheese; simmer for about 4 minutes.

4. Add fish back to pan and add salt and pepper. Simmer for 2 more minutes.

5. Serve over brown rice.

Exchanges

2 1/2 Starch	1/2 Fat
3 Very Lean Meat	

Calories 329
  Calories from Fat 62
Total Fat . . . . 7 g
  Saturated Fat . . . . 3 g
Cholesterol . . . . 42 mg
Sodium . . . . 340 mg
Total Carbohydrate . . . . . . 35 g
  Dietary Fiber . . . . 2 g
  Sugars . . . . 8 g
Protein . . . . 27 g

Chef's Tip: Steamed asparagus would be a great addition to this meal.

Cream of Broccoli Soup

Makes: 8 servings   *Serving Size: 1 cup*   *Prep Time: 10 minutes*

4 cups broccoli florets
1 tablespoon olive oil
1 cup finely diced onion
3 14.5-ounce cans fat-free, reduced-sodium chicken broth
2 tablespoons cornstarch
1 cup fat-free half-and-half
3/4 teaspoon salt (optional)
1/2 teaspoon ground black pepper

1. Coarsely chop broccoli florets in food processor or chopper.

2. Heat oil in a large soup pot over medium-high heat. Add broccoli and onions and cook for 3 minutes.

3. Add broth and bring to a boil. Reduce heat and simmer for 15 minutes or until broccoli and onions are soft.

4. In a small bowl, combine the cornstarch and half-and-half and whisk. Add this mixture (called a slurry) to the soup and bring back to a boil.

5. Reduce to a simmer for 5 more minutes; add salt and pepper.

Exchanges
1/2 Fat   1/2 Carbohydrate

Calories	72
Calories from Fat	21
Total Fat	2 g
Saturated Fat	0 g
Cholesterol	2 mg
Sodium	429 mg
Total Carbohydrate	9 g
Dietary Fiber	1 g
Sugars	4 g
Protein	4 g

Dietitian's Tip: Cream soups are typically higher in fat than broth-based soups, but fat-free half-and-half adds creaminess without fat in this recipe.

Cheesy Breadsticks

Makes: 12 servings   *Serving Size: 1 breadstick*   *Prep Time: 5 minutes*

Cooking spray
1 can ready-made refrigerated breadsticks (12 breadsticks)
1/2 cup shredded, reduced-fat cheddar cheese

1. Preheat oven to 375 degrees. Coat a large baking sheet with cooking spray. Place breadsticks on baking sheet and spray lightly with cooking spray.

2. Sprinkle cheese over each breadstick and bake for 15 minutes.

Exchanges

1 Starch

Calories	83
Calories from Fat	20
Total Fat	2 g
Saturated Fat	1 g
Cholesterol	3 mg
Sodium	224 mg
Total Carbohydrate	13 g
Dietary Fiber	0 g
Sugars	2 g
Protein	3 g

Chef's Tip: Reduced-fat versions of cheeses, rather than fat-free versions, work better in recipes like this because they melt better.

March ❖ Week 2

GROCERY LIST

Fresh Produce
Onions – 3
Lemons – 2
Tomato – 1
Cucumber – 1 large
Garlic – 1 head
Cantaloupe – 1 small
Strawberries – 1 pint
Green grapes – small
    bunch
Blueberries – 1/2 pint
Mushrooms – 1 pint
Carrots – small bag

Meat/Poultry/Fish
Boneless, skinless
    chicken breasts –
    2 pounds
Boneless beef tenderloin
    tips – 1 pound
Peeled, cooked shrimp –
    1 pound

Grains/Bread/Pasta
Lo mein noodles – 1 box
Whole-wheat pita
    pocket halves – 5
    (buy 3 whole)
No-boil lasagna
    noodles – 1 box
Egg noodles – 1 box

Dairy and Cheese
Egg substitute –
    4 ounces
Eggs
Plain, fat-free yogurt –
    8 ounces
Shredded, part-skim
    mozzarella
    cheese – 16 ounces
15-ounce container fat-
    free ricotta cheese –
    1 container
Grated Parmesan cheese
Fat-free sour cream –
    small container

Canned Goods and Sauces
14-ounce can bean
    sprouts – 1 can
14.5-ounce can fat-free,
    reduced-sodium
    chicken broth – 3 cans
14.5-ounce can fat-free,
    reduced-sodium beef
    broth – 1 can
15.5-ounce can Great
    Northern Beans –
    2 cans
4-ounce can mild green
    chilies – 1 can
1-pound jar marinara
    pasta sauce – 1 jar
Dijon mustard – 1 bottle
Lite soy sauce – 1 bottle

Frozen Foods
10-ounce box spinach –
    1 box

Staples/Seasonings/Baking Needs
Salt/ground black pepper
Cooking spray
All-purpose flour
Cornstarch
Sugar substitute
Dried oregano
Olive oil

Miscellaneous
Dry white wine

Shrimp Egg Fu Yung

Makes: 4 servings   *Serving Size: 1 patty*   *Prep Time: 10 minutes*

Cooking spray
1/4 cup minced onion
1 cup canned bean sprouts, drained and rinsed
4 ounces egg substitute
1 egg
3 tablespoons all-purpose flour
1 1/2 cups cooked shrimp, diced
1/2 teaspoon salt (optional)
1 tablespoon cornstarch
1 packet sugar substitute
1 tablespoon lite soy sauce
1 1/2 cups fat-free, reduced-sodium chicken broth

1. Coat a large nonstick skillet with cooking spray over medium heat. Add onion and bean sprouts. Sauté until onion turns clear. Set aside to cool.

2. In a medium bowl, whisk the egg substitute and egg together. Add flour, onion, bean sprouts, shrimp, and salt to eggs and stir well.

3. Over medium-high heat, pour batter by 1/2 cups into same pan to form patties and cook well on both sides until golden brown, about 4 minutes each side. Remove patties from pan and set aside

4. In a small bowl, combine cornstarch, sugar substitute, soy sauce, and chicken broth. Mix well. Add this mixture to the hot pan and bring to a boil; reduce heat and simmer 5 minutes to make a gravy.

5. Pour the gravy over patties and serve.

Exchanges
2 Very Lean Meat
1/2 Carbohydrate

Calories 123
Calories from Fat 16
Total Fat . . . . 2 g
Saturated Fat . . . . 1 g
Cholesterol . . . . 136 mg
Sodium . . . . 513 mg
Total Carbohydrate . . . . . . 10 g
Dietary Fiber . . . . 1 g
Sugars . . . . 2 g
Protein . . . . 16 g

Chef's Tip: Your dinner guests will never know this dish didn't come from a Chinese restaurant!

Chinese Noodles

Makes: 4 servings   *Serving Size: 1/2 cup*   *Prep Time: 10 minutes*

4 ounces uncooked lo mein noodles
Cooking spray
2 teaspoons lite soy sauce

1. Cook noodles according to package directions, omitting salt. Drain and cool for 5 minutes in the refrigerator.

2. Coat a large nonstick skillet with cooking spray. Over medium-high heat, add cooled noodles and sauté for 5 minutes.

3. Drizzle soy sauce over noodles and continue to sauté for 3 more minutes.

Exchanges

1 1/2 Starch

Calories	101
Calories from Fat	0
Total Fat	0 g
Saturated Fat	0 g
Cholesterol	0 mg
Sodium	101 mg
Total Carbohydrate	23 g
Dietary Fiber	1 g
Sugars	0 g
Protein	3 g

Chef's Tip: You can stir-fry any type of noodle for a little extra flavor and bite. Just be sure to cool the noodles completely before stir-frying, or you'll end up with a sticky mess!

Chicken Gyros

Makes: 5 servings   *Serving Size: 1 gyro*   *Prep Time: 15 minutes*

1/4 cup lemon juice
  1 teaspoon dried oregano
  1 pound boneless, skinless chicken breasts, thinly sliced into strips
    Cooking spray
1/4 teaspoon salt
1/4 teaspoon ground black pepper
  5 whole-wheat pocket pita halves
  1 cup diced tomato

SAUCE

  1 cup plain, fat-free yogurt
  1 cup peeled, seeded, and grated cucumber
  1 garlic clove, minced

1. In a medium bowl, combine lemon juice and oregano. Add chicken and marinate in the refrigerator for 15 minutes.

2. Remove the chicken from the marinade (reserve 1 tablespoon of the marinade).

3. Coat a large nonstick skillet with cooking spray and heat over medium-high heat. Add chicken strips and reserved marinade to pan and sauté for 4–5 minutes or until the chicken is done. Add salt and pepper.

4. In a medium bowl, combine all sauce ingredients.

5. Fill each pita with even amounts of chicken, tomatoes, and sauce.

Exchanges

2 Starch	3 Very Lean Meat

Calories 258
  Calories from Fat 32
Total Fat . . . . 4 g
  Saturated Fat . . . . 1 g
Cholesterol . . . . 56 mg
Sodium . . . . 315 mg
Total Carbohydrate . . . . . . 31 g
  Dietary Fiber . . . . 2 g
  Sugars . . . . 7 g
Protein . . . . 28 g

Chef's Tip: You can grate the peeled cucumber using the large hole on your cheese grater, or pulse the cucumber in a blender or food processor for 30 seconds.

Fruit Salad

Makes: 4 servings   *Serving Size: 1 cup*   *Prep Time: 15 minutes*

1 cup cubed cantaloupe
1 cup sliced strawberries
1 cup green grapes
1 cup blueberries

Combine all ingredients and toss gently.

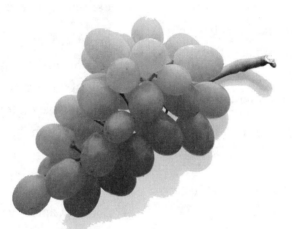

Exchanges
1 Fruit

Calories	75
Calories from Fat	6
Total Fat	1 g
Saturated Fat	0 g
Cholesterol	0 mg
Sodium	7 mg
Total Carbohydrate	18 g
Dietary Fiber	3 g
Sugars	13 g
Protein	1 g

Dietitian's Tip: Fruit is a sweet end to a great meal.

Spinach Lasagna

Makes: 10 servings   *Serving Size: 1 slice*   *Prep Time: 12 minutes*

Cooking spray

1 egg

2 cups shredded, part-skim mozzarella cheese, divided

1 15-ounce container fat-free ricotta cheese

1/4 cup grated Parmesan cheese

10-ounce package frozen chopped spinach, thawed and drained

5 cups jarred marinara pasta sauce

12 no-boil lasagna noodles

1. Preheat oven to 350 degrees. Coat a 13 × 9 × 2-inch glass baking dish with cooking spray.

2. In a medium bowl, mix together egg, 1 cup mozzarella, ricotta, and Parmesan cheese. Add spinach and mix well.

3. Spread 1 cup pasta sauce on bottom of baking dish. Arrange noodles side by side on top of sauce, overlapping slightly. Spread 1 cup spinach and cheese mixture on top of noodles.

4. Repeat layering with pasta sauce, noodles, and spinach and cheese mixture 3 more times.

5. Top with remaining 3 noodles and 1 cup sauce. Cover lasagna with foil and bake 25 minutes. Uncover; top with remaining 1 cup mozzarella cheese, and bake an additional 25–35 minutes or until cheese is light golden brown.

Exchanges

1 Starch	3 Vegetable
1 Lean Meat	1/2 Fat

Calories 242
　Calories from Fat 53
Total Fat . . . . 6 g
　Saturated Fat . . . . 3 g
Cholesterol . . . . 70 mg
Sodium . . . . 583 mg
Total Carbohydrate . . . . . . 30 g
　Dietary Fiber . . . . 4 g
　Sugars . . . . 10 g
Protein . . . . 19 g

Chef's Tip: Using no-boil noodles really saves time in this recipe.

Beef Stroganoff

Makes: 5 servings   *Serving Size: 1/5 recipe*   *Prep Time: 15 minutes*

5 ounces uncooked egg noodles

2 teaspoons olive oil

1 pound boneless beef tender-loin tips, sliced into 2-inch strips

1 1/2 cups sliced mushrooms

1/2 cup minced onion

1 tablespoon all-purpose flour

1/2 cup dry white wine

1 teaspoon Dijon mustard

1 14.5-ounce can fat-free, reduced-sodium beef broth

1/2 cup fat-free sour cream

1/4 teaspoon salt

1/4 teaspoon ground black pepper

1. Cook noodles according to package directions, omitting salt.

2. Add oil to a large sauté pan over high heat. Add meat and sauté for about 3 minutes. Remove meat from pan. Add mushrooms and onion and sauté for 5 minutes or until beginning to brown.

3. Add flour and cook for 1 minute. Add wine to deglaze pan; cook for 2 minutes. Add Dijon mustard and beef broth; bring to a boil. Reduce heat and simmer for 5 minutes.

4. Add beef and any juices back to broth and simmer for 3 more minutes. Add sour cream, salt, and pepper; simmer for 30 seconds.

5. Serve over egg noodles.

Exchanges

2 Starch	1/2 Fat
2 Lean Meat	

Calories 293
Calories from Fat 79
Total Fat . . . . 9 g
Saturated Fat . . . . 3 g
Cholesterol . . . . 77 mg
Sodium . . . . 364 mg
Total Carbohydrate . . . . . . 28 g
Dietary Fiber . . . . 1 g
Sugars . . . . 4 g
Protein . . . . 22 g

Chef's Tip: Save prep time by buying presliced mushrooms.

White Chicken Chili

Makes: 7 servings   *Serving Size: 1 cup*   *Prep Time: 10 minutes*

Cooking spray

1 pound boneless, skinless chicken breasts, cut into 1-inch cubes

1 medium onion, finely diced

2 medium carrots, finely diced

3 garlic cloves, minced

2 15.5-ounce cans Great Northern Beans, undrained

1 cup fat-free, reduced-sodium chicken broth

1 4-ounce can mild green chilies, diced

1/2 teaspoon ground black pepper

1. Coat a large soup pot with cooking spray. Add chicken and cook over medium-high heat until lightly brown. Remove chicken from pan and set aside.

2. Spray pan again with cooking spray. Sauté onion and carrots about 4 minutes until onion turns clear.

3. Add all remaining ingredients and chicken and stir. Bring to a boil, reduce heat, and simmer 15 minutes.

Exchanges

1 Starch	1 Vegetable
3 Very Lean Meat	

Calories 210
  Calories from Fat 24
Total Fat . . . . 3 g
  Saturated Fat . . . . 1 g
Cholesterol . . . . 39 mg
Sodium . . . . 588 mg
Total Carbohydrate . . . . . . 21 g
  Dietary Fiber . . . . 6 g
  Sugars . . . . 5 g
Protein . . . . 22 g

Chef's Tip: Canned green chilies are an easy way to add great flavor to recipes.

RECIPE LIST

DAY 1: Linguine with Red Clam Sauce **92**

DAY 2: Tuna Melt **93**

DAY 3: Turkey Divan with Broccoli **94**

DAY 4: Corned Beef Sandwich **95**
Irish Vegetables **96**

DAY 5: Spinach and Pine Nut-Stuffed
Chicken **97**
Rice Pilaf **98**

GROCERY LIST

Fresh Produce
Garlic – 1 head
Fresh basil – 1 bunch
Broccoli – 2 heads
Cabbage – 1 medium
head
Idaho potatoes – 4
medium
Carrots – small bag
Celery – small bag
Onion – 1

Meat/Poultry/Fish
Boneless, skinless
chicken breasts – 4
(4-ounce) breasts
Boneless, skinless
turkey breast – 1
pound
Thinly-sliced deli lean
corned beef –
12 ounces

Grains/Bread/Pasta
Linguine pasta – 1 box
English muffins – 1 box
Brown rice – 1 box
Rye bread – 1 loaf
White rice – 1 box

Dairy and Cheese
Shredded, reduced-fat
cheddar cheese –
2 bags
Fat-free milk
Grated Parmesan cheese

Canned Goods
and Sauces
14.5-ounce can fat-free,
reduced-sodium
chicken broth – 3 cans
6.5-ounce can minced
clams – 3 cans
28-ounce can crushed
tomatoes – 1 can
8-ounce can tomato
sauce – 1 can
6-ounce can tuna packed
in water – 2 cans
Light mayonnaise – 1 jar
Dijon mustard – 1 bottle
Horseradish – 1 bottle
Brown mustard –
1 bottle

Frozen Foods
10-ounce box spinach –
1 box

Staples/Seasonings/
Baking Needs
Salt/ground black pepper
Cooking spray
Olive oil
Crushed red pepper
flakes
Onion salt
All-purpose flour
Paprika
Dried thyme
Bay leaf

Miscellaneous
White wine
Pine nuts – small bag

Linguine with Red Clam Sauce

Makes: 8 servings   *Serving Size: 1 cup*   *Prep Time: 10 minutes*

16 ounces uncooked linguine
 2 teaspoons olive oil
 2 garlic cloves, minced
 3 6.5-ounce cans minced clams with juice (drain one can only)
1/2 cup white wine
 1 28-ounce can crushed tomatoes
1/4 teaspoon salt
1/4 teaspoon ground black pepper
1/4 teaspoon crushed red pepper flakes
 1 cup tomato sauce
 1 tablespoon chopped fresh basil

1. Cook pasta according to package directions, omitting salt. Drain.

2. Add oil to a large nonstick skillet over medium-high heat. Add garlic and sauté 30 seconds.

3. Add clams (with juice) and wine. Turn heat to high and cook for about 10 minutes or until liquid is reduced by half.

4. Add all remaining ingredients except basil and simmer 10 minutes. Remove from heat and add basil.

5. Serve sauce over linguine noodles.

Exchanges

3 Starch   2 Vegetable
1 Very Lean Meat

Calories 325
  Calories from Fat 27
Total Fat . . . . 3 g
  Saturated Fat . . . . 0 g
Cholesterol . . . . 22 mg
Sodium . . . . 626 mg
Total Carbohydrate . . . . . . 55 g
  Dietary Fiber . . . . 5 g
  Sugars . . . . 10 g
Protein . . . . 17 g

Chef's Tip: A green leaf or spinach salad would be a great addition to this meal.

Tuna Melt

Makes: 5 servings   *Serving Size: 1 tuna melt*   *Prep Time: 5 minutes*

2 6-ounce cans tuna packed in water, drained

1/4 cup light mayonnaise

1/4 teaspoon ground black pepper

1/4 teaspoon onion salt

2 teaspoons Dijon mustard

5 English muffin halves

2/3 cup shredded, reduced-fat cheddar cheese

1. Preheat oven to 400 degrees. In a medium mixing bowl, combine tuna, mayonnaise, pepper, onion salt, and Dijon mustard.

2. Spread 1/4 cup tuna mixture on top of each muffin half and top with about 2 tablespoons cheese.

3. Place muffins on baking sheet and bake 10 minutes.

Exchanges

1 Starch	1/2 Fat
2 Lean Meat	

Calories 223
  Calories from Fat 74
Total Fat . . . . 8 g
  Saturated Fat . . . . 3 g
Cholesterol . . . . 32 mg
Sodium . . . . 675 mg
Total Carbohydrate . . . . . . 14 g
  Dietary Fiber . . . . 1 g
  Sugars . . . . 1 g
Protein . . . . 22 g

Dietitian's Tip: A fruit salad would be a great side dish for this meal.

Turkey Divan with Broccoli

Makes: 6 servings   Serving Size: 1/6 recipe   Prep Time: 15 minutes

Cooking spray
4 cups broccoli florets
1 pound boneless, skinless turkey breast, cubed
2 cups cooked brown rice
2 cups fat-free milk
1 1/2 tablespoons all-purpose flour
3/4 cup shredded, reduced-fat cheddar cheese
1/2 teaspoon salt
1/4 teaspoon ground black pepper

1. Preheat oven to 350 degrees. Coat a 9 × 9-inch glass baking dish with cooking spray.

2. Steam broccoli florets until tender-crisp. In a large bowl, combine steamed broccoli, turkey breast, and rice and spread into the prepared baking dish.

3. Whisk together fat-free milk and flour in a small bowl. In a medium saucepan, bring milk and flour mixture to a boil. Reduce heat and add cheese, salt, and pepper. Simmer for 1 minute or until all cheese is melted.

4. Pour cheese sauce over turkey, broccoli, and rice mixture and stir. Bake for 30 minutes or until turkey is done and sauce is bubbly.

Exchanges

1 Starch	1 Vegetable
3 Very Lean Meat	1/2 Fat

Calories 245
  Calories from Fat 40
Total Fat . . . . 4 g
  Saturated Fat . . . . 2 g
Cholesterol . . . . 58 mg
Sodium . . . . 409 mg
Total Carbohydrate . . . . . . 23 g
  Dietary Fiber . . . . 3 g
  Sugars . . . . 5 g
Protein . . . . 28 g

Chef's Tip: This is a great dish to serve if you have enough turkey left over after Thanksgiving.

Corned Beef Sandwich

Makes: 4 servings   *Serving Size: 1 sandwich*   *Prep Time: 10 minutes*

4 teaspoons horseradish
2 tablespoons brown mustard
8 slices rye bread
12 ounces thinly sliced deli lean corned beef

1. Spread 1 teaspoon horseradish and 1 1/2 teaspoons brown mustard on 1 slice of bread. Add 3 ounces corned beef to each slice of bread. Top with a slice of bread.

2. Repeat process for remaining 3 sandwiches.

Exchanges

2 Starch	1/2 Fat
3 Very Lean Meat	

Calories 296
Calories from Fat 57
Total Fat . . . . 6 g
Saturated Fat . . . . 2 g
Cholesterol . . . . 45 mg
Sodium . . . . 1354 mg
Total Carbohydrate . . . . . . 33 g
Dietary Fiber . . . . 4 g
Sugars . . . . 3 g
Protein . . . . 27 g

Chef's Tip: Lean corned beef is a nice change from turkey.

Irish Vegetables

Makes: 4 servings   *Serving Size: 1/4 recipe*   *Prep Time: 10 minutes*

1 medium head cabbage, cut
  into 4 wedges
4 medium Idaho potatoes,
  peeled and quartered
4 large carrots, peeled and cut
  into large chunks
1 14.5-ounce can fat-free,
  reduced-sodium chicken broth
3 cups water
3 garlic cloves, sliced in half
1/2 teaspoon salt
1/2 teaspoon ground black pepper

1. In a large soup pot, add all ingredients. Bring to a boil; reduce heat and simmer 35 minutes or until cabbage is tender.

2. Serve vegetables in a bowl with 1/4 cup of liquid served over them.

Exchanges

2 Starch   3 Vegetable

Calories 220
  Calories from Fat 11
Total Fat . . . . 1 g
  Saturated Fat . . . . 0 g
Cholesterol . . . . 0 mg
Sodium . . . . 582 mg
Total Carbohydrate . . . . . . 48 g
  Dietary Fiber . . . . 11 g
  Sugars . . . . 13 g
Protein . . . . 8 g

Chef's Tip: These vegetables taste great with corned beef.

Spinach and Pine Nut-Stuffed Chicken

Makes: 4 servings   *Serving Size: 1 chicken breast*   *Prep Time: 15 minutes*

1/4 cup pine nuts

4 4-ounce boneless, skinless chicken breasts

3 tablespoons grated Parmesan cheese

1/2 cup frozen spinach, thawed and drained

2 garlic cloves, minced

1/2 teaspoon salt

1/2 teaspoon ground black pepper

1 teaspoon paprika
Cooking spray

1. Preheat oven to 350 degrees.

2. In a small nonstick sauté pan, sauté pine nuts over medium-high heat for 2–3 minutes to toast. Set aside.

3. Place one chicken breast on a cutting board and cover with plastic wrap. Pound meat with a meat tenderizer or rolling pin until it is about 1/4 inch thick. Repeat this process for the other 3 breasts. Set aside.

4. In a medium bowl, combine toasted pine nuts, Parmesan cheese, spinach, and garlic. Spread 3 tablespoons of this mixture on one side of the pounded chicken breast. Roll breast and secure the seam with a toothpick. Repeat procedure for remaining 3 chicken breasts.

5. Sprinkle all sides of rolled chicken breasts with salt, pepper, and paprika.

6. Coat a glass or metal baking dish with cooking spray and place chicken in dish seam side down. Bake for 30 minutes or until chicken is done.

7. To serve, remove toothpicks and slice each piece into 5 rounds. Serve over Rice Pilaf (see recipe, page 98).

Exchanges
4 Lean Meat

Calories 220
  Calories from Fat . . . 88
Total Fat . . . . 10 g
  Saturated Fat . . . . 3 g
Cholesterol . . . . 74 mg
Sodium . . . . 468 mg
Total Carbohydrate . . 4 g
  Dietary Fiber . . . . 1 g
  Sugars . . . . 1 g
Protein . . . . 31 g

Chef's Tip: For added flavor, bring 1 cup of balsamic vinegar to a boil and cook until it's reduced by half. Drizzle a little of the vinegar over each chicken breast after it has been sliced.

Rice Pilaf

Makes: 5 servings   *Serving Size: 2/3 cup*   *Prep Time: 10 minutes*

1 teaspoon olive oil
1 medium carrot, finely diced
2 medium celery stalks, finely diced
1 medium onion, finely diced
1 cup uncooked white rice
3 cups fat-free, reduced-sodium chicken broth
1/2 teaspoon dried thyme
1 bay leaf
1/2 teaspoon salt (optional)
1/4 teaspoon ground black pepper

1. Add oil to a medium saucepan. Sauté carrots, celery, and onion over medium-high heat for about 3 minutes or until onion begins to turn clear.

2. Add rice to the mixture and stir constantly over heat for 2 minutes. Add remaining ingredients except salt and pepper and bring to a boil.

3. Reduce heat to low and simmer, covered. Cook for 20 minutes. Add salt and pepper and remove bay leaf. Fluff rice with a fork.

Exchanges

2 Starch   1 Vegetable

Calories 174
  Calories from Fat 11
Total Fat . . . . 1 g
  Saturated Fat . . . . 0 g
Cholesterol . . . . 0 mg
Sodium . . . . 328 mg
Total Carbohydrate . . . . . . 35 g
  Dietary Fiber . . . . 2 g
  Sugars . . . . 4 g
Protein . . . . 5 g

Chef's Tip: You can use brown rice instead of white in this recipe to boost the fiber content. Just add 1 cup of water to the chicken broth and cook for 30–35 minutes.

March ❖ Week 4

GROCERY LIST

Fresh Produce
Mushrooms – 2 pints
Garlic – 1 head
Onions – 2 large
Romaine lettuce – 1 large
head or 6 cups prepack-
aged salad in a bag
Tomatoes – 2 large
Carrots – small bag
Celery – small bag
Red potatoes –
12–16 potatoes
Fresh parsley – 1 bunch
Iceberg lettuce – 1 head
Fresh rosemary – 1 sprig
Lemon – 1

Meat/Poultry/Fish
Beef tenderloin steaks – 4
(4-ounce) steaks
3-pound fryer chicken, cut
up into 8 pieces – 1
chicken
Whole chicken – 1
(3 pounds)
10-ounce package pre-
cooked, flavored chicken
breast strips – 1 package
Live mussels – 1/2 pound

Unpeeled shrimp –
1/2 pound
White fish (cod) –
1/2 pound

Grains/Bread/Pasta
16-ounce loaf French
bread – 1 loaf
Corn tortillas – 12
Farfalle pasta – 1 box

Dairy and Cheese
Egg substitute – 8 ounces
Eggs
Fat-free milk
Fat-free half-and-half –
1 pint
Grated Asiago cheese –
4 ounces
Grated Parmesan cheese
Shredded, reduced-fat ched-
dar or Colby cheese –
1 package (2 cups)
Fat-free sour cream –
small container
Corn oil stick margarine –
small package

Canned Goods and Sauces
14.5-ounce can fat-free,
reduced-sodium
chicken broth – 2 cans

10 3/4-ounce can low-fat
condensed cream of
chicken soup – 2 cans
4-ounce can chopped
green chilies – 2 cans
15-ounce can no-salt-
added diced tomatoes –
1 can
12–14-ounce can mush-
room stems and
pieces – 1 can
1-pound jar marinara
pasta sauce – 1 jar
Light Italian dressing –
1 bottle
Light Ranch dressing –
1 bottle

Staples/Seasonings/ Baking Needs
Salt/ground black pepper
Cooking spray
Paprika
Cayenne pepper
Chili powder
Cumin
Olive oil
Dried sage
Dried basil
Dried thyme
All-purpose flour
Baking powder
Sugar
Vanilla extract
Powdered sugar
Whole black peppercorns

Miscellaneous
White wine
Poppy seeds

Blackened Beef Tenderloin

Makes: 4 servings   *Serving Size: 1 steak*   *Prep Time: 5 minutes*

2 tablespoons paprika
1 teaspoon cayenne pepper
1 tablespoon chili powder
1 teaspoon cumin
1/2 teaspoon salt
1/2 teaspoon ground black pepper
4 4-ounce beef tenderloin steaks
     Cooking spray

1. In a small bowl combine first six ingredients and stir well.

2. Rub one side of each steak well with spice mixture.

3. Coat a large nonstick skillet with cooking spray. Over medium-high heat, place each steak spice side down and cook for 6 minutes on each side.

Exchanges

3 Lean Meat

Calories 160
  Calories from Fat 67
Total Fat . . . . 7 g
  Saturated Fat . . . . 3 g
Cholesterol . . . . 60 mg
Sodium . . . . 201 mg
Total Carbohydrate . . . . . . 2 g
  Dietary Fiber . . . . 1 g
  Sugars . . . . 1 g
Protein . . . . 20 g

Chef's Tip: If you like your steaks less spicy, reduce the cayenne pepper to 1/2 teaspoon.

Savory Mushroom Bread Pudding

Makes: 9 servings   *Serving Size: 1/3 cup*   *Prep Time: 25 minutes*

Cooking spray
2 teaspoons olive oil
4 cups chopped fresh mushrooms
2 garlic cloves, minced
1 teaspoon dried sage
1 teaspoon dried basil
1/2 teaspoon salt (optional)
1/4 teaspoon ground black pepper
1 cup egg substitute
1 egg
1/2 cup fat-free milk
2 cups fat-free half-and-half
1/3 cup grated Asiago cheese
1 16-ounce loaf French bread with crust, cut into 1-inch cubes (about 6 cups)
2 tablespoons grated Asiago cheese

1. Preheat oven to 350 degrees. Generously coat an 8 × 8-inch baking dish with cooking spray. Set aside.

2. In a large nonstick sauté pan, heat oil over medium-high heat. Add mushrooms and garlic. Sauté until all liquid evaporates and mushrooms begin to brown. Remove from heat.

3. Add dried herbs, salt, and pepper and mix well; set aside to cool.

4. In a medium bowl, whisk egg substitute and egg together. Add milk, half-and-half, and 1/3 cup grated cheese and whisk well. Add bread to egg mixture and stir to coat well. Let sit for 5 minutes.

5. Fold mushroom mixture into bread mixture. Pour into prepared pan. Sprinkle with 2 tablespoons grated cheese. Bake for 45 minutes or until pudding is brown and puffed.

Exchanges

2 Starch	1 Lean Meat

Calories	207
Calories from Fat	25
Total Fat	3 g
Saturated Fat	1 g
Cholesterol	29 mg
Sodium	458 mg
Total Carbohydrate	34 g
Dietary Fiber	1 g
Sugars	5 g
Protein	11 g

Chef's Tip: Just a touch of Asiago cheese adds great flavor to this bread pudding.

Chicken Cacciatore

Makes: 6 servings   *Serving Size: 1/6 recipe*   *Prep Time: 15 minutes*

1 3-pound fryer chicken, cut up into 8 pieces
  Cooking spray
1 1-pound jar marinara pasta sauce
1 cup sliced mushrooms
2 garlic cloves, minced
1/4 cup grated Parmesan cheese

1. Preheat oven to 350 degrees.

2. Remove skin from chicken and trim any excess fat.

3. Coat a 9-inch glass baking dish with cooking spray and place chicken in bottom of dish.

4. In a medium bowl, combine pasta sauce, mushrooms, and garlic. Pour sauce over chicken. Sprinkle chicken with Parmesan cheese.

5. Bake for 35 minutes.

 Go to www.diabetes.org to find out more about the American Diabetes Alert, a one-day call to action held on the fourth Tuesday of March for people to find out if they are at risk for diabetes. Go ahead—take the Risk Test!

Exchanges

3 Lean Meat	1 Vegetable

Calories 194
  Calories from Fat 63
Total Fat . . . . 7 g
  Saturated Fat . . . . 3 g
Cholesterol . . . . 69 mg
Sodium . . . . 365 mg
Total Carbohydrate . . . . 8 g
  Dietary Fiber . . . . 2 g
  Sugars . . . . 6 g
Protein . . . . 25 g

Chef's Tip: If you can't find a cut-up fryer in the meat department racks, the butcher will cut one up for you.

Enchilada Casserole

Makes: 12 servings *Serving Size: 1 slice* *Prep Time: 35 minutes*

1/2 cup chopped onion
1/2 cup chopped celery
  6 whole black peppercorns
     Sprig rosemary
  1 3-pound whole chicken
     Cooking spray
  1 large onion, chopped
  2 10 3/4-ounce cans low-fat condensed cream of chicken soup
  2 4-ounce cans chopped green chilies
  1 15-ounce can no-salt-added diced tomatoes, drained
  1 12–14 ounce can mushroom stems and pieces, undrained
10–12 corn tortillas, cut into eighths
  2 cups shredded, reduced-fat cheddar or Colby cheese

Exchanges

1 Starch	1 Vegetable
2 Lean Meat	1/2 Fat

Calories 227
Calories from Fat 76
Total Fat . . . . 8 g
Saturated Fat . . . . 4 g
Cholesterol . . . . 50 mg
Sodium . . . . 599 mg
Total Carbohydrate . . . . . . 20 g
Dietary Fiber . . . . 3 g
Sugars . . . . 4 g
Protein . . . . 18 g

1. Preheat oven to 350 degrees. Fill a large soup pot 2/3 full with water. Add onion, celery, peppercorns, and rosemary. Remove neck and giblet bag from cavity of chicken. Rinse chicken and place in the soup pot and cook over high heat until boiling. Reduce heat and simmer 30 minutes or until chicken is done.

2. Remove chicken and strain broth through colander. Remove fat from broth. Reserve 1 3/4 cups for use in this recipe. Save remaining broth for another use. Remove skin from chicken and pull meat from bones into chunks.

3. Coat a medium nonstick skillet with cooking spray over medium-high heat. Sauté remaining onion until onion is slightly brown.

4. In large bowl, combine chicken, reserved broth, soup, sautéed onion, green chilies, tomatoes, and mushrooms. Mix well.

5. Coat an extra-large casserole dish (at least 10 × 15) with cooking spray. Cover bottom of casserole with half of the tortillas. Spoon half of chicken mixture over the tortillas and top with 1 cup of cheese. Repeat process, ending with cheese. Bake for 45 minutes.

Chef's Tip: Serve this satisfying dish with salsa, fat-free sour cream, and black olives as garnishes.

Tossed Salad with Chicken and Pasta

Makes: 4 servings   *Serving Size: 1/4 recipe*   *Prep Time: 10 minutes*

2 1/2 cups cooked farfalle pasta

6 cups shredded romaine lettuce

1 large tomato, seeded and diced

1 10-ounce package precooked, flavored chicken breast strips (try lemon pepper or garlic herb)

1/4 cup light Italian dressing

In a large salad bowl, toss together all ingredients.

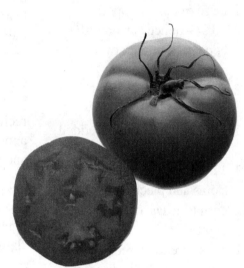

Exchanges

1 1/2 Starch	1 Vegetable
2 Very Lean Meat	

Calories 204
  Calories from Fat 26
Total Fat . . . . 3 g
  Saturated Fat . . . . 1 g
Cholesterol . . . . 32 mg
Sodium . . . . 383 mg
Total Carbohydrate . . . . . . 28 g
  Dietary Fiber . . . . 2 g
  Sugars . . . . 5 g
Protein . . . . 16 g

Chef's Tip: Precooked chicken breast strips are near the packaged lunch meats at most grocery stores. This product is higher in sodium than plain chicken breasts, though.

Seafood Stew

Makes: 6 servings   *Serving Size: 1 1/2 cups*   *Prep Time: 25 minutes*

1 tablespoon olive oil
1 cup diced carrot
1 cup diced celery
1 cup diced onion
2 garlic cloves, minced
3 cups unpeeled diced red
   potatoes
1/2 cup white wine
2 14.5-ounce cans fat-free,
   reduced-sodium chicken broth
1 teaspoon dried thyme
2 tablespoons chopped fresh
   parsley
1/2 teaspoon salt (optional)
1/2 teaspoon ground black pepper
1/2 pound live mussels, cleaned
   (see Chef's Tip)
1/2 pound shrimp, peeled and
   deveined
1/2 pound white fish (such as
   cod), cubed

1. Add oil to a large soup pot over medium-high heat. Add carrots, celery, onion, and garlic and sauté until onion turns clear.

2. Add potatoes and sauté for 2 more minutes. Add wine and cook until liquid is reduced by half.

3. Add chicken broth, thyme, parsley, salt, and pepper; bring to a boil.

4. Reduce heat to a simmer for 20 minutes or until potatoes are soft. Add mussels, shrimp, and fish; simmer for 5 minutes or until shrimp is done and mussels have opened.

Exchanges

| 1 Starch | 1 Vegetable |
| 2 Very Lean Meat | 1/2 Fat |

Calories 190
  Calories from Fat 30
Total Fat . . . . 3 g
  Saturated Fat . . . . 0 g
Cholesterol . . . . 52 mg
Sodium . . . . 478 mg
Total Carbohydrate . . . . . . 23 g
  Dietary Fiber . . . . 3 g
  Sugars . . . . 6 g
Protein . . . . 16 g

Chef's Tip: Live mussels in the shell should be closed when you purchase them from the store. Wash them under cold water and remove the beard (the stringy substance) attached to the shell. Discard any open mussels. The mussels will open when they are cooked.

Green Salad

1 head iceberg lettuce, quartered
1 large tomato, quartered
1/4 cup light Ranch dressing

1. Place 1/4 of iceberg lettuce and 1/4 tomato in a salad bowl.

2. Drizzle 1 tablespoon of Ranch dressing over the top.

3. Repeat for remaining quarters.

 National Doctor's Day is March 30 every year—thank your doctor for helping you feel better!

Exchanges

1 Vegetable	1 Fat

Calories 67	
Calories from Fat 35	
Total Fat . . . . 4 g	
Saturated Fat . . . . 0 g	
Cholesterol . . . . 0 mg	
Sodium . . . . 156 mg	
Total Carbohydrate . . . . . . 7 g	
Dietary Fiber . . . . 3 g	
Sugars. . . . . 3 g	
Protein . . . . 2 g	

Chef's Tip: Some people prefer bleu cheese dressing with this simple salad.

Lemon Poppy Seed Bundt Cake

Makes: 16 servings　　　　*Serving Size: 1 slice*　　　　*Prep Time: 25 minutes*

CAKE

    Cooking spray
 2 cups all-purpose flour
1 1/2 teaspoons baking powder
 1/4 teaspoon salt
1 1/2 cups sugar
 1/2 cup corn oil stick margarine,
     softened
 2 eggs
 1 egg white
1 1/2 teaspoons vanilla extract
 1 tablespoon lemon rind
 1 tablespoon lemon juice
 1/2 cup fat-free sour cream
 1/4 cup poppy seeds

GLAZE

 1/2 cup powdered sugar
 1 tablespoon lemon juice
 1 teaspoon water

1. Preheat oven to 325 degrees. Coat a bundt pan with cooking spray. In a medium bowl, sift together flour, baking powder, and salt. Set aside.

2. In a large bowl, beat sugar and margarine with an electric mixer at medium speed until well blended. Add eggs and egg white, one at a time. Beat well. Add vanilla, lemon rind, and lemon juice; beat 30 seconds.

3. Add part of flour mixture to sugar mixture and beat. Add part of sour cream to sugar mixture and beat. Continue alternating flour and sour cream to sugar mixture. Beat at low speed until well blended.

4. Stir in poppy seeds. Spoon batter in bundt pan and bake for 35 minutes or until toothpick inserted in center comes out clean. Let cool.

5. In a small bowl, whisk together powdered sugar, lemon juice, and water until glaze consistency is formed. Drizzle glaze over cooled cake.

Exchanges

1 Fat	2 1/2 Carbohydrate

Calories 222	
Calories from Fat 67	
Total Fat . . . . 7 g	
Saturated Fat . . . . 1 g	
Cholesterol . . . . 27 mg	
Sodium . . . . 159 mg	
Total Carbohydrate . . . . . . 36 g	
Dietary Fiber . . . . 1 g	
Sugars . . . . 23 g	
Protein . . . . 3 g	

Chef's Tip: Make sure this cake is completely cool before you drizzle the glaze over it; otherwise, the glaze will melt into the cake.

April

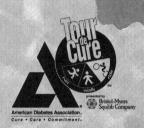

American Diabetes Association.
Cure • Care • Commitment.

Tour de Cure® is the ADA's
signature cycling fundraising
event, taking place in over
70 cities nationwide. Ride
a tour route that is breezy
and easy or challenging
and tough—you decide!
Call 1-888-DIABETES
for more info.

Spring into Health

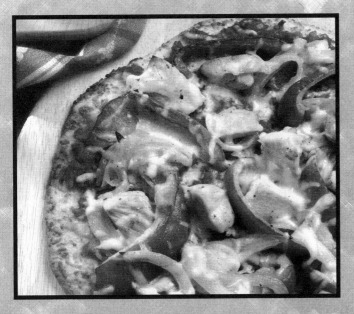

Chicken Fajita Pizza (page 150)
You could also make this delicious pizza with beef or
pork strips. The bell pepper adds a festive touch.

April ❖ Recipes

April ❖ Week 1

GROCERY LIST

Fresh Produce
12-ounce container
extra-firm tofu –
2 containers
Broccoli – 3 heads
Orange – 1
Shallots – 2
Idaho potatoes –
4 medium
Green bell pepper – 1
Red bell pepper – 1
Zucchini – 1 small
Yellow squash – 1 small
Fresh rosemary –
1 bunch
Garlic – 1 head
Asparagus – 1 bunch
(about 22 spears)
Scallions – 1 bunch

Meat/Poultry/Fish
Boneless, skinless
chicken breasts – 4
(4-ounce) breasts
Veal rib chops – 4
(6-ounce) chops
Tuna steaks – 4
(4-ounce) steaks

Grains/Bread/Pasta
Brown rice – 1 box
Orzo pasta – 1 box

Dairy and Cheese
Fat-free milk
Shredded, reduced-fat
cheddar cheese –
1 bag
9-ounce package cheese
tortellini – 1 package

Canned Goods and Sauces
14.5-ounce can fat-free,
reduced-sodium
chicken broth – 3 cans
Lite soy sauce – 1 bottle

Staples/Seasonings/Baking Needs
Salt/ground black pepper
Cooking spray
Olive oil
Sesame oil
Cornstarch
Crushed red pepper
flakes
Sugar
Apple cider vinegar
Garlic salt
Red wine vinegar
Honey

Miscellaneous
Orange juice
Sesame seeds

111

Broccoli Tofu Stir-Fry

Makes: 4 servings   *Serving Size: 2 cups*   *Prep Time: 10 minutes*

2 12-ounce packages extra-firm tofu, drained and cut into 1-inch squares
2 teaspoons olive oil, divided
2 teaspoons sesame oil, divided
2 tablespoons lite soy sauce
4 cups broccoli florets
2 teaspoons cornstarch
3 cups fat-free, reduced-sodium chicken broth
3 teaspoons sesame seeds, toasted
1/4 teaspoon crushed red pepper flakes
1/2 teaspoon salt (optional)
1/2 teaspoon ground black pepper
2 2/3 cups cooked white or brown rice

1. Sauté tofu pieces in 1 teaspoon olive oil and 1 teaspoon sesame oil in a wok or large sauté pan until golden brown on both sides. Add soy sauce and sauté for 1 more minute.

2. Remove tofu from pan and add remaining olive and sesame oil; sauté broccoli until tender-crisp.

3. In a small bowl, whisk together cornstarch and chicken broth.

4. Return tofu to the pan and add broth and the remaining ingredients except rice.

5. Simmer for 5–10 minutes or until sauce begins to thicken. Serve over white or brown rice.

Exchanges

2 1/2 Starch	1 Vegetable
1 Medium-Fat Meat	1/2 Fat

Calories 319
Calories from Fat 83
Total Fat . . . . 9 g
Saturated Fat . . . . 2 g
Cholesterol . . . . 0 mg
Sodium . . . . 786 mg
Total Carbohydrate . . . . . . 39 g
Dietary Fiber . . . . 3 g
Sugars . . . . 5 g
Protein . . . . 19 g

✔ *April is National Soy Foods Month.*

Chef's Tip: If you've never tried tofu, this is a great first recipe. The keys are to make sure the tofu isn't too thick, and to cook it until it's golden brown so the texture is just right.

Orange Chicken

Makes: 4 servings   *Serving Size: 1 chicken breast*   *Prep Time: 10 minutes*

Cooking spray
4 4-ounce boneless, skinless chicken breasts
3 tablespoons sugar
1/4 cup water
2 tablespoons apple cider vinegar
1 1/2 cups fresh orange juice
2 tablespoons grated orange peel
2 tablespoons shallots, minced (1 small shallot)
1 1/2 cups fat-free, reduced-sodium chicken broth

1. Preheat oven to 350 degrees.

2. Coat a shallow baking dish with cooking spray. Arrange chicken breasts in the bottom of the pan and bake for 30 minutes.

3. In a medium saucepan, mix sugar and water over medium heat until sugar dissolves. Bring to a boil and boil until syrup begins to caramelize, about 6 minutes. Whisk in vinegar, orange juice, orange peel, and shallots. Boil until reduced by half, about 15 minutes.

4. Add broth and boil another 20–25 minutes until reduced to about 1 cup liquid. Pour 1/4 cup sauce over each breast.

Exchanges
3 Very Lean Meat
1 1/2 Carbohydrate

Calories 224
 Calories from Fat 27
Total Fat . . . . 3 g
 Saturated Fat . . . . 1 g
Cholesterol . . . . 68 mg
Sodium . . . . 249 mg
Total Carbohydrate . . . . . . 21 g
 Dietary Fiber . . . . 0 g
 Sugars . . . . 19 g
Protein . . . . 27 g

Chef's Tip: Be sure when you grate the orange peel not to include any of the white part (pith) of the peel, which is bitter.

Twice-Baked Potatoes

Makes: 4 servings   *Serving Size: 1 potato*   *Prep Time: 5 minutes*

4 medium Idaho potatoes
1 cup fat-free milk, heated
1/3 cup shredded, reduced-fat,
  sharp cheddar cheese
3 scallions, minced
1/2 teaspoon salt
1/4 teaspoon ground black pepper

1. Preheat oven to 400 degrees.

2. Wash and dry potatoes. Poke each potato several times with a fork. Place potatoes on the middle rack in the oven. Bake for 45 minutes. Cool potatoes on a cooling rack until they are easy to touch.

3. Slice the top of each potato and scoop out insides into a large mixing bowl, leaving the skin intact. Add remaining ingredients to the potato mixture and beat with an electric mixer on high until smooth (about 5 minutes).

4. Using a spoon or pastry bag, fill each potato skin with filling, over-stuffing it a little so the potato does not completely seal. Place potatoes on a baking sheet and bake for 25 minutes.

Exchanges
2 1/2 Starch

Calories 205
  Calories from Fat 21
Total Fat . . . . 2 g
  Saturated Fat . . . . 1 g
Cholesterol . . . . 8 mg
Sodium . . . . 416 mg
Total Carbohydrate . . . . . . 41 g
  Dietary Fiber . . . . 4 g
  Sugars . . . . 6 g
Protein . . . . 9 g

Chef's Tip: If you're in a hurry, you can microwave these potatoes on high for 10–15 minutes and then bake them in the oven when stuffed.

Tortellini Primavera

Makes: 7 servings   *Serving Size: 1 cup*   *Prep Time: 15 minutes*

1 9-ounce package cheese tortellini
Cooking spray
2 tablespoons olive oil, divided
2 cups broccoli florets
1 medium green bell pepper, thinly sliced
1 medium red bell pepper, thinly sliced
1 small zucchini, thinly sliced
1 small yellow squash, thinly sliced
1 teaspoon garlic salt

1. Cook tortellini according to package directions. Drain.

2. Coat a large nonstick skillet with cooking spray. Add 1 tablespoon olive oil and heat over medium-high heat. Add broccoli, green pepper, red pepper, zucchini, and squash and sauté for 5–7 minutes or until peppers begin to soften.

3. Add cooked tortellini to skillet and sauté another 2 minutes. Drizzle 1 tablespoon olive oil over entire mixture and sprinkle with garlic salt. Toss well to coat.

Exchanges

1 Starch	1 Fat
1 Vegetable	

Calories 167
    Calories from Fat 58
Total Fat . . . . 6 g
    Saturated Fat . . . . 2 g
Cholesterol . . . . 14 mg
Sodium . . . . 355 mg
Total Carbohydrate . . . . . . 22 g
    Dietary Fiber . . . . 3 g
    Sugars . . . . 3 g
Protein . . . . 6 g

Dietitian's Tip: The color of a meal can usually reveal the quality of its nutrients.

Marinated Veal Chops

Makes: 4 servings   *Serving Size: 1 veal chop*   *Prep Time: 25 minutes*

2 tablespoons olive oil

2 tablespoons red wine vinegar

1 1/2 tablespoons chopped fresh rosemary (or 2 teaspoons dried rosemary)

2 large garlic cloves, minced

1/2 teaspoon salt

1/4 teaspoon ground black pepper

4 6-ounce, bone-in veal rib chops

1. Prepare an indoor or outdoor grill.

2. In a medium bowl, whisk all ingredients except chops. Place chops in shallow baking dish and pour marinade over chops.

3. Marinate for 20 minutes in the refrigerator.

4. Grill chops over medium-high heat about 5–6 minutes per side.

Exchanges

3 Lean Meat

Calories	179
Calories from Fat	91
Total Fat	10 g
Saturated Fat	2 g
Cholesterol	74 mg
Sodium	243 mg
Total Carbohydrate	1 g
Dietary Fiber	0 g
Sugars	0 g
Protein	20 g

Chef's Tip: Rosemary is the signature flavor in this dish, but you can use any other herb if you prefer.

Asparagus with Scallions

1 bunch asparagus
(about 22 spears), ends
trimmed
2 teaspoons olive oil
Cooking spray
2 garlic cloves, minced
3 scallions, chopped
1/4 teaspoon salt

1. Steam asparagus until tender-crisp.

2. Add oil and a generous amount of cooking spray to a large nonstick skillet over medium-high heat. Add garlic and scallions and sauté for 30 seconds.

3. Add asparagus and sauté 3 more minutes. Season with salt and serve hot.

Exchanges

1 Vegetable	1/2 Fat

Calories 42
  Calories from Fat 22
Total Fat . . . . 2 g
  Saturated Fat . . . . 0 g
Cholesterol . . . . 0 mg
Sodium . . . . 155 mg
Total Carbohydrate . . . . . . 4 g
  Dietary Fiber . . . . 1 g
  Sugars . . . . 2 g
Protein . . . . 2 g

Dietitian's Tip: Asparagus is a great source of folic acid.

Tuna Steak over Orzo Pasta

Makes: 4 servings *Serving Size: 1 tuna steak* *Prep Time: 10 minutes*
plus 1/2 cup orzo

Cooking spray
4 4-ounce tuna steaks
1/2 teaspoon salt
1/4 teaspoon ground black pepper
4 garlic cloves, minced
2 tablespoons honey
1 teaspoon olive oil
2 cups orzo pasta, cooked

1. Preheat oven to 350 degrees.

2. Coat a shallow baking dish with cooking spray. Season tuna steaks on both sides with salt and pepper. Set aside.

3. In blender, purée garlic, honey, and olive oil until smooth. Place tuna steaks in baking dish and brush garlic purée on top of each steak, coating generously. Bake for 20 minutes.

4. Serve each steak over 1/2 cup cooked orzo.

Exchanges

2 Starch	1 Fat
3 Very Lean Meat	

Calories 307
Calories from Fat 63
Total Fat . . . . 7 g
Saturated Fat . . . . 0 g
Cholesterol . . . . 42 mg
Sodium . . . . 335 mg
Total Carbohydrate . . . . . . 31 g
Dietary Fiber . . . . 1 g
Sugars . . . . 12 g
Protein . . . . 29 g

Chef's Tip: Orzo is pasta, not rice, so be sure not to overcook it. Also, be sure to use a fine mesh sieve when draining it or you could lose it all down the sink!

RECIPE LIST

DAY 1: Chicken and Vegetables with Cashews **120**

DAY 2: Herb-Rubbed Pork Tenderloin **121**
Basil Mashed Potatoes **122**

DAY 3: Pasta Spinach Carbonara **123**

DAY 4: Baked Ham **124**
Cauliflower Florets with Lemon Mustard Butter **125**

DAY 5: Ham Salad **126**

GROCERY LIST

Fresh Produce
Carrots – small bag
Celery – small bag
Pea pods – 2 cups (small bag)
Broccoli – 2 heads
Garlic – 1 head
Idaho potatoes – 4 medium
Fresh basil – 1 bunch
Silken firm tofu – 1 box
Lemon – 1
Scallions – 1 bunch
Cauliflower – 1 head

Meat/Poultry/Fish
Boneless, skinless chicken breasts – 1 pound
Pork tenderloin – 1 pound
Turkey bacon – 1 small package
3-pound fully cooked, bone-in ham – 1 ham

Grains/Bread/Pasta
Farfalle pasta – 1 box
Whole-wheat bread – 1 loaf

Dairy and Cheese
Fat-free milk
Grated Parmesan cheese
Margarine
Fat-free, plain yogurt – 8 ounces
Eggs

Canned Goods and Sauces
14.5-ounce can fat-free, reduced-sodium chicken broth – 1 can
Lite soy sauce – 1 bottle
Dijon mustard – 1 bottle
Light mayonnaise – 1 jar
Horseradish – 1 jar
Pickle relish – 1 jar

Frozen Foods
10-ounce box spinach – 1 box

Staples/Seasonings/Baking Needs
Salt/ground black pepper
Cooking spray
Sesame oil
Cornstarch
Crushed red pepper flakes
Apple cider vinegar or brandy
Olive oil
Dried tarragon
Brown sugar

Miscellaneous
Cashews – small bag
Orange juice – small container

Chicken and Vegetables with Cashews

Makes: 6 servings   *Serving Size: 1 cup*   *Prep Time: 10 minutes*

1 14.5-ounce can fat-free, reduced-sodium chicken broth
4 cups water
1 pound boneless, skinless chicken breasts
2 teaspoons sesame oil
  Cooking spray
2 medium carrots, sliced into thin sticks
2 medium celery stalks, chopped
2 cups pea pods
3 cups broccoli florets
1/4 cup cashews
2 tablespoons cold water
1 tablespoon cornstarch
1 tablespoon lite soy sauce
1/4 teaspoon crushed red pepper flakes
1/2 teaspoon salt

1. In a large soup pot, bring broth and water to a boil. Reduce to a low simmer and add chicken breast. Simmer the chicken breast for 20 minutes. Remove from liquid and reserve 1 cup of the broth.

2. Using a fork, shred the chicken meat and set aside.

3. Add sesame oil and a generous amount of cooking spray to a large nonstick nonstick skillet or wok over medium-high heat. Add carrots, celery, pea pods, and broccoli and stir-fry 3–4 minutes. Add cashews and chicken to skillet.

4. In a small bowl, whisk together cold water, cornstarch, soy sauce, crushed red pepper, and salt. Whisk in reserved chicken broth. Pour liquid over vegetables and chicken. Bring to a boil and reduce heat to simmer for 2 minutes.

5. Serve over rice or Chinese noodles.

Exchanges

2 Very Lean Meat	1 Fat
2 Vegetable	

Calories 175
  Calories from Fat 57
Total Fat . . . . 6 g
  Saturated Fat . . . . 1 g
Cholesterol . . . . 45 mg
Sodium . . . . 401 mg
Total Carbohydrate . . . . . . 10 g
  Dietary Fiber . . . . 3 g
  Sugars . . . . 4 g
Protein . . . . 20 g

Dietitian's Tip: You should be eating 3–5 servings of vegetables each day. One serving is 1/2 cup cooked or 1 cup raw vegetables.

Herb-Rubbed Pork Tenderloin

Makes: 4 servings　　　*Serving Size: 3–4 ounces*　　　*Prep Time: 5 minutes*

2 tablespoons olive oil

2 tablespoons brandy or apple cider vinegar

1 tablespoon tarragon, dried

2 garlic cloves, minced

1 pound pork tenderloin

1/2 teaspoon salt

1/4 teaspoon ground black pepper

1. Preheat oven to 350 degrees.

2. In a small bowl, whisk together olive oil, brandy (or vinegar), tarragon, and garlic. Season pork tenderloin with salt and pepper on all sides.

3. Place tenderloin in a shallow baking dish. Pour sauce over tenderloin and turn several times to coat. Bake for 25–30 minutes or until done.

Exchanges

3 Lean Meat	1/2 Fat

Calories	200
Calories from Fat	98
Total Fat	11 g
Saturated Fat	2 g
Cholesterol	65 mg
Sodium	339 mg
Total Carbohydrate	1 g
Dietary Fiber	0 g
Sugars	1 g
Protein	24 g

Chef's Tip: Brandy or cider vinegars are classic flavors used with pork. Try them in marinades or sauces for instant hits!

Basil Mashed Potatoes

Makes: 6 servings   *Serving Size: 1/6 recipe*   *Prep Time: 10 minutes*

4 medium Idaho potatoes, peeled and cut into chunks

1 cup fat-free milk, heated

1/4 cup grated Parmesan cheese

2 teaspoons olive oil

3 garlic cloves, peeled and sliced

1/2 teaspoon salt

1/4 teaspoon ground black pepper

1 cup basil leaves

1. Add potatoes to a large soup pot and cover with cold water. Bring to a boil and cook for 20 minutes or until potatoes are soft. Drain and return to the pot.

2. Pour fat-free milk over the potatoes and beat with an electric mixer on high until smooth (about 5 minutes).

3. Add remaining ingredients to a blender and purée until smooth. Fold basil mixture into potatoes.

Exchanges

1 1/2 Starch   1/2 Fat

Calories 128
Calories from Fat 28
Total Fat . . . . 3 g
Saturated Fat . . . . 1 g
Cholesterol . . . . 6 mg
Sodium . . . . 305 mg
Total Carbohydrate . . . . . . 21 g
Dietary Fiber . . . . 2 g
Sugars . . . . 4 g
Protein . . . . 5 g

See photo insert.

Chef's Tip: If you're out of time, use ready-made frozen or refrigerated mashed potatoes in this recipe. They taste almost as good as homemade!

Pasta Spinach Carbonara

Makes: 5 servings   *Serving Size: 1 cup*   *Prep Time: 15 minutes*

8 ounces uncooked farfalle pasta
6 ounces silken firm tofu
1/4 cup grated Parmesan cheese
1/4 teaspoon ground black pepper
2 teaspoons olive oil
1 10-ounce package frozen spinach, thawed and drained
2 garlic cloves, minced
7 slices turkey bacon, cooked and chopped

1. Cook pasta according to package directions, omitting salt. Drain.

2. Combine tofu, Parmesan cheese, and pepper in a blender or food processor and process until smooth. Set aside.

3. Add oil to a large nonstick skillet over medium-high heat. Add spinach and cook 3 minutes. Add garlic and turkey bacon and cook 30 seconds.

4. Pour the tofu mixture in with the spinach and cook 1–2 minutes. Pour the tofu mixture over cooked pasta and toss to coat.

Exchanges

2 Starch	1 Vegetable
1 Medium-Fat Meat	1/2 Fat

Calories 285
  Calories from Fat 80
Total Fat . . . . 9 g
  Saturated Fat . . . . 3 g
Cholesterol . . . . 21 mg
Sodium . . . . 394 mg
Total Carbohydrate . . . . . . 38 g
  Dietary Fiber . . . . 3 g
  Sugars . . . . 4 g
Protein . . . . 15 g

Chef's Tip: Tofu can be used in many recipes to make a cream sauce or to provide a creamy texture. Most people would be surprised to know this recipe contains tofu.

Baked Ham

Makes: 9 servings   *Serving Size: 3 ounces*   *Prep Time: 10 minutes*
(see Chef's Tip)

1/2 cup Dijon or brown mustard
2 teaspoons brown sugar
1 small garlic clove, minced
1/4 cup orange juice
 Dash ground black pepper
1 3-pound fully cooked, bone-in
 ham

1. Preheat oven to 325 degrees.

2. Line a large roasting pan with aluminum foil. In a small bowl, whisk together the first five ingredients. Using a sharp knife, score the ham in a 1-inch diamond pattern. Trim off any excess fat.

3. Place ham in prepared pan and spread mustard mixture over entire ham. Bake for 30 minutes or until meat thermometer registers 140 degrees.

Exchanges

3 Lean Meat

Calories	137
Calories from Fat	43
Total Fat	5 g
Saturated Fat	1 g
Cholesterol	42 mg
Sodium	1313 mg
Total Carbohydrate	3 g
Dietary Fiber	0 g
Sugars	3 g
Protein	20 g

Chef's Tip: Reserve a third of the ham for tomorrow's Ham Salad recipe.

Cauliflower Florets with Lemon Mustard Butter

Makes: 8 servings   *Serving Size: 1/2 cup*   *Prep Time: 10 minutes*

2 tablespoons margarine, room temperature

1 tablespoon Dijon mustard

2 teaspoons grated lemon peel

1/4 cup scallions, chopped

1/4 teaspoon salt

4 cups cauliflower florets

1. In a small bowl, whisk together the first five ingredients.

2. Steam cauliflower florets until tender-crisp.

3. In a large saucepan, add cauliflower and margarine mixture over low heat. Toss gently until cauliflower is coated.

Exchanges

1 Vegetable	1/2 Fat

Calories 41	
Calories from Fat 27	
Total Fat . . . . 3 g	
Saturated Fat . . . . 1 g	
Cholesterol . . . . 0 mg	
Sodium . . . . 166 mg	
Total Carbohydrate . . . . 3 g	
Dietary Fiber . . . . 1 g	
Sugars . . . . 1 g	
Protein . . . . 1 g	

Chef's Tip: This great-tasting, low-fat sauce really perks up cauliflower.

Ham Salad

Makes: 6 servings   *Serving Size: 1 sandwich*   *Prep Time: 10 minutes*

1/3 Baked Ham recipe (see page 124), cubed (9 ounces cooked ham)

2 tablespoons light mayonnaise

1/2 cup fat-free, plain yogurt

3 hard-boiled egg whites, chopped

1 tablespoon horseradish

1 tablespoon pickle relish

12 slices whole-wheat bread

1. In a medium bowl, combine first six ingredients in a food processor and purée until slightly chunky but completely mixed.

2. Scoop 1/6 of salad onto 1 slice of whole-wheat bread and top with another slice of bread. Repeat for remaining five sandwiches.

Exchanges

2 Starch	1/2 Fat
1 Lean Meat	

Calories 247
  Calories from Fat 58
Total Fat . . . . 6 g
  Saturated Fat . . . . 1 g
Cholesterol . . . . 23 mg
Sodium . . . . 1065 mg
Total Carbohydrate . . . . . . 31 g
  Dietary Fiber . . . . 4 g
  Sugars . . . . 7 g
Protein . . . . 18 g

Chef's Tip: This is a great way to use up leftover ham!

April ❖ Week 3

GROCERY LIST

Fresh Produce
Orange – 1 medium
Garlic – 1 head
Lemon – 1
Onions – 2
Portabello mushrooms – 2 large
12.3-ounce box silken soft tofu – 2 boxes
Avocado – 1 small
Banana – 1
Mushrooms – 1 pint
Red bell pepper – 1
Roma (plum) tomatoes – 2
Broccoli – 1 large head
Mixed salad greens – 1 bag
Green bell pepper – 1

Meat/Poultry/Fish
Bone-in, center-cut pork chops – 4 (5-ounce) chops
Boneless, skinless chicken breasts – 4 (4-ounce) breasts
Lean ground turkey – 1 pound
Lean lamb stew meat – 1 1/2 pounds
Reduced-fat salami – 6 slices

Grains/Bread/Pasta
Whole-wheat hamburger buns – 6 buns (1 1/2 ounces each)

Dairy and Cheese
Fat-free half-and-half – 1 pint
Grated Parmesan cheese
1-ounce slices pepper-jack cheese – 6 slices
Fat-free milk

Canned Goods and Sauces
14.5-ounce can fat-free, reduced-sodium chicken broth – 2 cans
15-ounce can crushed tomatoes – 1 can
15-ounce can artichoke hearts – 1 can
Salsa – small jar
Dijon mustard – 1 jar

Frozen Foods
9-ounce bag lima beans – 2 bags
Corn – 1 large bag
Strawberries (unsweetened) – 1 bag
Blueberries – 1 bag
Peas – 1 bag

Staples/Seasonings/Baking Needs
Salt/ground black pepper
Cooking spray
Olive oil
Dried rosemary
Garlic salt
Sugar substitute
Red wine vinegar
All-purpose flour
Honey

Miscellaneous
Golden raisins – small box

Citrus Honey Pork Chops

Makes: 4 servings   *Serving Size: 1 pork chop*   *Prep Time: 25 minutes*

4 5-ounce bone-in, center-cut pork chops (about 1 inch thick)

1/2 teaspoon salt

1/4 teaspoon ground black pepper

1 tablespoon olive oil

3 tablespoons honey

1/4 cup orange juice (juice of one medium orange)

1 tablespoon lemon juice

2 garlic cloves, minced

2 teaspoons dried rosemary

1. Prepare an indoor or outdoor grill. Season pork chops with salt and pepper.

2. In a small bowl, whisk together remaining ingredients. Place chops in marinade and refrigerate for 20 minutes.

3. Remove chops from marinade and grill 5 minutes on each side over medium-high heat or until done.

Exchanges

3 Lean Meat   1/2 Carbohydrate

Calories 200
  Calories from Fat 74
Total Fat . . . . 8 g
  Saturated Fat . . . . 3 g
Cholesterol . . . . 59 mg
Sodium . . . . 336 mg
Total Carbohydrate . . . . . . 11 g
  Dietary Fiber . . . . 0 g
  Sugars . . . . 10 g
Protein . . . . 21 g

Chef's Tip: Fruit and citrus sauces go very well with pork, so don't be afraid to be creative.

Succotash

Makes: 8 servings   *Serving Size: 1/2 cup*   *Prep Time: 5 minutes*

2 9-ounce bags frozen lima beans
1 small onion, chopped
2 cups frozen corn
1/4 cup fat-free half-and-half
1/2 teaspoon salt
  Dash of ground black pepper

1. Add lima beans and onion to a large saucepan and cover with cold water. Bring to a boil; reduce heat and simmer, covered, for 5 minutes.

2. Stir in corn and simmer, covered, for 4 more minutes. Drain and return to pan.

3. Add half-and-half, salt, and pepper to pan and heat over medium heat, stirring occasionally until hot (about 2 minutes).

Exchanges
1 1/2 Starch

Calories 113
  Calories from Fat 5
Total Fat . . . . 1 g
  Saturated Fat . . . . 0 g
Cholesterol . . . . 1 mg
Sodium . . . . 196 mg
Total Carbohydrate . . . . . . 23 g
  Dietary Fiber . . . . 5 g
  Sugars. . . . . 3 g
Protein . . . . 6 g

Dietitian's Tip: Lima beans are tasty! Although they are high in carb, they are loaded with fiber.

Chicken with Portabello Tofu Sauce

Makes: 4 servings   *Serving Size: 1 chicken breast   Prep Time: 5 minutes*
plus 1/2 cup sauce

1 tablespoon olive oil
2 large Portabello mushrooms, diced
2 garlic cloves, minced
3/4 cup fat-free, reduced-sodium chicken broth, divided
1 12.3-ounce box silken soft tofu
4 4-ounce boneless, skinless chicken breasts
2 tablespoons grated Parmesan cheese
Cooking spray
1/2 teaspoon salt (optional)
1/4 teaspoon ground black pepper

1. Preheat oven to 350 degrees.

2. In a large nonstick sauté pan, heat oil over medium heat. Add mushrooms and garlic and sauté for 2 minutes. Add 1/4 cup chicken broth and simmer for 5 minutes.

3. In a blender purée the tofu and 1/2 cup chicken broth until smooth. Pour tofu mixture over mushrooms. Add Parmesan cheese and simmer 2 minutes, stirring consistently.

4. Coat a glass baking dish with cooking spray. Line chicken breasts along the pan. Pour the tofu and mushroom mixture over the top. Sprinkle with salt and pepper and bake for 20–25 minutes. Serve with brown rice.

Exchanges

4 Lean Meat   1/2 Carbohydrate

Calories 240
Calories from Fat 88
Total Fat . . . . 10 g
Saturated Fat . . . . 2 g
Cholesterol . . . . 71 mg
Sodium . . . . 215 mg
Total Carbohydrate . . . . 5 g
Dietary Fiber . . . . 1 g
Sugars. . . . . 3 g
Protein . . . . 33 g

Chef's Tip: There are two main types of tofu sold. Water-packed (extra-firm or firm) is solid and dense and works well in stir-frys, soups, or on the grill. Silken tofu (extra-firm, firm, soft, or reduced-fat) is a creamy, custard-like product and works well in puréed or blended dishes and smoothies.

Southwest Turkey Burger

Makes: 6 servings *Serving Size: 1 burger* *Prep Time: 5 minutes*

1 pound lean ground turkey
1/2 cup salsa, divided
1/2 cup frozen corn
1/2 teaspoon garlic salt
1/4 teaspoon ground black pepper
1/2 small avocado
6 whole-wheat hamburger buns
(1 1/2 ounces each)

1. Prepare an indoor or outdoor grill.

2. In a large bowl, combine ground turkey, 6 tablespoons salsa, frozen corn, garlic salt, and pepper. Mix well. Divide into six equal portions and form into 1/2-inch-thick patties.

3. Place patties on grill rack; grill 7 minutes on each side or until done. (Or coat a large nonstick skillet with cooking spray and cook patties over medium heat for 3–4 minutes per side, or until juices run clear.)

4. In a small bowl, combine avocado and 2 tablespoons salsa and mash with a fork.

5. Place one patty and 1 tablespoon avocado mixture on a whole-wheat bun. Repeat for remaining five burgers.

Exchanges

1 1/2 Starch	1 Fat
2 Lean Meat	

Calories 282
  Calories from Fat 109
Total Fat . . . . 12 g
  Saturated Fat . . . . 3 g
Cholesterol . . . . 56 mg
Sodium . . . . 421 mg
Total Carbohydrate . . . . . . 24 g
  Dietary Fiber . . . . 3 g
  Sugars . . . . 4 g
Protein . . . . 20 g

Chef's Tip: You can also blend the avocado and salsa mixture in a blender or food processor for a smoother consistency.

Fruit Smoothies

Makes: 4 servings   *Serving Size: about 1 cup*   *Prep Time: 5 minutes*

1   2.3-ounce box silken firm tofu, drained
1 1/2   cups frozen strawberries (unsweetened)
1/2   cup frozen blueberries
1   medium banana
1 1/2   cups soy or fat-free milk
4–6   packets sugar substitute

Add all ingredients to a blender and purée on high until smooth.

 April is National Alcohol Awareness Month. If you enjoy a glass of beer or wine, that's fine . . . just avoid over indulging!

Exchanges
1 Lean Meat
1 1/2 Fruit

Calories 150
  Calories from Fat 32
Total Fat . . . . 4 g
  Saturated Fat . . . . 1 g
Cholesterol . . . . 0 mg
Sodium . . . . 84 mg
Total Carbohydrate . . . . . . 21 g
  Dietary Fiber . . . . 3 g
  Sugars . . . . 14 g
Protein . . . . 10 g

Dietitian's Tip: This smoothie makes a quick, nutrient-packed breakfast.

Antipasto Salad

Makes: 6 servings *Serving Size: 1 cup* *Prep Time: 20 minutes*

DRESSING

- **2** tablespoons olive oil
- **1/2** cup red wine vinegar
- **1** tablespoon Dijon mustard
- **1/2** cup water
- **1** tablespoon honey
- **1/2** teaspoon salt (optional)
- **1/4** teaspoon ground black pepper

SALAD

- **2** cups mushrooms, stemmed and quartered
- **1** medium red bell pepper, sliced into thin strips
- **1** 15-ounce can artichoke hearts, drained and quartered
- **2** Roma (plum) tomatoes, diced
- **2** cups broccoli florets
- **6** slices reduced-fat salami, chopped
- **4** cups mixed salad greens

1. In a medium bowl, whisk together dressing ingredients. Set aside.

2. In a large salad bowl, toss together remaining ingredients except salad greens. Drizzle dressing over vegetables. Cover and refrigerate for 15 minutes.

3. Serve vegetables over salad greens.

Exchanges

1 Lean Meat	1 Fat
2 Vegetable	

Calories	142
Calories from Fat	71
Total Fat	8 g
Saturated Fat	1 g
Cholesterol	21 mg
Sodium	482 mg
Total Carbohydrate	13 g
Dietary Fiber	3 g
Sugars	7 g
Protein	8 g

Dietitian's Tip: You can still enjoy the great taste of salami— just buy the reduced-fat version (2.5 grams of fat or less per serving).

Lamb Stew

Makes: 6 servings   *Serving Size: 1/6 recipe*   *Prep Time: 15 minutes*

1 1/2 pounds lean lamb stew meat, cut into 1-inch pieces
1 tablespoon all-purpose flour
Cooking spray
1 tablespoon olive oil
1 large green bell pepper, chopped
1 medium onion, chopped
2 garlic cloves, minced
1 15-ounce can crushed tomatoes
1 14.5-ounce can fat-free, reduced-sodium chicken broth
1 cup frozen peas
1/2 cup golden raisins
1/2 teaspoon salt
1/4 teaspoon ground black pepper

1. Place lamb in a large bowl. Sprinkle with flour and toss to coat. Coat a large soup pot with cooking spray and add oil. Add lamb and sauté over high heat until browned well.

2. Stir in pepper and onion and cook until onion turns clear. Add garlic, tomato, and broth and bring to a boil while scraping the brown bits at the bottom of the pan.

3. Reduce heat and simmer, covered, for 50 minutes. Stir in peas, raisins, salt, and pepper and simmer 15 more minutes.

Exchanges
3 Lean Meat   1 1/2 Carbohydrate

Calories 287
  Calories from Fat 77
Total Fat . . . . 9 g
  Saturated Fat . . . . 2 g
Cholesterol . . . . 73 mg
Sodium . . . . 631 mg
Total Carbohydrate . . . . . . 25 g
  Dietary Fiber . . . . 5 g
  Sugars . . . . 16 g
Protein . . . . 27 g

Chef's Tip: If you can't find lamb stew meat at your grocery store, ask your butcher to cube some lamb chops for you. Most butchers are happy to help!

April ❖ Week 4

RECIPE LIST

DAY 1: Mediterranean Shrimp Wrap **136**

DAY 2: Corn Chowder **137**

DAY 3: Chicken Fajitas **138**

DAY 4: Bleu Cheese-Crusted Steak **139**
Garlic Butter Mushrooms **140**

DAY 5: Breaded Catfish **141**
"Buttery" Peas **142**

DESSERT OF THE MONTH: Caramel
Brownie Sundae **143**

GROCERY LIST

Fresh Produce
Lemon – 1
Romaine lettuce –
1 large head
Red bell pepper – 2
Carrots – small bag
Celery – small bag
Onions – 2
Jalapeño pepper – 1
12.3-ounce box silken
soft tofu – 1 box
Limes – 2
Green bell pepper – 1
Button mushrooms –
1 pint
Garlic – 1 head

Meat/Poultry/Fish
Peeled, cooked shrimp –
12 ounces
Boneless, skinless
chicken breasts –
1 pound
Tenderloin steaks – 4
(4-ounce) steaks
Catfish filets – 4
(4-ounce) filets

Grains/Bread/Pasta
10-inch flour tortillas – 4
6-inch flour tortillas – 8
Bread crumbs – small
container

Dairy and Cheese
Feta cheese – 4 ounces
Bleu cheese – 4 ounces
Margarine
Egg substitute –
4 ounces
Eggs

Canned Goods and Sauces
14.5-ounce can fat-free,
reduced-sodium
chicken broth – 3 cans
Unsweetened apple-
sauce – 8 ounces

Frozen Foods
Corn – 2 bags
Peas – 1 bag (1 pound)
Fat-free, no-sugar added
or light vanilla ice
cream – 1 carton

Staples/Seasonings/Baking Needs
Salt/ground black pepper
Cooking spray
Olive oil
Garlic salt
Chili powder
Canola oil
All-purpose flour
Dried thyme
19.8-ounce box fudge
brownie mix
(1.5 grams fat per
serving) – 1 box

Miscellaneous
Caramel sauce (light if
available)

Mediterranean Shrimp Wrap

Makes: 4 servings *Serving Size: 1 wrap* *Prep Time: 10 minutes*

DRESSING

- **1** tablespoon olive oil
- **2** tablespoons lemon juice
- **1/4** teaspoon garlic salt
  Dash ground black pepper

WRAPS

- **4** 10-inch flour tortillas
- **4** cups romaine lettuce, chopped
- **12** ounces cooked, peeled shrimp, chilled
- **1** red bell pepper, sliced into strips
- **1/4** cup crumbled feta cheese

1. In a small bowl, whisk together dressing ingredients.

2. Fill each tortilla with 1 cup romaine lettuce, about 8 shrimp, 1/4 of the peppers, 1 tablespoon feta cheese, and 1/2 tablespoon dressing. Fold left and right sides of tortillas in until they touch and roll from the bottom to make the wrap.

Exchanges

2 1/2 Starch	1 Vegetable
2 Lean Meat	1 Fat

Calories	381
Calories from Fat	98
Total Fat	11 g
Saturated Fat	3 g
Cholesterol	171 mg
Sodium	689 mg
Total Carbohydrate	43 g
Dietary Fiber	3 g
Sugars	4 g
Protein	26 g

Chef's Tip: Buy cooked, peeled shrimp—it really saves time!

Corn Chowder

Makes: 9 servings   *Serving Size: 1 cup*   *Prep Time: 10 minutes*

Cooking spray
1 teaspoon olive oil
2 carrots, finely diced
2 celery stalks, finely diced
1 small onion, finely diced
1 jalapeño pepper, seeded and minced
3 14.5-ounce cans fat-free, reduced-sodium chicken broth
6 cups frozen corn
1/2 teaspoon chili powder
1 12.3-ounce box silken soft tofu
1/2 teaspoon salt (optional)
1/4 teaspoon ground black pepper

1. Coat a large soup pot with cooking spray. Add oil and heat over medium-high heat. Add carrots, celery, onion, and jalapeño pepper and sauté for 4 minutes or until onion begins to turn clear.

2. Add broth, corn, and chili powder and bring to a boil; reduce heat and simmer for 20 minutes.

3. In a blender (or with an immersion blender), blend 1 quart of soup and tofu. Add back to soup and simmer for 2 minutes. Season with salt (if using) and pepper.

Exchanges

1 1/2 Starch   1 Vegetable

Calories	140
Calories from Fat	19
Total Fat	2 g
Saturated Fat	0 g
Cholesterol	0 mg
Sodium	371 mg
Total Carbohydrate	27 g
Dietary Fiber	4 g
Sugars	5 g
Protein	8 g

Chef's Tip: Serve with a handful of crushed baked tortilla chips over each serving.

Chicken Fajitas

Makes: 4 servings   *Serving Size: 2 fajitas*   *Prep Time: 20 minutes*

1 pound boneless, skinless chicken breasts, sliced into 1-inch strips
1/4 cup fresh lime juice
2 garlic cloves, minced
1/2 teaspoon salt
1/4 teaspoon ground black pepper
Cooking spray
1 tablespoon canola oil
1 large onion, thickly sliced
1 large red bell pepper, thickly sliced
1 large green bell pepper, thickly sliced
8 6-inch flour tortillas

1. Add chicken to a large bowl and drizzle with lime juice. Add garlic, salt, and pepper and toss to coat. Marinate in the refrigerator for 15 minutes.

2. Coat a large nonstick skillet or wok with cooking spray and add oil. Heat over high heat and add chicken. Sauté 5–6 minutes until done or beginning to brown.

3. Remove chicken from pan and spray pan generously again with cooking spray. Add onion and peppers and sauté for 5 minutes. Add chicken back to pan and toss with vegetables. Serve in warm tortillas.

Exchanges

2 1/2 Starch   2 Vegetable
3 Lean Meat

Calories 410
  Calories from Fat 97
Total Fat . . . . 11 g
  Saturated Fat . . . . 2 g
Cholesterol . . . . 68 mg
Sodium . . . . 567 mg
Total Carbohydrate . . . . . . 45 g
  Dietary Fiber . . . . 5 g
  Sugars . . . . 8 g
Protein . . . . 32 g

Chef's Tip: Garnish these fajitas with fat-free sour cream and salsa.

Bleu Cheese-Crusted Steak

Makes: 4 servings   *Serving Size: 1 steak*   *Prep Time: 2 minutes*

4 4-ounce tenderloin steaks
1/2 teaspoon salt
1/4 teaspoon ground black pepper
    Cooking spray
2 tablespoons bleu cheese

1. Preheat oven to 400 degrees. Season both sides of steak well with salt and pepper.

2. Coat a large oven-safe skillet with cooking spray. Sear steaks over high heat for 2 minutes on each side and transfer to oven. Bake for 10 minutes.

3. Remove from oven and sprinkle 1/2 tablespoon cheese on top of each steak. Return to oven and bake 2 more minutes.

Exchanges
3 Lean Meat

Calories	163
Calories from Fat	72
Total Fat	8 g
Saturated Fat	3 g
Cholesterol	63 mg
Sodium	385 mg
Total Carbohydrate	0 g
Dietary Fiber	0 g
Sugars	0 g
Protein	21 g

See photo insert.

Dietitian's Tip: Although bleu cheese is high in fat, you only need to use a small amount because of its strong flavor.

Garlic Butter Mushrooms

Makes: 4 servings *Serving Size: 1/3 cup* *Prep Time: 5 minutes*

Cooking spray
1 tablespoon margarine
1 pint button mushrooms, stemmed and halved
3 garlic cloves, minced
3 tablespoons water
1/2 teaspoon salt

1. Coat a large nonstick skillet with cooking spray and add margarine; melt over medium-low heat.

2. Add mushrooms, stirring constantly. Cook for 2 minutes. Add garlic and water and sauté 10 more minutes or until almost all the liquid is evaporated and the mushrooms are cooked through. Add salt and serve.

✔ *National Volunteer Week is the last week of April . . . give of yourself this year. You'll get more back!*

Exchanges

1 Vegetable	1/2 Fat

Calories 42
Calories from Fat 28
Total Fat . . . . 3 g
Saturated Fat . . . . 1 g
Cholesterol . . . . 0 mg
Sodium . . . . 326 mg
Total Carbohydrate . . . . 3 g
Dietary Fiber . . . . 1 g
Sugars . . . . 1 g
Protein . . . . 1 g

Chef's Tip: This recipe also makes a great appetizer.

Breaded Catfish

1/3 cup all-purpose flour
1/2 cup egg substitute
1/2 teaspoon dried thyme
1/2 teaspoon salt
1/4 teaspoon ground black pepper
1/2 cup bread crumbs
   4 4-ounce catfish filets
    Cooking spray

1. Preheat oven to 350 degrees.

2. Place flour in a shallow dish. Place egg substitute in another shallow dish. Add thyme, salt, and pepper to bread crumbs and place in a third shallow dish.

3. Dredge one filet in flour, coating all sides. Dip into egg substitute and roll in bread crumb mixture, coating well. Repeat for remaining three filets.

4. Coat a baking dish with cooking spray and line the bottom of pan with prepared filets. Spray each filet with more cooking spray. Bake for 25 minutes.

Exchanges

1 Starch	3 Lean Meat

Calories 235
  Calories from Fat 80
Total Fat . . . . 9 g
  Saturated Fat . . . . 2 g
Cholesterol . . . . 65 mg
Sodium . . . . 433 mg
Total Carbohydrate . . . . . . 14 g
  Dietary Fiber . . . . 1 g
  Sugars . . . . 1 g
Protein . . . . 23 g

Dietitian's Tip: This recipe is a great replacement for traditional fried catfish. The fat content is reduced dramatically with baking, but the great flavor still remains.

"Buttery" Peas

Cooking spray
1 tablespoon margarine
1 pound frozen peas
1/2 teaspoon garlic salt

1. Coat a large nonstick skillet with cooking spray and melt margarine over medium-high heat.

2. Add frozen peas and sauté for 5 minutes. Add garlic salt.

Exchanges

1/2 Starch	1/2 Fat

Calories 60
 Calories from Fat 16
Total Fat . . . . 2 g
 Saturated Fat . . . . 0 g
Cholesterol . . . . 0 mg
Sodium . . . . 161 mg
Total Carbohydrate . . . . . . 8 g
 Dietary Fiber . . . . 3 g
 Sugars . . . . 3 g
Protein . . . . 3 g

Chef's Tip: You can substitute fresh peas for frozen in this recipe.

Caramel Brownie Sundae

Makes: 20 servings   Serving Size: 1 brownie sundae   Prep Time: 5 minutes

Cooking spray
1 19.8-ounce package fudge brownie mix (1.5 grams fat per serving)
1/4 cup water
1/4 cup canola oil
1/4 cup unsweetened applesauce
1 egg
2 egg whites
7 cups fat-free, no-sugar-added or light vanilla ice cream
3/4 cup caramel sauce topping

1. Preheat oven to 350 degrees. Coat an 11 × 7-inch pan with cooking spray.

2. In a large bowl, stir in brownie mix, water, oil, applesauce, egg, and egg whites until well blended.

3. Spread in pan and bake 30–40 minutes or until toothpick inserted 2 inches from side of pan comes out almost clean. Cool.

4. Cut brownies into 20 slices. Put 1 brownie in bowl and top with 1/3 cup ice cream and 2 teaspoons caramel sauce. Repeat for remaining servings.

Exchanges

1/2 Fat   3 Carbohydrate

Calories 239
  Calories from Fat 48
Total Fat . . . . 5 g
  Saturated Fat . . . . 1 g
Cholesterol . . . . 11 mg
Sodium . . . . 160 mg
Total Carbohydrate . . . . . . 46 g
  Dietary Fiber . . . . 0 g
  Sugars . . . . 27 g
Protein . . . . 4 g

Chef's Tip: This is a fun dessert to make with kids. Let them assemble the sundaes after the brownies have been cooled and cut.

May

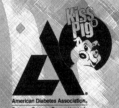

American Diabetes Association.
Cure • Care • Commitment.

To honor the pig, which helped us discover that people with diabetes need insulin, participants raise money for research, and the winner gets to kiss a pig! If you know the perfect candidate for this event, call your local ADA office.

Happy Cinco de Mayo

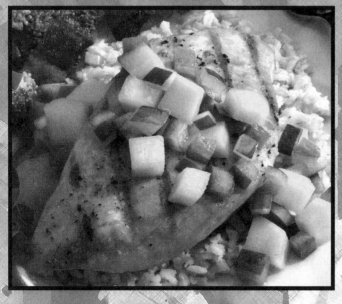

Mango Salsa Chicken over Rice (page 190)
This dish, with its great blend of flavors, is fun to make outside on the grill when the weather gets warm. Serve it with
steamed fresh green beans and some fruit sorbet for dessert!

May ❖ Recipes

May ❖ Week 1

RECIPE LIST

DAY 1: Butterfly Steak   **148**
Berry Compote   **149**

DAY 2: Chicken Fajita Pizza   **150**

DAY 3: Tortilla Soup   **151**

DAY 4: Farfalle Pasta with Asiago Cheese
Sauce   **152**

DAY 5: Crab Cakes   **153**
Wilted Lettuce Salad   **154**

GROCERY LIST

Fresh Produce
Lemon – 1
Fresh mint leaves –
1 bunch
Mixed berries (strawber-
ries, blueberries, rasp-
berries) – 4 cups
Green bell peppers – 2
Onions – 3
Garlic – 1 head
Boston or Bibb lettuce –
1 large bag

Meat/Poultry/Fish
Tenderloin steaks – 4
(4-ounce) steaks
Boneless, skinless
chicken breasts –
1/2 pound
Turkey bacon – 1 small
package

Grains/Bread/Pasta
Prepackaged 12-inch
pizza crust – 1
Farfalle pasta – 1 box
Bread crumbs – 1 box or
package

Dairy and Cheese
Shredded, part-skim
mozzarella cheese –
1 bag
Fat-free milk
Shredded Asiago
cheese – 4 ounces
Eggs

Canned Goods and Sauces
15-ounce can no-salt-
added diced
tomatoes – 1 can
14.5-ounce can fat-free,
reduced-sodium
chicken broth – 4 cans
6-ounce can lump crab-
meat – 2 cans
Salsa – 1 small jar
4-ounce can chopped
green chilies – 1 can

Staples/Seasonings/Baking Needs
Salt/ground black pepper
Cooking spray
Sugar
Vanilla extract
Olive oil
Dried oregano
Dried red chilies
All-purpose flour
Crushed red pepper
flakes
Apple cider vinegar
Hot pepper sauce

Miscellaneous
Baked tortilla chips –
small bag

Butterfly Steak

Makes: 4 servings   *Serving Size: 1 steak*   *Prep Time: 5 minutes*

4 4-ounce tenderloin steaks
   (about 1 1/2–2 inches thick)
1/2 teaspoon salt
1/4 teaspoon ground black pepper

1. Prepare an indoor or outdoor grill. Using a sharp knife, slice through steak lengthwise, leaving about 1/4 inch from the edge. Do not cut all the way through the steak. Fold steaks open at slit and season well with salt and pepper.

2. Grill over medium-high heat, about 5 minutes each side. Place steak on a plate cut side up. Serve with Berry Compote on the side (see recipe, page 149).

Exchanges

3 Lean Meat

Calories	150
Calories from Fat	63
Total Fat	7 g
Saturated Fat	3 g
Cholesterol	60 mg
Sodium	336 mg
Total Carbohydrate	0 g
Dietary Fiber	0 g
Sugars	0 g
Protein	20 g

Chef's Tip: Using a sharp knife is especially important in this recipe. A properly sharpened knife should slide right through your meat. And give the Berry Compote a try—it's really good with the steak!

Berry Compote

1/2 cup water
1/4 cup sugar
  1 tablespoon lemon juice
  1 tablespoon fresh mint leaves, chopped
  1 teaspoon vanilla extract
  4 cups mixed berries (strawberries, blueberries, and raspberries)

1. In a medium saucepan, bring water and sugar to a boil; add lemon juice, mint, and vanilla and whisk.

2. Stir in berries and reduce to a simmer. Simmer for 10 minutes or until berries are broken down.

3. Serve with Butterfly Steak (see recipe, page 148).

✔ *May is National Arthritis Month . . . ask your doctor about taking nutritional supplements to help you feel better.*

Exchanges
2 Carbohydrate

Calories	114
Calories from Fat	6
Total Fat	1 g
Saturated Fat	0 g
Cholesterol	0 mg
Sodium	4 mg
Total Carbohydrate	28 g
Dietary Fiber	5 g
Sugars	20 g
Protein	1 g

Dietitian's Tip: These berries are packed with vitamin C and are a great source of fiber, not to mention incredible flavor!

Chicken Fajita Pizza

Makes: 8 servings   *Serving Size: 1 slice*   *Prep Time: 15 minutes*

Cooking spray
1/2 pound boneless, skinless chicken breasts, cut into chunks
1/4 teaspoon ground black pepper
1 green bell pepper, sliced into 1-inch strips
1/2 large onion, sliced
12-inch prepackaged pizza crust
1 1/2 cups salsa
1 1/2 cups shredded, part-skim mozzarella cheese

1. Preheat oven to 450 degrees. Coat a medium nonstick skillet with cooking spray and sauté chicken over medium-high heat for 5–6 minutes. Season with black pepper.

2. When chicken is lightly brown, add green pepper and onion and sauté another 3 minutes.

3. Place pizza crust on baking sheet. Spread salsa over pizza crust.

4. Spoon chicken mixture over pizza crust and distribute evenly. Top with cheese. Bake 10 minutes or until pizza crust is crisp and cheese is melted.

Exchanges

1 1/2 Starch   1 Vegetable
2 Lean Meat

Calories 249
Calories from Fat 69
Total Fat . . . . 8 g
Saturated Fat . . . . 3 g
Cholesterol . . . . 29 mg
Sodium . . . . 520 mg
Total Carbohydrate . . . . . . 27 g
Dietary Fiber . . . . 2 g
Sugars . . . . 3 g
Protein . . . . 17 g

See photo insert.

Chef's Tip: For a great vegetarian version of this recipe, simply omit the chicken.

Tortilla Soup

- **1** tablespoon olive oil
- **1** medium onion, chopped
- **1** 15-ounce can no-salt-added diced tomatoes with juice
- **4** garlic cloves, minced
- **1** 4-ounce can chopped green chilies
- **2** dried red chilies
- **1/2** teaspoon dried oregano
- **3** 14.5-ounce cans fat-free, reduced-sodium chicken broth
- **1/2** teaspoon salt (optional)
- **1/4** teaspoon ground black pepper
- **3 1/2** cups coarsely crushed baked tortilla chips

1. Add oil to a large soup pot over medium-high heat. Add onion and sauté for 4–5 minutes or until onion turns clear. Add tomatoes, garlic, and green chilies. Sauté for 2–3 minutes.

2. Add red chilies, oregano, chicken broth, salt, and pepper. Bring to a boil. Reduce heat and simmer for 15 minutes. Remove red chilies from soup and discard. Serve each serving of soup with 1/2 cup crushed tortilla chips.

✓ *Have a great Cinco de Mayo, the Mexican Independence Day!*

Exchanges

1 1/2 Starch	1 Vegetable

Calories 143
Calories from Fat 26
Total Fat . . . . 3 g
Saturated Fat . . . . 0 g
Cholesterol . . . . 0 mg
Sodium . . . . 683 mg
Total Carbohydrate . . . . . . 26 g
Dietary Fiber . . . . 3 g
Sugars . . . . 4 g
Protein . . . . 5 g

Chef's Tip: Serve this soup with a Mexican side salad: shredded lettuce, black beans, reduced-fat shredded Mexican cheese, and a mixture of light Ranch dressing and salsa.

Farfalle Pasta with Asiago Cheese Sauce

Makes: 5 servings   *Serving Size: 1 cup*   *Prep Time: 5 minutes*

8 ounces uncooked farfalle pasta
1 tablespoon all-purpose flour
1 cup fat-free milk
Cooking spray
1 garlic clove, minced
1/4 teaspoon crushed red pepper flakes
1/4 teaspoon salt
1/8 teaspoon ground black pepper
1/2 cup shredded Asiago cheese

1. Cook pasta according to package directions, omitting salt; drain.

2. In a small bowl, whisk together flour and milk. Set aside.

3. Coat a medium saucepan generously with cooking spray. Add garlic and sauté for 30 seconds over low heat. Add crushed red pepper and stir for a few seconds.

4. Add flour and milk mixture and bring to a boil, whisking constantly; reduce to a simmer for 7–8 minutes, whisking occasionally. Stir in salt and pepper.

5. Toss cream sauce with cooked pasta. Sprinkle with Asiago cheese and toss.

Exchanges

2 1/2 Starch   1/2 Fat

Calories 238
Calories from Fat 33
Total Fat . . . . 4 g
Saturated Fat . . . . 2 g
Cholesterol . . . . 11 mg
Sodium . . . . 245 mg
Total Carbohydrate . . . . . . 39 g
Dietary Fiber . . . . 2 g
Sugars . . . . 6 g
Protein . . . . 11 g

Chef's Tip: The crushed red pepper flakes add just the right amount of zing for most people, but you can leave them out if you prefer.

Crab Cakes

Makes: 6 servings   *Serving Size: 1 cake*   *Prep Time: 10 minutes*

Cooking spray
1/4 cup onion, minced
1/4 cup minced green bell pepper
2 6-ounce cans lump crabmeat, drained
1/2 cup bread crumbs
1 egg
1 egg white
1/2 teaspoon hot pepper sauce
1/2 teaspoon salt
1/4 teaspoon ground black pepper
1 tablespoon olive oil

✔ *National Running and Fitness Week is in May. Try walking first, then gradually increase your speed and distance until you are actually—yes—running!*

1. Coat a small nonstick skillet with cooking spray over medium-high heat. Add onion and green pepper and sauté 2–3 minutes or until onion is clear. Set aside to cool.

2. In a medium bowl, combine crabmeat, bread crumbs, egg, egg white, hot pepper sauce, salt, and pepper. Mix well. Stir in cooled onion and green pepper.

3. Form crab mixture into 1/2-inch-thick patties with your hands using a heaping 1/4 cup mixture for each patty.

4. Add oil and a generous amount of cooking spray to a large nonstick skillet over medium-high heat. Fry crab cakes about 4–5 minutes on each side or until golden brown.

5. If desired, serve each crab cake over a bed of Wilted Lettuce Salad (see recipe, page 154).

Exchanges

1/2 Starch	1 Lean Meat
1/2 Fat	

Calories	114
Calories from Fat	36
Total Fat	4 g
Saturated Fat	1 g
Cholesterol	70 mg
Sodium	425 mg
Total Carbohydrate	8 g
Dietary Fiber	0 g
Sugars	1 g
Protein	11 g

Chef's Tip: You can mix a little hot sauce with low-fat or fat-free mayonnaise to make a nice sauce for crab cakes. Just serve a little dollop of the sauce on top of each cake.

Wilted Lettuce Salad

Makes: 6 servings   *Serving Size: 1/2 cup*   *Prep Time: 10 minutes*

7 cups Boston or Bibb lettuce, torn into pieces
4 slices turkey bacon
1 tablespoon olive oil
4 tablespoons apple cider vinegar
1 teaspoon sugar
1/4 cup fat-free, reduced-sodium chicken broth
1/4 teaspoon salt
Dash ground black pepper

1. Place lettuce in a large salad bowl.

2. In a small nonstick sauté pan, cook bacon over medium heat until crisp. Remove bacon from pan and chop into small pieces. Toss bacon with lettuce.

3. In a small bowl, whisk together remaining ingredients. In the bacon skillet, add dressing and bring to a boil. Reduce heat and simmer for 8–10 minutes or until slightly thickened.

4. Pour hot dressing over salad and toss well to coat.

Exchanges

1 Vegetable	1 Fat

Calories 56	
Calories from Fat 37	
Total Fat . . . . 4 g	
Saturated Fat . . . . 1 g	
Cholesterol . . . . 7 mg	
Sodium . . . . 237 mg	
Total Carbohydrate . . . . 3 g	
Dietary Fiber . . . . 1 g	
Sugars. . . . . 2 g	
Protein . . . . 2 g	

Chef's Tip: Most people think wilted lettuce is a bad thing, but try this delicious salad!

May ❖ Week 2

RECIPE LIST

DAY 1: Smokin' Turkey Sandwich **156**

DAY 2: Mexican Meat Loaf **157**
Spicy Sweet Potato Fries **158**

DAY 3: Chicken Tostadas **159**

DAY 4: Sweet Onion Salmon **160**
Melon Salad **161**

DAY 5: Broccoli and Cheese-Stuffed
Potatoes **162**

GROCERY LIST

Fresh Produce
Garlic – 1 head
Onions – 4
Field greens – 1 bag
Sweet potatoes – 2 large
Lettuce – 1 small head
Tomatoes – 2
Idaho potatoes –
4 medium
Broccoli – 2 heads
Cantaloupe – 1 small
Honeydew – 1 small
Mint leaves – small
bunch

Meat/Poultry/Fish
Thinly sliced, oven-
roasted, deli turkey –
1/2 pound
Lean ground beef –
1 pound
Boneless, skinless
chicken breasts –
1 pound
Salmon filets – 4
(4-ounce) filets

Grains/Bread/Pasta
Italian-style bread –
1 loaf
Bread crumbs – 1 box or
package
Tostada shells – 8 shells

Dairy and Cheese
Shredded reduced-fat
Mexican cheese –
1 package
Eggs
Shredded, reduced-fat
cheddar cheese –
2 bags
Fat-free milk

Canned Goods and Sauces
16-ounce can black
beans – 1 can
15-ounce can crushed
tomatoes – 1 can
16-ounce can fat-free
refried beans – 1 can
Canned chipotle peppers
in adobe sauce –
1 small can
Light mayonnaise – 1 jar
Salsa – small jar
Light sugar-free apricot
preserves – 1 jar

Frozen Foods
Corn – small bag

Staples/Seasonings/Baking Needs
Salt/ground black pepper
Cooking spray
Olive oil
Cayenne pepper
Cumin
Chili powder
Garlic salt
Cornstarch
Rice wine vinegar
Honey

Smokin' Turkey Sandwich

Makes: 4 servings   *Serving Size: 1 sandwich*   *Prep Time: 10 minutes*

1/4 cup light mayonnaise

2 teaspoons canned chipotle peppers packed in adobe sauce

1 garlic clove, sliced

8 1-ounce slices Italian-style bread, lightly toasted

8 ounces thinly sliced, oven-roasted deli turkey

2 ounces shredded reduced-fat Mexican cheese

1 medium onion, thinly sliced

2 cups mixed field greens

1. Blend the first three ingredients in a blender or food processor until smooth.

2. Spread 1 tablespoon mayonnaise mixture onto 1 slice of bread. Add 2 ounces turkey breast, 1/2 ounce cheese, onion, and lettuce. Top with another slice of bread.

3. Repeat procedure for remaining three sandwiches.

✔ *National Women's Health Week is the second week of May . . . go to www.4woman.gov/whw to find out where to get free health screenings in your neighborhood!*

Exchanges

2 Starch	1 Vegetable
2 Lean Meat	1 Fat

Calories 334
  Calories from Fat 107
Total Fat . . . . 12 g
  Saturated Fat . . . . 4 g
Cholesterol . . . . 41 mg
Sodium . . . . 1078 mg
Total Carbohydrate . . . . . . 36 g
  Dietary Fiber . . . . 3 g
  Sugars . . . . 6 g
Protein . . . . 22 g

Chef's Tip: Chipotle peppers have a great smoky flavor that complements roasted turkey well.

Mexican Meat Loaf

Makes: 6 servings   *Serving Size: 1/6 recipe*   *Prep Time: 10 minutes*

1 pound lean ground beef
1 cup canned black beans,
   rinsed and drained
1 cup salsa, divided
1/2 cup frozen corn
1 egg
1/2 cup bread crumbs
   Cooking spray

1. Preheat oven to 400 degrees.

2. In a medium bowl, add all ingredients except cooking spray, using 3/4 cup salsa, and mix well. Coat a 5 × 9-inch loaf pan with cooking spray. Spread mixture evenly in a loaf pan.

3. Bake for 50–60 minutes. Remove from oven and let sit for 15 minutes. Top with 1/4 cup salsa.

Exchanges

1 Starch	3 Lean Meat

Calories	224
Calories from Fat	70
Total Fat	8 g
Saturated Fat	3 g
Cholesterol	81 mg
Sodium	281 mg
Total Carbohydrate	18 g
Dietary Fiber	4 g
Sugars	2 g
Protein	20 g

Chef's Tip: Meat loaf certainly doesn't have to be boring, as this recipe proves. You can have fun inventing your own meat loaf recipes. For example, try adding roasted red peppers, chopped garbanzo beans, and fresh oregano to ground turkey to make a Mediterranean-style meat loaf. It's easy and fun to create your own recipes!

Spicy Sweet Potato Fries

Makes: 4 servings   *Serving Size: 1/4 recipe*   *Prep Time: 20 minutes*

2 large sweet potatoes, peeled and cut into 2-inch wedges
1 tablespoon olive oil
1/2 teaspoon cayenne pepper
1 teaspoon cumin
1 teaspoon chili powder
1 teaspoon garlic salt
1/2 teaspoon salt (optional)

1. Preheat oven to 400 degrees.

2. Place potato wedges in a bowl and add oil; toss to coat.

3. In a small bowl, combine remaining ingredients.

4. Sprinkle spice mixture over potatoes and toss to coat.

5. Place on a baking sheet and bake for 30 minutes or until potatoes are soft.

 May is Older Americans Month. Pay tribute to an older American in your community today!

Exchanges

1 1/2 Starch	1/2 Fat

Calories	127
Calories from Fat	33
Total Fat	4 g
Saturated Fat	0 g
Cholesterol	0 mg
Sodium	337 mg
Total Carbohydrate	23 g
Dietary Fiber	3 g
Sugars	10 g
Protein	2 g

See photo insert.

Chef's Tip: If you prefer a sweeter sweet potato fry, omit the cayenne pepper, cumin, and chili powder from this recipe. It'll still taste great!

Chicken Tostadas

Makes: 8 servings   *Serving Size: 1 tostada*   *Prep Time: 15 minutes*

1 pound boneless, skinless chicken breasts, cooked and shredded

1 15-ounce can crushed tomatoes

1/2 tablespoon chili powder

1 teaspoon cumin

1/4 teaspoon cayenne pepper

8 tostada shells

1 16-ounce can fat-free refried beans

1 cup shredded, reduced-fat cheddar cheese

1 cup shredded lettuce

2 tomatoes, diced

1. Preheat oven to 350 degrees.

2. In a medium bowl, combine shredded chicken, tomatoes, chili powder, cumin, and cayenne pepper.

3. Place tostada shells on a large baking sheet. Spread 1/4 cup refried beans on each tostada, top with 1/4 cup chicken mixture, and sprinkle with 2 tablespoons cheese.

4. Bake for 15–20 minutes or until heated through and cheese is melted. Remove from oven and top with lettuce and tomato.

Exchanges

1 Starch	1 Vegetable
2 Lean Meat	1/2 Fat

Calories 236
  Calories from Fat 64
Total Fat . . . . 7 g
  Saturated Fat . . . . 3 g
Cholesterol . . . . 44 mg
Sodium . . . . 570 mg
Total Carbohydrate . . . . . . 22 g
  Dietary Fiber . . . . 5 g
  Sugars . . . . 4 g
Protein . . . . 21 g

Chef's Tip: To cook shredded chicken, place chicken breasts in a shallow baking dish and bake in a 350-degree oven for 30–35 minutes. Remove the chicken from the oven and shred the meat with a fork.

Sweet Onion Salmon

Makes: 4 servings   *Serving Size: 1 filet*   *Prep Time: 5 minutes*

4 4-ounce salmon filets
1 tablespoon olive oil
3 small onions, sliced into thin rings
1 tablespoon honey
1/4 cup rice wine vinegar
1 tablespoon light sugar-free apricot preserves

1. Preheat oven to 350 degrees.

2. Place salmon filets on a medium baking sheet and bake for 10–12 minutes.

3. Meanwhile, heat oil in a medium nonstick skillet over medium-high heat. Add onions and sauté 7–10 minutes or until onions are caramelized.

4. In a small bowl, whisk together honey, vinegar, and apricot preserves. Pour over onions in pan and sauté for 2 more minutes. Serve onions over filets.

✔ *Are you up for the American Diabetes Association's Tour de Cure, a great bicycle event that helps raise money to find a cure for diabetes? Sign up today at www.diabetes.org!*

Exchanges
3 Lean Meat   1 Carbohydrate
1/2 Fat

Calories 270
  Calories from Fat 119
Total Fat . . . . 13 g
  Saturated Fat . . . . 2 g
Cholesterol . . . . 77 mg
Sodium . . . . 61 mg
Total Carbohydrate . . . . . . 12 g
  Dietary Fiber . . . . 1 g
  Sugars . . . . 9 g
Protein . . . . 25 g

Chef's Tip: The slight sweetness of the onion is a nice complement to the rich flavor of salmon.

Melon Salad

3 cups cubed cantaloupe

3 cups cubed honeydew melon

1 tablespoon chopped mint leaves

1 tablespoon honey

1. Place melon in a medium bowl.

2. Sprinkle with mint leaves and honey and toss gently to coat.

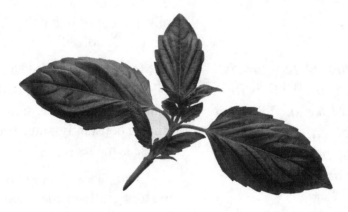

Exchanges
1 Fruit

Calories 69
  Calories from Fat 3
Total Fat . . . . 0 g
  Saturated Fat . . . . 0 g
Cholesterol . . . . 0 mg
Sodium . . . . 16 mg
Total Carbohydrate . . . . . . 17 g
  Dietary Fiber . . . . 1 g
  Sugars . . . . 16 g
Protein . . . . 1 g

Chef's Tip: This is a quick, delicious summer dessert.

Broccoli and Cheese-Stuffed Potatoes

Makes: 4 servings   *Serving Size: 1 stuffed potato*   *Prep Time: 10 minutes*

4 medium Idaho potatoes
4 cups broccoli florets
1 cup fat-free milk
1 tablespoon cornstarch
1 cup shredded, reduced-fat
    cheddar cheese
1/2 teaspoon salt
1/4 teaspoon ground black pepper

 National Osteoporosis Prevention Week is in May. Make sure you get enough calcium and weight-bearing exercise every day!

1. Wash and dry potatoes. Poke each potato several times with a fork. Place on plate and microwave on high for 15 minutes or until soft, or bake in a 400-degree oven for 45 minutes.

2. Steam broccoli until tender-crisp; set aside.

3. In a small bowl, whisk together milk and cornstarch until all the cornstarch is dissolved.

4. In a medium saucepan, bring milk and cornstarch to a boil. Reduce heat to a simmer. Add cheese, salt, and pepper. Stirring constantly, simmer until all cheese is melted.

5. Pour cheese sauce over broccoli and toss gently to coat. Remove potatoes from oven. Slice potatoes open and fluff flesh with a fork. Fill each potato with 1/2 cup broccoli mixture.

Exchanges

2 1/2 Starch   1 Vegetable
1 Lean Meat

Calories 279
  Calories from Fat 60
Total Fat . . . . 7 g
  Saturated Fat . . . . 4 g
Cholesterol . . . . 21 mg
Sodium . . . . 598 mg
Total Carbohydrate . . . . . . 43 g
  Dietary Fiber . . . . 6 g
  Sugars . . . . 6 g
Protein . . . . 15 g

Dietitian's Tip: You can add protein to this meal by stirring in tuna or low-fat cottage cheese with the broccoli mixture.

May ❖ Week 3

GROCERY LIST

Fresh Produce
Granny Smith apples – 2
Red bell pepper – 1
Field greens – 1 bag
Garlic – 1 head
Red new potatoes –
  1 pound
Baby carrots – 1 pound
Lettuce – 1 head
Tomatoes – 3

Meat/Poultry/Fish
Pork tenderloin –
  1 pound
Boneless, skinless
  chicken breasts –
  2 pounds

Sirloin steak – 1 pound
Extra lean thinly sliced
  deli ham – 8 ounces

Grains/Bread/Pasta
Egg bread or other
  sturdy bread – 1 loaf
6-inch flour tortillas – 8

Dairy and Cheese
Bleu cheese – 2 ounces
Fat-free half-and-half –
  1 pint
Egg substitute –
  8 ounces
Fat-free milk
1-ounce slices reduced-
  fat Swiss cheese –
  4 slices

Shredded, reduced-fat
  cheddar cheese –
  1 bag

Canned Goods and Sauces
16-ounce can black
  beans – 1 can
16-ounce can fat-free
  refried beans – 1 can
Canned chipotle
  peppers – 1 small can
Salsa – 1 small jar
Dijon mustard – 1 jar

Staples/Seasonings/Baking Needs
Salt/ground black pepper
Cooking spray
Apple cider vinegar
Dried sage
Olive oil
Cornstarch
Dried tarragon
Chili powder
Cumin
Cayenne pepper
Honey

Pork and Apple Salad

Makes: 6 servings   *Serving Size: 1/6 recipe*   *Prep Time: 15 minutes*

SALAD

- **1** tablespoon Dijon mustard
- **2** tablespoons apple cider vinegar
- **1** tablespoon honey
- **1** tablespoon dried sage
- **1** pound pork tenderloin
- **2** medium Granny Smith apples, cored and sliced into rings (1/4-inch thick)
- **1** large red bell pepper, sliced into thin strips
- **4** cups field greens
- **1** tablespoon bleu cheese

DRESSING

- **2** teaspoons olive oil
- **2** tablespoons apple cider vinegar
- **1** tablespoon honey
- **1/4** teaspoon salt

Exchanges

2 Lean Meat   1 Carbohydrate

Calories	174
Calories from Fat	45
Total Fat	5 g
Saturated Fat	1 g
Cholesterol	44 mg
Sodium	211 mg
Total Carbohydrate	17 g
Dietary Fiber	2 g
Sugars	13 g
Protein	17 g

1. Preheat broiler.

2. In a medium bowl, whisk together Dijon mustard, cider vinegar, honey, and sage. Reserve 2 tablespoons of this mixture. Add pork tenderloin to bowl and marinate in the refrigerator for 15 minutes.

3. Arrange apples on a baking sheet and brush all sides of apples with reserved Dijon mixture. Place apples under broiler for 2 minutes. Turn apples and return to broiler for 2 more minutes. Remove from broiler and set aside to cool.

4. Remove tenderloin from marinade and broil for 12–15 minutes, turning once. Remove from broiler and slice into thin pieces.

5. In a large salad bowl, toss together red pepper, field greens, and bleu cheese.

6. Whisk dressing ingredients in a small bowl and drizzle over salad; toss to coat. Arrange salad greens on a plate. Lay apple slices and pork slices over top of salad (pork should still be warm).

Chef's Tip: Pork and applesauce is a classic combination, but you've probably never had pork and apple salad before! Try it; it's great.

Black Bean Salsa Chicken

Makes: 4 servings   *Serving Size: 1 breast*   *Prep Time: 5 minutes*

Cooking spray
4 4-ounce boneless, skinless
   chicken breasts
1 cup canned black beans,
   rinsed and drained
1 cup salsa
1/2 teaspoon salt (optional)
1/4 teaspoon ground black pepper

1. Preheat oven to 350 degrees.

2. Coat a shallow baking dish with cooking spray. Arrange chicken breasts in bottom of pan. Bake for 20–25 minutes or until done.

3. In a medium bowl, combine remaining ingredients.

4. Coat a medium nonstick skillet with cooking spray. Add beans and salsa mixture to pan and cook over medium-high heat. Sauté for 5–6 minutes. While sautéing, use a spoon or spatula to slightly mash beans.

5. Serve bean and salsa mixture over chicken breasts.

Exchanges

1 Starch	1/2 Fat
3 Very Lean Meat	

Calories 206
  Calories from Fat 29
Total Fat . . . . 3 g
  Saturated Fat . . . . 1 g
Cholesterol . . . . 68 mg
Sodium . . . . 283 mg
Total Carbohydrate . . . . . . 13 g
  Dietary Fiber . . . . 4 g
  Sugars . . . . 3 g
Protein . . . . 30 g

Chef's Tip: You can also grill the chicken breasts instead of baking them.

Sirloin Steak with Chipotle Cream Sauce

Makes: 4 servings   *Serving Size: 4 ounces*   *Prep Time: 5 minutes*

1	pound sirloin steak
1/2	teaspoon salt
1/4	teaspoon ground black pepper
1/2	cup fat-free half-and-half
1 1/2	tablespoons cornstarch
1	garlic clove, minced
1	tablespoon canned chipotle peppers, puréed

1. Preheat broiler.

2. Season steaks with salt and pepper. Place in broiler and broil for 10–12 minutes, turning once.

3. In a small bowl, whisk together half-and-half and cornstarch until cornstarch is dissolved. Add mixture to a small saucepan and bring to a boil.

4. Reduce heat to a simmer and add garlic and chipotle pepper purée. Simmer for 5 minutes and serve sauce over each steak.

✔ *National Women's Checkup Day is this month . . . be sure to get yours!*

Exchanges

3 Lean Meat   1/2 Carbohydrate

Calories	176
Calories from Fat	49
Total Fat	5 g
Saturated Fat	2 g
Cholesterol	66 mg
Sodium	416 mg
Total Carbohydrate	7 g
Dietary Fiber	0 g
Sugars	2 g
Protein	23 g

Chef's Tip: Using canned chili peppers reduces the chances of burning your eyes with raw peppers!

Smashed Potatoes

1 pound red new potatoes, washed and quartered

4 garlic cloves, peeled

1/2 cup fat-free half-and-half, heated

1/2 teaspoon salt

1/4 teaspoon ground black pepper

1. Add potatoes and garlic cloves to a large soup pot. Cover with cold water and bring to a boil. Cook for 20 minutes or until potatoes are soft. Drain and return to pot.

2. Add remaining ingredients, and using a potato masher or sturdy whisk, smash potatoes and garlic until blended but still lumpy.

Exchanges
1 1/2 Starch

Calories 118
  Calories from Fat 5
Total Fat . . . . 1 g
  Saturated Fat . . . . 0 g
Cholesterol . . . . 2 mg
Sodium . . . . 339 mg
Total Carbohydrate . . . . . . 26 g
  Dietary Fiber . . . . 2 g
  Sugars . . . . 4 g
Protein . . . . 3 g

Dietitian's Tip: Leaving the skin on these potatoes increases the fiber content of the dish.

Monte Cristo

Makes: 4 servings   *Serving Size: 1 sandwich*   *Prep Time: 10 minutes*

1 cup egg substitute
1/2 cup fat-free milk
8 slices egg bread or other sturdy bread
Cooking spray
1/4 cup Dijon mustard
8 ounces extra lean thinly-sliced deli ham
4 1-ounce slices reduced-fat Swiss cheese

1. In a medium bowl, whisk together egg substitute and milk. Dip each piece of bread in mixture until soaked through.

2. Coat a large nonstick skillet with cooking spray over medium heat. Working in batches, place soaked bread slices in pan and fry about 4 minutes on each side until browned and cooked through. Set aside.

3. Spread 1 tablespoon Dijon mustard on 1 slice of the toasted bread. Top with 2 ounces ham, 1 slice cheese, and 1 slice toasted bread. Repeat for remaining three sandwiches.

✔ *National Employer Health and Fitness Day is May 21—find out what your company is doing to participate!*

Exchanges

2 1/2 Starch   3 Lean Meat

Calories 348	
Calories from Fat 75	
Total Fat . . . . 8 g	
Saturated Fat . . . . 3 g	
Cholesterol . . . . 66 mg	
Sodium . . . . 1357 mg	
Total Carbohydrate . . . . . . 34 g	
Dietary Fiber . . . . 2 g	
Sugars . . . . 7 g	
Protein . . . . 32 g	

Dietitian's Tip: By simply substituting a few low-fat ingredients, you can still enjoy a classic favorite.

Honey Tarragon Carrots

Makes: 4 servings   *Serving Size: 1/2 cup*   *Prep Time: 3 minutes*

1 pound baby carrots
1 cup water
2 tablespoons honey
1 teaspoon tarragon, dried
1/4 teaspoon salt
1/4 teaspoon ground black pepper

1. In a medium sauté pan, simmer carrots in water, covered, for 10 minutes.

2. Remove lid and add remaining ingredients.

3. Turn flame to high and cook until all liquid is reduced.

4. Sauté carrots until caramelized (golden brown).

Exchanges
2 Vegetable   1/2 Carbohydrate

Calories 81
  Calories from Fat 2
Total Fat . . . . 0 g
  Saturated Fat . . . . 0 g
Cholesterol . . . . 0 mg
Sodium . . . . 186 mg
Total Carbohydrate . . . . . . 20 g
  Dietary Fiber . . . . 3 g
  Sugars . . . . 15 g
Protein . . . . 1 g

See photo insert.

Chef's Tip: This is an excellent and quick side dish that can be served with a variety of entrees.

Chicken Tacos

Makes: 8 servings   *Serving Size: 1 taco*   *Prep Time: 10 minutes*

1 tablespoon olive oil
Cooking spray
1 pound boneless, skinless chicken breasts, sliced into 2-inch strips
1 tablespoon chili powder
1 teaspoon cumin
1/4 teaspoon cayenne pepper
3 tablespoons water
8 6-inch flour tortillas, heated
1 16-ounce can fat-free refried beans, heated
2 cups shredded lettuce
2 cups diced tomatoes
1 cup shredded, reduced-fat cheddar cheese

1. Add oil and a generous amount of cooking spray to a large nonstick skillet over high heat. Add chicken and sauté until beginning to brown. Stir in chili powder, cumin, cayenne pepper, and water. Sauté until all liquid evaporates.

2. Fill each tortilla with 1/4 cup refried beans, 1/4 cup chicken, 1/4 cup lettuce, 1/4 cup tomatoes, and 2 tablespoons cheese.

✔ *May is National High Blood Pressure Month. Make sure you're taking your medication and watching sodium intake if you have high blood pressure.*

Exchanges

2 Starch	2 Lean Meat

Calories 281
Calories from Fat 78
Total Fat . . . . 9 g
Saturated Fat . . . . 3 g
Cholesterol . . . . 44 mg
Sodium . . . . 528 mg
Total Carbohydrate . . . . . . 28 g
Dietary Fiber . . . . 5 g
Sugars . . . . 3 g
Protein . . . . 22 g

Chef's Tip: To make this dish a little spicier, stir in 1/2 cup salsa with the rest of the spices.

May ❖ Week 4

RECIPE LIST

DAY 1: Chicken Hash **172**
Spanish Rice **173**

DAY 2: Black Bean Burritos **174**

DAY 3: Baked Ravioli **175**

DAY 4: Spicy Shrimp Tacos **176**
Fried Corn **177**

DAY 5: Beef Barley Soup **178**

DESSERT OF THE MONTH: Pretzel and
Strawberry Delight **179**

GROCERY LIST

Fresh Produce
Onions – 6
Green bell pepper –1
Red bell pepper –1
Garlic – 1 head
Celery – 1 bag
Carrots – 1 bag
Button mushrooms –
8 ounces
Strawberries – 1 pint

Meat/Poultry/Fish
Boneless, skinless
chicken breasts –
1/2 pound
Unpeeled shrimp –
1 pound
Top round steak –
1/2 pound

Grains/Bread/Pasta
10-inch flour tortillas – 4
Corn tortillas – 8
Brown rice – 1 box or bag
White rice – 1 box or bag
Barley –1 box

Dairy and Cheese
Shredded, reduced-fat
cheddar cheese – 1 bag
Shredded, reduced-fat
mozzarella cheese –
1 bag
Margarine
8-ounce package light
cream cheese –
1 package
9-ounce package
reduced-fat cheese
ravioli – 2 packages

Canned Goods and Sauces
14.5-ounce can fat-free,
reduced-sodium
chicken broth – 2 cans
16-ounce can black
beans – 1 can
8-ounce can tomato
sauce – 1 can
15-ounce can crushed
tomatoes – 1 can
15-ounce can no-salt-
added diced
tomatoes – 1 can
14.5-ounce can fat-free,
reduced-sodium beef
broth – 3 cans
1-pound jar marinara
pasta sauce – 1 jar
Canned chipotle
peppers – 1 small can

Frozen Foods
1-pound bag hash
browns –1 bag
Corn – 1 large bag
8-ounce container light
whipped topping –
1 container

Staples/Seasonings/Baking Needs
Salt/ground black pepper
Cooking spray
Olive oil
Cumin
Garlic salt
Paprika
Canola oil
Chili powder
Crushed red pepper
flakes
Cayenne pepper
Hot pepper sauce
Dried basil
All-purpose flour
Bay leaf
Sugar
0.6-ounce package sugar-
free strawberry gelatin
mix – 1 package

Miscellaneous
Thin pretzels – medium-
size bag

Chicken Hash

Makes: 7 servings   *Serving Size: 1 cup*   *Prep Time: 10 minutes*

Cooking spray
2 teaspoons olive oil
1/2 pound boneless, skinless chicken breasts, cubed
1 medium onion, chopped
1 medium green bell pepper, chopped
1 medium red bell pepper, chopped
1 1-pound bag frozen or refrigerated hash browns
1 cup fat-free, reduced-sodium chicken broth
1/2 teaspoon hot pepper sauce
1/4 teaspoon ground black pepper
1/2 teaspoon cumin
1/2 teaspoon garlic salt
1 teaspoon paprika
1 cup shredded, reduced-fat cheddar cheese

1. Preheat oven to 375 degrees. Coat a 9 × 13-inch baking dish with cooking spray.

2. Add oil to a large nonstick skillet and heat over high heat. Add chicken and sauté for 3–4 minutes. Add onion, green pepper, and red pepper and sauté another 4 minutes or until onion begins to turn clear. Stir in hash browns; set aside.

3. In a small bowl, combine broth, hot pepper sauce, black pepper, cumin, garlic salt, and paprika.

4. Pour chicken/hash brown mixture into baking dish. Pour broth mixture over the chicken and bake for 20 minutes. Sprinkle the cheese over the top and bake for 5 more minutes or until cheese is melted.

Exchanges

1 Starch	1 Vegetable
1 Lean Meat	1/2 Fat

Calories 175
 Calories from Fat 54
Total Fat . . . . 6 g
 Saturated Fat . . . . 3 g
Cholesterol . . . . 31 mg
Sodium . . . . 333 mg
Total Carbohydrate . . . . . . 17 g
 Dietary Fiber . . . . 2 g
 Sugars . . . . 3 g
Protein . . . . 14 g

Dietitian's Tip: Hash is traditionally made with high-fat corned beef, but this recipe uses chicken for a healthy and tasty twist on this old diner favorite.

Spanish Rice

Makes: 6 servings   *Serving Size: 1/2 cup*   *Prep Time: 10 minutes*

Cooking spray
1 tablespoon olive oil
1 small onion, finely diced
1 cup uncooked white rice
1 cup canned crushed tomatoes
3/4 cup fat-free, reduced-sodium chicken broth
1/2 teaspoon salt
1/4 teaspoon ground black pepper
1/8 teaspoon cayenne pepper

1. Coat a large saucepan with cooking spray and heat oil over medium-high heat. Add onion and sauté until onion turns clear. Add rice and sauté 2 more minutes.

2. Add remaining ingredients and bring to a boil. Reduce heat and simmer, covered, for 20–25 minutes. Fluff with a fork and serve.

 National Senior Health and Fitness Day is May 28. Start by taking a walk this morning to wake yourself up!

Exchanges
2 Starch

Calories 158
  Calories from Fat 23
Total Fat . . . . 3 g
  Saturated Fat . . . . 0 g
Cholesterol . . . . 0 mg
Sodium . . . . 372 mg
Total Carbohydrate . . . . . . 30 g
  Dietary Fiber . . . . 2 g
  Sugars . . . . 3 g
Protein . . . . 3 g

Chef's Tip: Serve this zesty rice with other dishes as well. It goes great with fish, chicken, and steak.

Black Bean Burritos

Makes: 4 servings   *Serving Size: 1 burrito*   *Prep Time: 10 minutes*

Cooking spray

1 tablespoon canola oil

1 medium onion, finely diced

2 garlic cloves, minced

1 16-ounce can black beans, rinsed and drained

1/2 cup tomato sauce

1 teaspoon chili powder

1/2 teaspoon cumin

1/4 teaspoon crushed red pepper flakes

1/2 teaspoon salt

1/4 teaspoon ground black pepper

4 10-inch flour tortillas

2 cups cooked brown rice

1. Coat a large nonstick skillet with cooking spray. Add oil and heat over medium-high heat. Add onion and sauté about 4–5 minutes, or until onion turns clear. Add all ingredients except tortillas and rice and bring to a boil. Reduce heat and simmer 10 minutes.

2. Lay tortilla on a dry, flat surface. Fill tortilla with 1/2 cup rice and 1/4 of the bean mixture. Fold left and right sides of tortillas to the center and roll from the bottom to form burrito. Repeat procedure for remaining three burritos.

Exchanges

5 Starch	1 Fat
1 Vegetable	

Calories 474
Calories from Fat 89
Total Fat . . . . 10 g
Saturated Fat . . . . 2 g
Cholesterol . . . . 0 mg
Sodium . . . . 610 mg
Total Carbohydrate . . . . . . 82 g
Dietary Fiber . . . . 11 g
Sugars . . . . 8 g
Protein . . . . 15 g

Dietitian's Tip: These burritos are quite high in carb, so be sure to account for the total in your meal plan . . . or only have half of the burrito, for 41 grams total carb.

Baked Ravioli

Makes: 5 servings   *Serving Size: 1 cup*   *Prep Time: 5 minutes*

Cooking spray

2 9-ounce packages reduced-fat cheese ravioli, cooked

1 1-pound jar marinara pasta sauce

2 garlic cloves, minced

1 teaspoon dried basil

1/2 cup shredded, reduced-fat mozzarella cheese (optional)

1. Preheat oven to 375 degrees.

2. Coat a medium casserole dish with cooking spray. Line the bottom of dish with ravioli.

3. In a medium bowl, combine pasta sauce, garlic, and basil. Pour sauce over ravioli and stir. Bake for 30 minutes.

4. Sprinkle cheese (if using) over the top of ravioli and return to oven; bake an additional 10 minutes or until cheese is melted.

Exchanges

3 Starch   1 Vegetable
1 Lean Meat

Calories	321
Calories from Fat	55
Total Fat	6 g
Saturated Fat	4 g
Cholesterol	35 mg
Sodium	654 mg
Total Carbohydrate	52 g
Dietary Fiber	4 g
Sugars	11 g
Protein	17 g

Chef's Tip: This ravioli is great served with a mixed green salad.

Spicy Shrimp Tacos

Makes: 8 servings   *Serving Size: 1 taco*   *Prep Time: 10 minutes*

2 teaspoons olive oil

2 small onions, thinly sliced

2 tablespoons canned chipotle
  peppers, chopped

1 15-ounce can no-salt-added
  diced tomatoes, drained

2 tablespoons water

1 pound shrimp, peeled and
  deveined

1/2 teaspoon salt

8 corn tortillas, warmed

1. Add oil to a large nonstick skillet over medium heat. Sauté onion for 4 minutes or until onion is clear. Stir in peppers, tomatoes, and water and bring to a simmer for 10 minutes.

2. Add shrimp and cook, covered, for an additional 4 minutes or until shrimp are done. Season with salt.

3. Serve 1/8 of shrimp mixture on each tortilla.

Exchanges

1 Starch	1 Very Lean Meat

Calories 120
  Calories from Fat 21
Total Fat . . . . 2 g
  Saturated Fat . . . . 0 g
Cholesterol . . . . 73 mg
Sodium . . . . 313 mg
Total Carbohydrate . . . . . . 15 g
  Dietary Fiber . . . . 2 g
  Sugars . . . . 3 g
Protein . . . . 10 g

Chef's Tip: If you want to add even more kick to this spicy dish, add another tablespoon of chopped chipotle peppers.

Fried Corn

Makes: 6 servings   *Serving Size: 1/4 cup*   *Prep Time: 5 minutes*

1/2 cup water
1 tablespoon all-purpose flour
1/2 teaspoon salt
Dash pepper
3 cups frozen corn, thawed
Cooking spray
1 tablespoon margarine

1. In a medium bowl, whisk together water, flour, salt, and pepper. Add corn and toss to coat. Set aside.

2. Coat a medium nonstick skillet with cooking spray; add margarine and melt over high heat. Add corn and fry for 10–12 minutes.

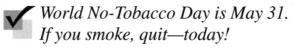 *World No-Tobacco Day is May 31. If you smoke, quit—today!*

Exchanges
1 Starch

Calories 87
Calories from Fat 20
Total Fat . . . . 2 g
Saturated Fat . . . . 0 g
Cholesterol . . . . 0 mg
Sodium . . . . 220 mg
Total Carbohydrate . . . . . . 17 g
Dietary Fiber . . . . 2 g
Sugars . . . . 2 g
Protein . . . . 2 g

Dietitian's Tip: Work the carb in this corn dish into your daily meal plan along with any other starchy vegetables, bread, pasta, or sweets.

Beef Barley Soup

Makes: 6 servings   *Serving Size: 1 cup*   *Prep Time: 10 minutes*

2 teaspoons canola oil

1/2 pound top round steak, finely diced

3 medium celery stalks, finely diced

2 medium carrots, finely diced

1 small onion, finely diced

8 ounces button mushrooms, sliced

3 14.5-ounce cans fat-free, reduced-sodium beef broth

1/2 teaspoon salt (optional)

1/4 teaspoon ground black pepper
Bay leaf

1/2 cup uncooked barley

1. Add oil to a large soup pot and heat over high heat. Add beef and sauté for 7–8 minutes; brown well. Stir in celery, carrots, and onion and sauté an additional 7–8 minutes or until vegetables begin to caramelize.

2. Add mushrooms and sauté for 5 more minutes. Add remaining ingredients and bring to a boil. Reduce heat and simmer for 45 minutes. Remove bay leaf and serve.

Exchanges

1 Starch	1 Vegetable
1 Lean Meat	

Calories 150
  Calories from Fat 34
Total Fat . . . . 4 g
  Saturated Fat . . . . 1 g
Cholesterol . . . . 19 mg
Sodium . . . . 424 mg
Total Carbohydrate . . . . . . 18 g
  Dietary Fiber . . . . 5 g
  Sugars . . . . 4 g
Protein . . . . 11 g

Chef's Tip: Barley, a heartier grain than rice, is very filling and helps make this soup a satisfying meal.

Pretzel and Strawberry Delight

Makes: 16 servings　　　*Serving Size: 1/16 recipe*　　　*Prep Time: 40 minutes*

2 cups thin pretzels, crushed

2 tablespoons margarine, melted

1/2 cup plus 1 tablespoon sugar

1 8-ounce package light cream cheese, softened

1 8-ounce container light whipped topping, thawed

1 0.6-ounce package sugar-free strawberry gelatin mix

3 cups fresh strawberries, thinly sliced

> The ADA recommends eating only a small amount of saturated fat every day. This recipe is higher in saturated fat, so try to balance it by eating foods low in saturated fat at your other meals today.

Exchanges

| 1 Fat | 1 Carbohydrate |

Calories 135

　Calories from Fat . . . 57

Total Fat . . . . 6 g

　Saturated Fat . . . . 4 g

Cholesterol . . . . 10 mg

Sodium . . . . 168 mg

Total Carbohydrate . . 16 g

　Dietary Fiber . . . . 1 g

　Sugars . . . . 10 g

Protein . . . . 3 g

1. Preheat oven to 400 degrees.

2. In a medium bowl, mix together pretzels, margarine, and 1 tablespoon sugar. Pour mixture into a 9 × 13-inch glass baking dish and press to cover bottom of pan. Bake 8–10 minutes. Remove from oven and let cool.

3. In a medium bowl, beat 1/2 cup sugar and cream cheese with electric mixer on high until creamy and smooth. Fold in whipped topping. Pour cream cheese mixture around edge of pretzel layer in baking dish and use a flat spatula to spread mixture evenly and gently toward the center. Refrigerate.

4. In a large bowl, add 2 cups boiling water to gelatin mix and stir constantly for 2 minutes or until dissolved. Stir in 1 cup cold water and refrigerate 30 minutes. Remove gelatin from refrigerator and stir in strawberries; refrigerate another 30 minutes.

5. Pour gelatin over cream cheese layer and refrigerate dessert 2–3 hours.

Chef's Tip: When you spread the cream cheese mixture over the pretzel layer, be sure to use a flat spatula and slowly spread the mixture toward the center. This will prevent the pretzel layer from mixing in with the cream cheese layer.

June

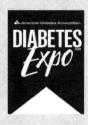

Fruits of the Harvest

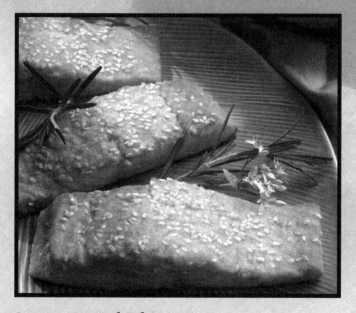

Sesame-Crusted Salmon (page 204)
Searing this fish on both sides seals in its natural
juices and enhances the flavor of the sesame seeds.
It's delicious with broccoli and steamed rice.

June ❖ Recipes

June ❖ Week 1

RECIPE LIST

DAY 1: Pesto Pasta Salad   **184**

DAY 2: Grilled Ham and Veggie
Sandwich   **185**
Tortellini Salad   **186**

DAY 3: Grilled Pork Chops with Peach
Compote   **187**

DAY 4: Grilled Halibut   **188**
Grilled Eggplant   **189**

DAY 5: Mango Salsa Chicken over
Rice   **190**

GROCERY LIST

Fresh Produce
Fresh basil – 1 bunch
Portabello mushrooms –
2
Broccoli – 1 small head
Grape tomatoes –
1 container
Yellow pepper – 1
Peaches – 4 large
Fresh marjoram –
1 bunch
Garlic – 1 head
Eggplant – 1 medium
Mango – 1
Red onion – 1
Green bell pepper – 1

Meat/Poultry/Fish
Extra lean, thinly sliced
deli ham – 8 ounces
Bone-in, center-cut pork
chops – 4 (5-ounce)
chops
Halibut filets – 4
(4-ounce) filets
Boneless, skinless
chicken breasts – 4
(4-ounce) breasts

Grains/Bread/Pasta
Farfalle pasta – 1 box
2-ounce Kaiser rolls – 4
Brown rice –1 box

Dairy and Cheese
Plain, fat-free yogurt –
8 ounces
Grated Parmesan cheese
3/4-ounce slices
reduced-fat
mozzarella cheese –
4 slices
9-ounce package three-
cheese tortellini –
1 package

Canned Goods
and Sauces
Light mayonnaise – 1 jar
Roasted red peppers –
1 jar
Fat-free Italian
dressing – 1 bottle

Staples/
Seasonings/Baking
Needs
Salt/ground black pepper
Garlic salt
Red wine vinegar
Olive oil
Balsamic vinegar
Dried sage
Hot pepper sauce
Honey
Rice wine vinegar

Miscellaneous
Pine nuts – small bag

Pesto Pasta Salad

Makes: 6 servings   *Serving Size: 1 cup*   *Prep Time: 13 minutes*

12 ounces uncooked farfalle pasta
1 cup fresh basil leaves
2 tablespoons pine nuts
1/3 cup light mayonnaise
1/3 cup plain, fat-free yogurt
1/2 teaspoon garlic salt
1 tablespoon red wine vinegar
3 tablespoons grated Parmesan cheese

1. Cook pasta according to package directions, omitting salt. Rinse under cold water to cool.

2. In a food processor, add basil and pine nuts and purée.

3. In a large mixing bowl, whisk together mayonnaise, yogurt, garlic salt, red wine vinegar, and Parmesan cheese. Add basil and pine nuts and mix well.

4. Add cooled pasta to bowl; toss lightly to coat. Refrigerate.

Exchanges

3 Starch   1 1/2 Fat

Calories	297
Calories from Fat	73
Total Fat	8 g
Saturated Fat	2 g
Cholesterol	8 mg
Sodium	293 mg
Total Carbohydrate	45 g
Dietary Fiber	2 g
Sugars	4 g
Protein	11 g

Dietitian's Tip: The fat-free yogurt in this recipe provides creaminess without changing the flavor of the salad. Try using plain, fat-free yogurt mixed with light mayonnaise in many mayonnaise-based salads, such as tuna or chicken salad.

Grilled Ham and Veggie Sandwich

Makes: 4 servings   *Serving Size: 1 sandwich*   *Prep Time: 8 minutes*

4 tablespoons light mayonnaise

2 teaspoons hot pepper sauce

4 2-ounce Kaiser rolls

2 portabello mushrooms, sliced in half

4 roasted red pepper halves (jarred)

8 ounces extra lean, thinly sliced deli ham

4 3/4-ounce slices reduced-fat mozzarella cheese

1. Preheat oven to 350 degrees. In a small bowl, whisk together mayonnaise and hot pepper sauce.

2. Spread 1 tablespoon mayonnaise mixture onto bottom half of Kaiser roll and top with 1/2 portabello mushroom, 1 red pepper half, 2 ounces ham, 1 slice mozzarella cheese, and top half of roll.

3. Repeat procedure for remaining three sandwiches.

4. Place sandwiches on baking sheet and bake for 13–15 minutes until cheese is melted.

Exchanges

2 Starch	1 Vegetable
2 Lean Meat	1 Fat

Calories 349
 Calories from Fat 106
Total Fat . . . . 12 g
 Saturated Fat . . . . 4 g
Cholesterol . . . . 42 mg
Sodium . . . . 1125 mg
Total Carbohydrate . . . . . . 37 g
 Dietary Fiber . . . . 2 g
 Sugars . . . . 6 g
Protein . . . . 23 g

Chef's Tip: Roasted red peppers add zing to this tasty sandwich.

Tortellini Salad

Makes: 6 servings   *Serving Size: 1 cup*   *Prep Time: 8 minutes*

1 9-ounce package three-cheese tortellini
1 cup broccoli florets
3/4 cup grape tomatoes, halved
1/2 cup yellow bell pepper strips
1/2 cup fat-free Italian dressing

1. Cook tortellini according to package directions; drain.

2. Toss all ingredients in a large salad bowl. Serve immediately or refrigerate until ready to serve.

Exchanges

1 1/2 Starch	1/2 Fat

Calories 148
Calories from Fat 26
Total Fat . . . . 3 g
Saturated Fat . . . . 1 g
Cholesterol . . . . 16 mg
Sodium . . . . 404 mg
Total Carbohydrate . . . . . . 24 g
Dietary Fiber . . . . 2 g
Sugars . . . . 5 g
Protein . . . . 7 g

Chef's Tip: Feel free to experiment with this recipe by adding more of your favorite vegetables.

Grilled Halibut

Makes: 4 servings   *Serving Size: 1 filet*   *Prep Time: 10 minutes*

1/2 cup finely chopped fresh marjoram (or 2 tablespoons dried marjoram)

4 garlic cloves, minced

1 teaspoon olive oil

1/2 teaspoon salt

1/4 teaspoon ground black pepper

4 4-ounce halibut filets

1. Prepare an indoor or outdoor grill.

2. In a small bowl, combine marjoram, garlic, olive oil, salt, and pepper.

3. Rub 2 tablespoons of marjoram mixture on non-skin side of filet.

4. Grill filets over medium heat for 3 minutes on each side.

Exchanges

3 Very Lean Meat	1/2 Fat

Calories	144
Calories from Fat	34
Total Fat	4 g
Saturated Fat	0 g
Cholesterol	37 mg
Sodium	355 mg
Total Carbohydrate	2 g
Dietary Fiber	1 g
Sugars	1 g
Protein	24 g

Chef's Tip: If you can't find halibut, try flounder, haddock, or perch in this recipe instead.

Grilled Pork Chops with Peach Compo

Makes: 4 servings   *Serving Size: 1 pork chop and 1/4 cup compote*   *Prep Time: 10 mi*

- **4** 5-ounce bone-in, center-cut pork chops
- **1/2** teaspoon salt
- **1/4** teaspoon ground black pepper
- **3** cups peaches, peeled, pitted, and chopped (about 4 large peaches)
- **1** teaspoon olive oil
- **1** teaspoon honey
- **3** teaspoons balsamic vinegar
- **1/4** teaspoon dried sage

1. Prepare an indoor or outdoor g
Season pork chops with salt and pe
on both sides. Grill pork chops ove
medium heat until done.

2. Meanwhile, in a medium nons
skillet, sauté peaches in olive oil ar
honey over medium heat for 7 min
Add balsamic vinegar and sage; sa
for another 2 minutes.

3. Serve 1/4 cup peach compote
each pork chop.

Exchanges

3 Lean Meat	1 Fruit

Calories 226	
Calories from Fat 64	
Total Fat . . . . 7 g	
Saturated Fat . . . . 2 g	
Cholesterol . . . . 59 mg	
Sodium . . . . 335 mg	
Total Carbohydrate . . . . . . 20 g	
Dietary Fiber . . . . 3 g	
Sugars . . . . 16 g	
Protein . . . . 22 g	

Chef's Tip: June is the best month to buy peaches. Check out your local farmer's market f the best selection. And make sure the peaches are very ripe for this recipe.

Grilled Eggplant

Makes: 4 servings　　　*Serving Size: 2 slices*　　　*Prep Time: 3 minutes*

1 tablespoon olive oil
1 medium eggplant
1/2 teaspoon salt
1/4 teaspoon ground black pepper

1. Prepare an indoor or outdoor grill.

2. Cut the ends off eggplant and thinly slice lengthwise. Brush eggplant slices with olive oil. Sprinkle with salt and pepper.

3. Grill eggplant slices over medium-high heat for about 3 minutes for each side.

Exchanges

1 Vegetable   1/2 Fat

Calories. 58
　Calories from Fat. 32
Total Fat . . . . 4 g
　Saturated Fat . . . . 0 g
Cholesterol . . . . 0 mg
Sodium . . . . 293 mg
Total Carbohydrate. . . . . . . 7 g
　Dietary Fiber . . . . 3 g
　Sugars. . . . . 4 g
Protein. . . . . 1 g

Chef's Tip: The best time to buy eggplant is in the summer. Stop by your local farmer's market and pick up the plumpest eggplant you can find.

Mango Salsa Chicken over Rice

Makes: 4 servings   *Serving Size: 1 chicken breast*   *Prep Time: 10 minutes*
and 1/2 cup brown rice

4 4-ounce boneless, skinless chicken breasts

1/2 teaspoon salt

1/4 teaspoon ground black pepper

1 teaspoon olive oil

1 tablespoon rice wine vinegar

1 mango, finely diced (1 cup)

1/2 cup finely diced red onion

1 green bell pepper, finely diced

2 cups brown rice, cooked

1. Prepare an indoor or outdoor grill.

2. Season chicken breasts with salt and pepper on both sides. Grill chicken breasts over medium heat for about 5 minutes on each side or until juices run clear.

3. In a small bowl, whisk olive oil and vinegar. Add remaining ingredients except rice and toss to coat.

4. Pour mango salsa over grilled chicken breasts. Serve each chicken breast over 1/2 cup brown rice.

Exchanges

1 1/2 Starch	1/2 Fruit
3 Very Lean Meat	1/2 Fat
1 Vegetable	

Calories 298
  Calories from Fat 46
Total Fat . . . . 5 g
  Saturated Fat . . . . 1 g
Cholesterol . . . . 68 mg
Sodium . . . . 358 mg
Total Carbohydrate . . . . . . 34 g
  Dietary Fiber . . . . 4 g
  Sugars . . . . 9 g
Protein . . . . 28 g

See photo insert.

Dietitian's Tip: Mangoes are a good source of vitamin C. They taste great in smoothies, too!

June ❖ Week 2

GROCERY LIST

Fresh Produce
Fresh basil – 1 bunch
Garlic – 1 head
Broccoli – 3 heads
Red onion – 1
Tomato – 1 large
Red bell peppers – 3
Napa cabbage – 1 head
Scallions – 1 bunch
Sugar-snap peas –
   1 small bag (2 cups)
Carrots – 1 bag
Zucchini – 3 large
Garlic – 1 head
Button mushrooms –
   1 pint
Yellow squash – 1 large
Red potatoes – 12
Onion – 1

Meat/Poultry/Fish
Boneless, skinless
   chicken breasts – 4
   (4-ounce) breasts
Turkey bacon – 1 package
Thinly sliced, smoked
   deli turkey –
   12 ounces
Pork tenderloin –
   1 pound
Beef tenderloin –
   1 pound

Grains/Bread/Pasta
2-ounce French (sub)
   rolls – 4
3-ounce package ramen-
   style noodles –
   2 packages
Angel hair pasta – 1 box

Dairy and Cheese
Plain, fat-free yogurt –
   8 ounces
Egg substitute – 12
   ounces
Shredded, part-skim
   mozzarella cheese –
   1 bag

Canned Goods and Sauces
14-ounce can artichoke
   hearts – 1 can
15-ounce can no-salt-
   added diced
   tomatoes – 1 can
Light mayonnaise – 1 jar
Lite soy sauce – 1 bottle
Teriyaki sauce – 1 bottle
Fat-free Italian
   dressing – 1 bottle

Staples/Seasonings/ Baking Needs
Salt/ground black pepper
Cooking spray
Balsamic vinegar
Sugar
Apple cider vinegar
Garlic powder
Rice wine vinegar
Olive oil
Sesame oil
Dried basil
Dried rosemary
Hot pepper sauce
Honey

Miscellaneous
Golden raisins – small
   box
Bamboo skewers

191

Marinated Grilled Chicken

Makes: 4 servings　　　*Serving Size: 1 chicken breast*　　　*Prep Time: 5 minutes*

1 tablespoon olive oil
1/4 cup balsamic vinegar
1 tablespoon honey
3 tablespoons fresh basil, coarsely chopped
3 garlic cloves, minced
4 4-ounce boneless, skinless chicken breasts

1. Prepare an indoor or outdoor grill.

2. In a large bowl, whisk oil, balsamic vinegar, honey, basil, and garlic together. Add chicken breasts and coat well. Marinate in the refrigerator for 15–30 minutes.

3. Grill chicken breasts over medium heat for about 5 minutes on each side or until juices run clear.

Exchanges

3 Very Lean Meat	1/2 Fat
1/2 Carbohydrate	

Calories	174
Calories from Fat	46
Total Fat	5 g
Saturated Fat	1 g
Cholesterol	68 mg
Sodium	61 mg
Total Carbohydrate	5 g
Dietary Fiber	0 g
Sugars	5 g
Protein	25 g

Dietitian's Tip: Marinating meats and vegetables can be a great way to add flavor without adding fat.

Broccoli Salad with Raisins

Makes: 7 servings   *Serving Size: 1 cup*   *Prep Time: 15 minutes*

SALAD

8 slices turkey bacon, cut into 1-inch pieces, cooked
6 cups broccoli florets
1/3 cup finely diced red onion
1/3 cup golden raisins

DRESSING

1/3 cup light mayonnaise
1/4 cup plain, fat-free yogurt
1 tablespoon sugar
1 tablespoon apple cider vinegar

1. In a large salad bowl, toss together salad ingredients.

2. In a small bowl, whisk together dressing ingredients.

3. Drizzle dressing over broccoli salad and toss well to coat.

✔ *Dairy Month is in June. Try all the delicious fat-free and reduced-fat milk products on the market today! Your family recipes will taste just as delicious as they used to, and be healthier for you, too.*

Exchanges

1 Vegetable	1 1/2 Fat
1/2 Fruit	

Calories 125
Calories from Fat 63
Total Fat . . . . 7 g
Saturated Fat . . . . 2 g
Cholesterol . . . . 16 mg
Sodium . . . . 311 mg
Total Carbohydrate . . . . . . 13 g
Dietary Fiber . . . . 2 g
Sugars . . . . 9 g
Protein . . . . 5 g

See photo insert.

Chef's Tip: To quickly cook the bacon pieces, microwave them on high for 2 minutes.

Turkey and Artichoke Sandwich

Makes: 4 servings   *Serving Size: 1 sandwich*   *Prep Time: 10 minutes*

1 14-ounce can artichoke hearts, drained
1/3 cup light mayonnaise
1 teaspoon garlic powder
4 2-ounce French (sub) rolls
12 ounces thinly-sliced, smoked deli turkey
1 large tomato, sliced

1. In a food processor or blender, purée artichoke hearts, mayonnaise, and garlic powder to form a spread.

2. Spread 2 1/2 tablespoons of artichoke mixture on a French roll. Add 3 ounces turkey breast and 1–2 tomato slices.

3. Repeat procedure for remaining three sandwiches.

Exchanges

2 Starch	1 Vegetable
2 Very Lean Meat	1 1/2 Fat

Calories 320
 Calories from Fat 81
Total Fat . . . . 9 g
 Saturated Fat . . . . 2 g
Cholesterol . . . . 52 mg
Sodium . . . . 1427 mg
Total Carbohydrate . . . . . . 35 g
 Dietary Fiber . . . . 2 g
 Sugars. . . . . 6 g
Protein. . . . . 23 g

Chef's Tip: Don't be afraid to try this delicious flavor combination.

Asian Noodle Salad with Shredded Pork

Makes: 8 servings   *Serving Size: 1/8 recipe*   *Prep Time: 30 minutes*

SALAD

- 2 tablespoons lite soy sauce
- 1 teaspoon hot pepper sauce
- 1 pound pork tenderloin
- 2 3-ounce packages ramen-style noodles (discard seasoning packet)
- 1 red bell pepper, sliced into strips
- 1 1/2 cups Napa cabbage, shredded
- 2 scallions, chopped
- 2 cups sugar snap peas
- 1 cup carrots, shredded

DRESSING

- 1/4 cup rice wine vinegar
- 1 tablespoon olive oil
- 1 tablespoon sesame oil
- 1 tablespoon teriyaki sauce
- 1/2 teaspoon hot pepper sauce

1. Preheat oven to 400 degrees. In a small bowl, whisk together soy sauce and 1 teaspoon hot pepper sauce. Brush entire pork tenderloin with soy sauce mixture and place in a medium baking dish. Roast for 20–25 minutes or until done.

2. While pork is roasting, cook noodles according to package directions, omitting salt; drain and run under cold water to cool.

3. In a large salad bowl, toss together cooled noodles and all vegetables. In a small bowl, whisk together all dressing ingredients. Drizzle dressing over salad; toss to coat.

4. Remove pork from oven and shred the meat with a fork. Toss the shredded pork with the salad and serve.

Exchanges

1 Starch	1 Vegetable
1 Lean Meat	1 1/2 Fat

Calories 221	
Calories from Fat 86	
Total Fat . . . . 10 g	
Saturated Fat . . . . 3 g	
Cholesterol . . . . 32 mg	
Sodium . . . . 336 mg	
Total Carbohydrate . . . . . . 19 g	
Dietary Fiber . . . . 2 g	
Sugars . . . . 3 g	
Protein . . . . 15 g	

Chef's Tip: If you can't find Napa, or Chinese, cabbage for this recipe, regular cabbage will work just fine.

Italian Garden Frittata

Makes: 8 servings   *Serving Size: 1/8 recipe*   *Prep Time: 15 minutes*

8 ounces uncooked angel hair pasta, broken in half
  Cooking spray
2 zucchini, diced
1 15-ounce can no-salt-added diced tomatoes, drained
3 garlic cloves, minced
1 teaspoon dried basil
1/2 teaspoon salt
12 ounces egg substitute
1/2 cup shredded, part-skim mozzarella cheese

1. Preheat oven to 300 degrees. Cook pasta according to package directions, omitting salt. Drain.

2. Coat a large oven-safe skillet with cooking spray and sauté zucchini over medium-high heat for about 8 minutes. Stir frequently.

3. Add diced tomatoes, garlic, basil, and salt. Add cooked pasta and cook 1 minute, tossing to coat.

4. Add egg substitute and cheese and mix well to distribute eggs evenly. Cook 3–5 more minutes.

5. Place in oven and bake for 15 minutes

Exchanges

1 1/2 Starch   1 Vegetable
1 Very Lean Meat

Calories 159
  Calories from Fat 16
Total Fat . . . . 2 g
  Saturated Fat . . . . 1 g
Cholesterol . . . . 4 mg
Sodium . . . . 288 mg
Total Carbohydrate . . . . . . 25 g
  Dietary Fiber . . . . 3 g
  Sugars . . . . 4 g
Protein . . . . 11 g

Dietitian's Tip: Pasta is a delicious addition to this frittata.

Beef Kabobs

Makes: 4 servings   *Serving Size: 2 skewers*   *Prep Time: 20 minutes*

1 pint button mushrooms

1 large zucchini, sliced into 1/2-inch-thick rounds

1 large yellow squash, sliced into 1/2-inch-thick rounds

2 red bell peppers, sliced into 1-inch chunks

1 pound beef tenderloin, cut into 1-inch cubes

1/2 cup fat-free Italian dressing

8 bamboo skewers, soaked in warm water

1. Prepare an indoor or outdoor grill.

2. Assemble kabobs by alternating mushrooms, zucchini, squash, peppers, and beef on each skewer.

3. Brush all sides of kabobs with Italian dressing. Grill over medium heat for 10 minutes, turning occasionally.

✔ *June is Headache Awareness Month. Did you know hidden food allergies can cause headaches? Try keeping a food diary to figure out if something you're eating is causing the headaches.*

Exchanges

3 Lean Meat	3 Vegetable

Calories 222	
Calories from Fat 68	
Total Fat . . . . 8 g	
Saturated Fat . . . . 3 g	
Cholesterol . . . . 60 mg	
Sodium . . . . 362 mg	
Total Carbohydrate . . . . . . 15 g	
Dietary Fiber . . . . 4 g	
Sugars . . . . 9 g	
Protein . . . . 23 g	

Chef's Tip: If you don't soak these skewers before using them, they can catch fire on the grill!

Herb-Grilled Potatoes

Makes: 6 servings   *Serving Size: 2 potatoes*   *Prep Time: 10 minutes*
(8 quarters)

12 small red potatoes, cut into quarters

1/2 teaspoon ground black pepper

3/4 teaspoon salt

1 small onion, thinly sliced

3 garlic cloves, minced

1 tablespoon olive oil

2 teaspoons dried rosemary
Cooking spray

1. Prepare an indoor or outdoor grill.

2. In a large bowl, toss together all ingredients.

3. Cut aluminum foil into six 8 × 8-inch pieces. Spray foil with cooking spray. Put 2 cups of potato mixture into one foil piece and fold together to create a packet.

4. Repeat procedure for remaining five aluminum foil pieces.

5. Place aluminum foil packets on grill and cook over medium-high heat for 30–40 minutes.

Exchanges

2 Starch

Calories 141
  Calories from Fat 21
Total Fat . . . . 2 g
  Saturated Fat . . . . 0 g
Cholesterol . . . . 0 mg
Sodium . . . . 302 mg
Total Carbohydrate . . . . . . 27 g
  Dietary Fiber . . . . 3 g
  Sugars . . . . 4 g
Protein . . . . 4 g

Chef's Tip: Cooking potatoes in a foil packet is a great way to enhance their flavor.

RECIPE LIST

DAY 1: Harvest Beef Burrito **200**

DAY 2: Lemon Chicken with Bell
Peppers **201**

DAY 3: Vegetable Quesadillas **202**
Fruit with Dip **203**

DAY 4: Sesame-Crusted Salmon **204**
Stir-Fried Vegetables **205**

DAY 5: Egg Salad Sandwich **206**

GROCERY LIST

Fresh Produce

Broccoli – 4 heads
Red bell peppers – 3
Green bell peppers – 3
Lemon – 1
Onion – 1
Tomatoes – 2 small
Watermelon – small
 (1 cup cubes)
Cantaloupe – small
 (1 cup cubes)
Honeydew – small
 (1 cup cubes)
Strawberries – 1 pint
Bananas – 2
Apples – 2
Pea pods – 1 bag
 (2 cups)
Carrots – 1 small bag
Silken firm tofu – 1 box

Meat/Poultry/Fish

Flank steak – 1 pound
Boneless, skinless
 chicken breasts – 4
 (4-ounce) breasts
Salmon filets – 4
 (4-ounce) filets

Grains/Bread/Pasta

Brown rice – 1 box
10-inch flour
 tortillas – 10
Whole-wheat bread –
 1 loaf

Dairy and Cheese

Shredded, reduced-fat
 mozzarella cheese –
 1 bag
Fat-free sour cream –
 small container
Sugar-free vanilla
 pudding – 1 cup
Eggs

Canned Goods and Sauces

16-ounce can black
 beans – 1 can
14.5-ounce can fat-free,
 reduced-sodium
 chicken broth – 1 can
Salsa – 1 jar
Lite soy sauce –1 bottle
Dijon mustard – 1 jar
Light mayonnaise – 1 jar
4-ounce can tomato
 paste – 1 can

Frozen Foods

8-ounce container light
 whipped topping –
 1 container

Staples/Seasonings/Baking Needs

Salt/ground black pepper
Cooking spray
Olive oil
Chili powder
Cayenne pepper
Cumin
Dried oregano
Vanilla extract
All-purpose flour
Sesame seeds
Sesame oil
Canola oil

Harvest Beef Burrito

Makes: 6 servings   *Serving Size: 1 burrito*   *Prep Time: 15 minutes*

1 teaspoon olive oil
1 pound flank steak, sliced into
   1-inch pieces
1 tablespoon chili powder
1 teaspoon cayenne pepper
1 teaspoon cumin
4 cups broccoli florets
1 cup canned black beans,
   rinsed and drained
1/2 teaspoon salt
1 cup brown rice, cooked
6 10-inch flour tortillas

1. Heat oil in a large sauté pan and sear beef over high heat. Reduce heat to medium.

2. Add chili powder, cayenne pepper, cumin, broccoli, beans, and salt and cook 5 more minutes. Remove from heat. Add brown rice to mixture and mix well.

3. Place even amounts of meat and brown rice mixture in tortilla and wrap.

4. Repeat for remaining five tortillas.

> The ADA recommends eating only a small amount of saturated fat every day. This recipe is higher in saturated fat, so try to balance it by eating foods low in saturated fat at your other meals today.

Exchanges

4 Starch	2 Lean Meat

Calories 439
  Calories from Fat 110
Total Fat . . . . 12 g
  Saturated Fat . . . . 4 g
Cholesterol . . . . 36 mg
Sodium . . . . 636 mg
Total Carbohydrate . . . . . . 57 g
  Dietary Fiber . . . . 7 g
  Sugars . . . . 3 g
Protein . . . . 26 g

Dietitian's Tip: This dish can be made just as easily with chicken pieces, further reducing its fat content.

Lemon Chicken with Bell Peppers

Makes: 4 servings   *Serving Size: 1 chicken breast*   *Prep Time: 15 minutes*

4 4-ounce boneless, skinless chicken breasts
1 1/2 teaspoons dried oregano
1/2 teaspoon salt
1/4 teaspoon ground black pepper
1/4 teaspoon cayenne pepper
Cooking spray
1 1/2 cups red bell pepper strips
1 1/2 cups green bell pepper strips
1 tablespoon grated lemon rind
1/2 cup fresh lemon juice
1/2 cup fat-free, reduced-sodium chicken broth
1 tablespoon tomato paste

1. Season the chicken with oregano, salt, black pepper, and cayenne pepper.

2. Heat a large sauté pan coated with cooking spray over medium-high heat. Add chicken and sear on one side for 3 minutes or until lightly browned.

3. Turn chicken over; top with bell peppers, lemon rind, and juice.

4. Cover, reduce heat, and simmer 15 minutes or until chicken is done.

5. Combine broth and tomato paste in a small bowl. Stir tomato mixture into pan; bring to a boil. Serve pepper mixture with chicken. Serve over rice or noodles.

Exchanges

3 Very Lean Meat	1/2 Fat
1 Vegetable	

Calories 168
Calories from Fat 28
Total Fat . . . . 3 g
Saturated Fat . . . . 1 g
Cholesterol . . . . 68 mg
Sodium . . . . 423 mg
Total Carbohydrate . . . . 8 g
Dietary Fiber . . . . 2 g
Sugars . . . . 3 g
Protein . . . . 26 g

Chef's Tip: Be sure to grate only the yellow rind (the zest) of the lemon. The white part, or pith, is bitter.

Vegetable Quesadillas

Makes: 4 servings   *Serving Size: 1 quesadilla*   *Prep Time: 8 minutes*

Cooking spray
1 cup diced red bell pepper
1 cup diced green bell pepper
1/2 cup diced onion
2 small tomatoes, cut into
  6 slices
4 10-inch flour tortillas
3/4 cup shredded, reduced-fat
  mozzarella cheese
6 tablespoons fat-free sour
  cream
1 cup salsa

1. Spray a large nonstick skillet with cooking spray. Over medium-high heat, sauté red peppers, green peppers, and onion for about 4 minutes. Add tomatoes and sauté for 1 more minute.

2. Remove vegetables from pan. Spray pan again with cooking spray and add one tortilla to pan. Top tortilla with 3 tablespoons mozzarella cheese. Add 2/3 cup veggie mixture over cheese. Fold tortilla in half. Grill about 2 minutes each side.

3. Top quesadilla with 2 tablespoons sour cream and 1/4 cup salsa.

4. Repeat procedure for remaining three quesadillas.

Exchanges

3 Starch	2 Vegetable
1 Fat	

Calories 347
  Calories from Fat 76
Total Fat . . . . 8 g
  Saturated Fat . . . . 3 g
Cholesterol . . . . 13 mg
Sodium . . . . 686 mg
Total Carbohydrate . . . . . . 54 g
  Dietary Fiber . . . . 5 g
  Sugars . . . . 9 g
Protein . . . . 15 g

Chef's Tip: Feel free to experiment with this dish by adding more of your favorite vegetables.

Fruit with Dip

Makes: 10 servings   *Serving Size: 1/10 recipe*   *Prep Time: 15 minutes*

DIP

1 cup sugar-free vanilla pudding

4 ounces light whipped topping

1 teaspoon vanilla extract

FRUIT

1 cup cubed watermelon

1 cup cubed cantaloupe

1 cup cubed honeydew

1 cup strawberries, stems cut off

2 bananas, sliced

2 apples, sliced with skin on

1. In a medium bowl, combine dip ingredients and mix well.

2. Arrange fruit on a platter with dip bowl in middle. Provide toothpicks.

Exchanges
1 Fruit   1/2 Carbohydrate

Calories 103
  Calories from Fat 16
Total Fat . . . . 2 g
  Saturated Fat . . . . 1 g
Cholesterol . . . . 0 mg
Sodium . . . . 7 mg
Total Carbohydrate . . . . . . 20 g
  Dietary Fiber . . . . 2 g
  Sugars . . . . 13 g
Protein . . . . 2 g

Chef's Tip: This is a wonderful dish to serve at a picnic. It looks beautiful on a platter, and the dip tastes so great it's hard to believe it's low-fat.

Sesame-Crusted Salmon

Makes: 4 servings　　　*Serving Size: 1 filet*　　　*Prep Time: 10 minutes*

1/4 cup all-purpose flour
1/4 cup sesame seeds
1/2 teaspoon salt
1/4 teaspoon ground black pepper
4 4-ounce salmon filets
1 teaspoon sesame oil
　Cooking spray
2 teaspoons canola oil

1. In a medium bowl, combine flour, sesame seeds, salt, and pepper. Brush one side of each filet with sesame oil. Press oiled side of fish into sesame mixture.

2. Coat a medium nonstick skillet with cooking spray. Heat canola oil over medium-high heat. Place salmon filets crust side down into the hot pan.

3. Cook on both sides for 3–4 minutes.

Exchanges

3 Lean Meat　　1/2 Carbohydrate
1 1/2 Fat

Calories 282
　Calories from Fat 149
Total Fat . . . . 17 g
　Saturated Fat . . . . 3 g
Cholesterol . . . . 77 mg
Sodium . . . . 280 mg
Total Carbohydrate . . . . . . 6 g
　Dietary Fiber . . . . 1 g
　Sugars . . . . 1 g
Protein . . . . 26 g

See photo insert.

Chef's Tip: This recipe is also good with tuna or halibut.

Stir-Fried Vegetables

Makes: 4 servings   *Serving Size: 1/4 recipe*   *Prep Time: 10 minutes*

Cooking spray
1 teaspoon sesame oil
3 cups broccoli florets
2 cups pea pods
2 medium carrots, sliced into thin sticks
2 tablespoons lite soy sauce

1. Coat a large nonstick skillet with cooking spray and heat oil over medium heat. Add the broccoli, pea pods, and carrots. Stir-fry for 6–7 minutes.

2. Drizzle soy sauce over vegetables and continue to stir-fry for 1 more minute.

Exchanges

2 Vegetable

Calories 58
  Calories from Fat 13
Total Fat . . . . 1 g
  Saturated Fat . . . . 0 g
Cholesterol . . . . 0 mg
Sodium . . . . 332 mg
Total Carbohydrate . . . . . . 10 g
  Dietary Fiber . . . . 4 g
  Sugars . . . . 5 g
Protein . . . . 3 g

Dietitian's Tip: You can make a meal out of these vegetables by adding chicken or beef and serving them over rice.

Egg Salad Sandwich

Makes: 4 servings   *Serving Size: 1 sandwich*   *Prep Time: 5 minutes*

5 hard-boiled eggs, peeled and mashed

8 ounces silken firm tofu, patted dry

1 tablespoon Dijon mustard

2 tablespoons light mayonnaise

1/4 teaspoon salt

1/4 teaspoon ground black pepper

8 slices whole-wheat bread

1. In a medium bowl, combine all ingredients except bread and mix well.

2. Spoon 1/2 cup egg salad onto 1 slice whole-wheat bread and top with slice of whole-wheat bread.

3. Repeat for remaining three sandwiches.

Exchanges

2 Starch   2 Medium-Fat Meat

Calories 293
  Calories from Fat 116
Total Fat . . . . 13 g
  Saturated Fat . . . . 4 g
Cholesterol . . . . 269 mg
Sodium . . . . 689 mg
Total Carbohydrate . . . . . . 29 g
  Dietary Fiber . . . . 4 g
  Sugars . . . . 5 g
Protein . . . . 18 g

Chef's Tip: This a great recipe to try if you've never eaten tofu. The consistency of tofu is similar to that of hard-boiled egg whites. Tofu picks up the flavor of foods it's mixed with—you'll barely know it's there.

June ❖ Week 4

RECIPE LIST

DAY 1: Shrimp Skewers with Pineapple and
Peppers **208**
Green Bean Tomato Salad **209**

DAY 2: Stir-Fried Beef and Noodles **210**

DAY 3: Pork Tenderloin with Black Bean
and Corn Salsa **211**

DAY 4: Chicken Guacamole Salad **212**

DAY 5: Angel Hair Pasta with Tomato
Cream Sauce **213**
Caprese Salad **214**

DESSERT OF THE MONTH: Banana Split
Cake **215**

GROCERY LIST

Fresh Produce
Green bell peppers – 3
Cherry tomatoes –
1 container
Tomatoes – 6
Avocado – 1 large
Onion – 1
Red onion – 1
Fresh cilantro – 1 bunch
Garlic – 1 head
Fresh basil – 1 bunch
Bananas – 4 medium

Meat/Poultry/Fish
Unpeeled shrimp –
1 pound
Flank steak – 1 pound
Pork tenderloin – 1 pound
Boneless, skinless chicken
breasts – 1 pound

Grains/Bread/Pasta
Chow mein noodles –
1 package
Angel hair pasta – 1 box

Graham crackers – 1 small
box

Dairy and Cheese
Fat-free sour cream –
1 container
Grated Parmesan cheese
Fat-free half-and-half –
1 pint
Fresh mozzarella –
3 ounces
Fat-free milk
8-ounce package light
cream cheese – 1 package

Canned Goods and Sauces
14.5-ounce can fat-free,
reduced-sodium
chicken broth – 2 cans
15-ounce can black
beans – 1 can
14.5-ounce can tomato
purée – 1 can
10-ounce can crushed
pineapple packed in
juice – 1 can

Pineapple chunks packed
in juice – 1 can
Fat-free Italian dressing
–1 bottle
Dijon mustard – 1 jar
Lite soy sauce – 1 bottle

Frozen Foods
16-ounce bag cut green
beans – 1 bag
Corn – 1 bag
8-ounce container light
whipped topping –
1 container

Staples/Seasonings/ Baking Needs
Salt/ground black pepper
Apple cider vinegar
Dried basil
Sugar
Canola oil
Dried thyme
Dried sage
Dried tarragon
Dry mustard
Hot pepper sauce
Olive oil
Balsamic vinegar
1-ounce package sugar-
free instant vanilla pud-
ding mix – 1 package

Miscellaneous
White wine
Slivered almonds – small
bag
Pecans, chopped – small
bag
Creamy peanut butter –
small container
Bamboo skewers

207

Shrimp Skewers with Pineapple and Peppers

Makes: 5 servings   *Serving Size: 2 skewers*   *Prep Time: 10 minutes*

1 pound shrimp, peeled and deveined

1 16-ounce can pineapple chunks packed in juice, drained (reserve 1/4 cup juice)

3 green bell peppers, cut into 1-inch chunks

3 tablespoons fat-free Italian dressing

10 bamboo skewers, soaked in warm water

1. Prepare an indoor or outdoor grill.

2. Assemble skewers by alternating shrimp, pineapple, and green peppers on each skewer.

3. In a small bowl, whisk together reserved 1/4 cup pineapple juice and Italian dressing.

4. Brush all sides of shrimp skewers with dressing. Sprinkle with salt and pepper. Grill over medium heat for 5 minutes, turning occasionally.

Exchanges

1 Very Lean Meat   1 Fruit
1 Vegetable

Calories	124
Calories from Fat	8
Total Fat	1 g
Saturated Fat	0 g
Cholesterol	117 mg
Sodium	230 mg
Total Carbohydrate	16 g
Dietary Fiber	2 g
Sugars	13 g
Protein	14 g

Chef's Tip: Make this dish even more beautiful by using different colored bell peppers, such as red, yellow, and orange.

Green Bean Tomato Salad

Makes: 7 servings   *Serving Size: 1/7 recipe*   *Prep Time: 20 minutes*

16 ounces frozen cut green beans

2 tablespoons olive oil

1/4 cup apple cider vinegar

1/2 teaspoon salt

2 teaspoons sugar

1/8 teaspoon dried basil

1 teaspoon Dijon mustard

3 tablespoons slivered almonds, toasted

2 cups cherry tomatoes, halved

1. Cook green beans according to package directions.

2. In a salad bowl, whisk together olive oil, vinegar, salt, sugar, basil, and mustard. Add green beans, almonds, and tomatoes and toss well.

3. Serve warm or cover and chill 30 minutes.

Exchanges

2 Vegetable   1 Fat

Calories 86
Calories from Fat 53
Total Fat . . . . 6 g
Saturated Fat . . . . 1 g
Cholesterol . . . . 0 mg
Sodium . . . . 193 mg
Total Carbohydrate . . . . 8 g
Dietary Fiber . . . . 3 g
Sugars . . . . 4 g
Protein . . . . 2 g

Chef's Tip: You can use fresh green beans in this salad if you wish.

Stir-Fried Beef and Noodles

Makes: 6 servings   *Serving Size: 1/6 recipe*   *Prep Time: 15 minutes*

8 ounces uncooked chow mein noodles

2 tablespoons creamy peanut butter

1/4 cup canned fat-free, reduced-sodium chicken broth

1 tablespoon lite soy sauce

1/4 teaspoon hot pepper sauce

2 teaspoons canola oil

1 pound flank steak, sliced into thin strips against the grain

1. Cook chow mein noodles according to directions.

2. In a small bowl, whisk together peanut butter, chicken broth, soy sauce, and hot pepper sauce. Set aside.

3. Add oil to a medium sauté pan over high heat. Add beef strips and stir-fry for 4 minutes. Add peanut sauce to meat and stir-fry 2 more minutes.

4. Drain noodles and toss with the beef.

Exchanges

2 Starch	1/2 Fat
2 Lean Meat	

Calories 291
Calories from Fat 93
Total Fat . . . . 10 g
Saturated Fat . . . . 3 g
Cholesterol . . . . 36 mg
Sodium . . . . 424 mg
Total Carbohydrate . . . . . . 27 g
Dietary Fiber . . . . 2 g
Sugars . . . . 1 g
Protein . . . . 21 g

Chef's Tip: Peanut butter is the secret ingredient in this recipe. It adds flavor, richness, and creaminess to the sauce.

Pork Tenderloin with Black Bean and Corn Salsa

Makes: 4 servings   *Serving Size: 4 ounces*   *Prep Time: 10 minutes*

1 cup canned black beans, drained and rinsed

1 cup frozen corn, thawed

1 cup diced tomato

1/2 cup chopped red onion

1 tablespoon dried thyme

1 tablespoon dried sage

1 tablespoon dried tarragon

2 teaspoons dry mustard

1/4 teaspoon salt

1/4 teaspoon ground black pepper

1 pound pork tenderloin, trimmed of fat

1. Preheat oven to 350 degrees. In a small bowl, toss together beans, corn, tomatoes, and onion.

2. Combine thyme, sage, tarragon, mustard, salt, and pepper in a small bowl and transfer onto a plate, spreading evenly.

3. Roll pork tenderloin in mixture and coat well.

4. Bake for 30 minutes or until juices run clear. Serve pork sliced with salsa.

Exchanges

1 1/2 Starch	1/2 Fat
3 Very Lean Meat	

Calories	241
Calories from Fat	45
Total Fat	5 g
Saturated Fat	2 g
Cholesterol	65 mg
Sodium	184 mg
Total Carbohydrate	21 g
Dietary Fiber	6 g
Sugars	3 g
Protein	29 g

Chef's Tip: This recipe is also great with beef tenderloin.

Chicken Guacamole Salad

Makes: 5 servings   *Serving Size: 1/5 recipe*   *Prep Time: 35 minutes*

1   14.5-ounce can fat-free, reduced-sodium chicken broth
1   can water
1   pound boneless, skinless chicken breasts
1   medium avocado, finely diced
1   small onion, finely diced (about 1/2 cup)
2   small tomatoes, diced
2   tablespoons chopped fresh cilantro
2   tablespoons fat-free sour cream
1/2   teaspoon salt
1/4   teaspoon ground black pepper

1. In a medium saucepan, bring chicken broth and 1 can water to a boil. Add chicken breasts and simmer over low heat for about 20 minutes.

2. Remove chicken and chop into small chunks. Cool in a medium bowl for 10 minutes. Add remaining ingredients and mix well.

3. Serve on toasted whole-wheat tortillas or pitas.

✔ *National Prevention of Eye Injuries Awareness Week is the last week of June. Keep your eyes safe!*

Exchanges

3 Very Lean Meat	1 Fat
1 Carbohydrate	

Calories 178
  Calories from Fat 63
Total Fat . . . . 7 g
  Saturated Fat . . . . 1 g
Cholesterol . . . . 52 mg
Sodium . . . . 305 mg
Total Carbohydrate . . . . 7 g
  Dietary Fiber . . . . 3 g
  Sugars . . . . 3 g
Protein . . . . 22 g

Chef's Tip: You can use grilled steak strips instead of chicken in this recipe if you wish.

Angel Hair Pasta with Tomato Cream Sauce

Makes: 5 servings　　　*Serving Size: 1/5 recipe*　　　*Prep Time: 10 minutes*

8 ounces uncooked angel hair pasta
2 teaspoons olive oil
1 14.5-ounce can tomato purée
1 teaspoon dried basil
3 garlic cloves, minced
1/4 cup white wine
1 cup fat-free half-and-half
3 tablespoons grated Parmesan cheese

1. Cook pasta according to package directions, omitting salt.

2. Heat oil in a large nonstick skillet over medium heat. Add tomato purée, basil, garlic, and white wine. Bring to a boil. Reduce heat and simmer for 10 minutes.

3. In a small saucepan or in the microwave, heat half-and-half for 1 minute or until it simmers. Pour heated half-and-half into tomato sauce. Add Parmesan and stir constantly until cheese is incorporated.

4. Toss sauce with drained pasta.

Exchanges

2 1/2 Starch	1 Fat
1 Vegetable	

Calories	275
Calories from Fat	42
Total Fat	5 g
Saturated Fat	2 g
Cholesterol	8 mg
Sodium	160 mg
Total Carbohydrate	46 g
Dietary Fiber	3 g
Sugars	9 g
Protein	11 g

Dietitian's Tip: Lycopene, an antioxidant found in tomato products, may help protect you against cancer.

Caprese Salad

3 ounces fresh mozzarella
2 medium tomatoes, sliced into 8 slices
8 fresh basil leaves
1/4 teaspoon salt
1/8 teaspoon ground black pepper
1 tablespoon balsamic vinegar

1. Slice mozzarella into eight 1/4-inch-thick slices. Layer tomato, basil leaves, and cheese into stacks starting with tomato and ending with cheese (tomato, basil, cheese, tomato, basil, cheese), making 4 stacks.

2. Sprinkle each stack with salt and pepper. Drizzle balsamic vinegar lightly over each stack.

Exchanges

1 Medium-Fat Meat	1/2 Fat
1 Vegetable	

Calories 106
    Calories from Fat 44
Total Fat . . . . 5 g
    Saturated Fat . . . . 2 g
Cholesterol . . . . 17 mg
Sodium . . . . 167 mg
Total Carbohydrate . . . . 4 g
    Dietary Fiber . . . . 1 g
    Sugars . . . . 3 g
Protein . . . . 4 g

Chef's Tip: Fresh mozzarella cheese comes packed in water. You can usually find it in your grocer's deli or near the cheese aisle. Its texture is much different than the mozzarella you find on your pizza.

Veggie Lasagna Roulades, page 240;
Green Salad with Raspberry Vinaigrette, page 428

Veggie Pizza, page 48;
Chicken Fajita Pizza, page 150

Italian Sausage with Pepper Medley, page 389;
Spicy Sweet Potato Fries, page 158

Bleu Cheese-Crusted Steak, page 139;
Basil Mashed Potatoes, page 122;
Honey Tarragon Carrots, page 169

esame-Crusted Salmon,
age 204; Roasted Parmesan
ucchini, page 78

Mango Salsa Chicken over Rice, page 190; Broccoli Salad with Raisins, page 193

Veggie Chili, page 350;
Jalapeño Corn Muffins,
page 54

Tiramisu, page 287;
Raspberry Almond Layer
Cake, page 431;
Cherry Tarts, page 251

Banana Split Cake

Makes: 16 servings *Serving Size: 1 slice* *Prep Time: 15 minutes*

6 1/2 graham cracker sheets (two
1 1/2-inch squares per sheet)

1 ounce sugar-free, instant
vanilla pudding mix

2 cups fat-free milk

8 ounces light cream cheese

10 ounces canned crushed
pineapple packed in juice,
drained

4 medium bananas, sliced
8-ounce container light
whipped topping

3 tablespoons pecans,
chopped

1. Cover the bottom of a 9 × 13-inch pan with graham cracker sheets.

2. In a medium bowl, prepare pudding with 2 cups fat-free milk according to package directions. Add cream cheese to pudding and whip together. Spread pudding mixture over graham crackers.

3. Spread the crushed pineapple over the pudding layer and top with bananas, then whipped topping. Sprinkle pecans on top.

> The ADA recommends eating only a small amount of saturated fat every day. This recipe is higher in saturated fat, so try to balance it by eating foods low in saturated fat at your other meals today.

Exchanges

1 Fat	1 1/2 Carbohydrate

Calories 156
Calories from Fat 58
Total Fat . . . . 6 g
Saturated Fat . . . . 4 g
Cholesterol . . . . 11 mg
Sodium . . . . 194 mg
Total Carbohydrate . . . . . . 21 g
Dietary Fiber . . . . 1 g
Sugars . . . . 11 g
Protein . . . . 3 g

Chef's Tip: You can add sliced fresh strawberries on top of this cake if you like.

July

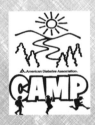

Kids and teenagers with diabetes
love diabetes camps, where they
can meet friends, have fun, and
learn something along the way!
To find a diabetes camp
sponsored by the ADA
near you, see the website
at www.diabetes.org.

Happy Birthday, America!

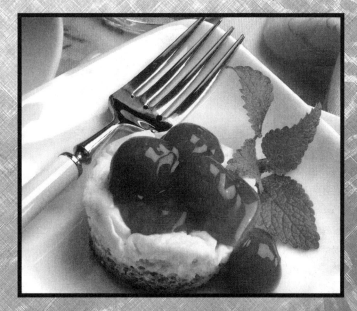

Cherry Tarts (page 251)
This month's festive dessert couldn't get much easier to
make. These tarts look beautiful and taste even better, with
a mixture of cream cheese, vanilla wafers, and cherries.

July ❖ Recipes

July ❖ Week 1

RECIPE LIST

DAY 1: Honey Lime Chicken **220**
Grilled Fruit **221**

DAY 2: Shrimp Salad **222**

DAY 3: Grilled Pizza **223**

DAY 4: Turkey Club **224**

DAY 5: Apple and Raisin-Stuffed Pork
Chops **225**
Grilled Tomatoes **226**

GROCERY LIST

Fresh Produce
Limes – 2
Garlic – 1 head
Strawberries – 1 pint
Mangoes – 2 small
Granny Smith apples – 4
Broccoli – 2 heads
Carrots – small bag
Romaine lettuce –
2 heads
Spinach – 1 bunch
Tomatoes – 5
Red onion – 1 small

Meat/Poultry/Fish
Boneless, skinless
chicken breasts – 4
(4-ounce) breasts
Cooked shrimp –
12 ounces

Thinly sliced deli turkey
breast – 12 ounces
Turkey bacon –
1 package
Center-cut pork chops –
4 (4-ounce) chops

Grains/Bread/Pasta
Prepackaged 12-inch
pizza crust
Whole-wheat bread –
8 slices

Dairy and Cheese
Feta cheese –
1 container

Canned Goods
and Sauces
16-ounce can pineapple
chunks in juice –
1 can
Lite soy sauce – small
bottle

Light mayonnaise – 1 jar
Dijon mustard – small
bottle
14.5-ounce can fat-free,
reduced-sodium
chicken broth – 1 can

Staples/Seasonings/
Baking Needs
Salt/ground black pepper
Cooking spray
Rice wine vinegar
Olive oil
Balsamic vinegar
Crushed red pepper
flakes
Canola oil
Apple cider vinegar or
brandy
Ground nutmeg
Ground cinnamon
Dried sage
Cayenne pepper
Hot pepper sauce
Honey

Miscellaneous
Bamboo skewers
Sun-dried tomatoes –
small package (not
packed in oil)
Orange juice – small
carton
Raisins – 1 small box

Honey Lime Chicken

Makes: 4 servings   *Serving Size: 1 chicken breast*   *Prep Time: 5 minutes*

1/3 cup lime juice
  3 tablespoons honey
  3 garlic cloves, minced
  1 tablespoon lite soy sauce
  4 4-ounce boneless, skinless
    chicken breasts

1. In a medium bowl, whisk together lime juice, honey, garlic, and soy sauce. Place chicken in bowl and marinate in the refrigerator for at least 20 minutes (or longer, if possible).

2. Prepare an indoor or outdoor grill. Remove chicken from marinade and cook over medium heat until done.

Exchanges

3 Very Lean Meat	1/2 Fat
1/2 Carbohydrate	

Calories	163
Calories from Fat	26
Total Fat	3 g
Saturated Fat	1 g
Cholesterol	68 mg
Sodium	138 mg
Total Carbohydrate	8 g
Dietary Fiber	0 g
Sugars	7 g
Protein	25 g

Chef's Tip: You can substitute lemon juice for lime juice if you prefer.

Grilled Fruit

Makes: 8 servings   *Serving Size: 1 skewer*   *Prep Time: 20 minutes*

1 pint strawberries, stemmed and halved

2 small mangoes, peeled and cut into 1-inch chunks
   16-ounce can pineapple chunks packed in juice, drained

2 Granny Smith apples, peeled, cored, and sliced into eighths

8 bamboo skewers, soaked in warm water

2 tablespoons honey

1. Prepare an indoor or outdoor grill.

2. Assemble kabobs by alternating strawberries, mango, pineapple, and apple on each skewer.

3. Brush all sides of kabobs with honey. Grill over medium heat for 6 minutes, turning occasionally.

Exchanges

2 Fruit

Calories 104
  Calories from Fat 4
Total Fat . . . . 0 g
  Saturated Fat . . . . 0 g
Cholesterol . . . . 0 mg
Sodium . . . . 2 mg
Total Carbohydrate . . . . . . 27 g
  Dietary Fiber . . . . 3 g
  Sugars. . . . . 24 g
Protein . . . . 1 g

Chef's Tip: Grilling fruit is a unique way to bring out its natural sweetness.

Shrimp Salad

| Makes: 6 servings | Serving Size: 2 cups | Prep Time: 15 minutes |

SALAD

12 ounces medium shrimp, peeled, deveined, and cooked (about 3 cups)
1/4 cup crumbled feta cheese
1/4 cup chopped sun-dried tomatoes
4 cups broccoli florets
1 1/2 cups carrots, sliced into rounds (about 3 medium carrots)
1 large head romaine lettuce, chopped

DRESSING

1/2 cup orange juice
2 tablespoons rice wine vinegar
2 tablespoons olive oil
1/2 teaspoon hot pepper sauce
1/4 teaspoon salt
1/4 teaspoon ground black pepper

1. In a large salad bowl, toss together all salad ingredients.

2. In a medium bowl, whisk together all dressing ingredients.

3. Drizzle dressing over salad and toss well to coat.

Exchanges

| 1 Lean Meat | 1 Fat |
| 2 Vegetable | |

Calories 146	
Calories from Fat 58	
Total Fat . . . . 6 g	
Saturated Fat . . . . 1 g	
Cholesterol . . . . 77 mg	
Sodium . . . . 266 mg	
Total Carbohydrate . . . . 11 g	
Dietary Fiber . . . . 3 g	
Sugars. 7 g	
Protein. . . . . 12 g	

Chef's Tip: This recipe has a lot of ingredients, but it's so easy to make!

Grilled Pizza

Makes: 4 servings   *Serving Size: 2 slices*   *Prep Time: 10 minutes*

SAUCE

1/4 cup balsamic vinegar
1 tablespoon Dijon mustard
1/2 tablespoon honey
1/4 teaspoon crushed red pepper flakes

TOPPING

1 teaspoon olive oil
1/4 cup chopped sun-dried tomatoes
4 cups chopped fresh spinach
2 garlic cloves, minced
1/4 teaspoon salt (optional)
1/4 teaspoon ground black pepper
1 12-inch prepackaged pizza crust
1/4 cup crumbled feta cheese

1. Prepare an indoor or outdoor grill and spray grill with cooking spray. In a small bowl, whisk together sauce ingredients.

2. Heat oil in a large nonstick skillet over medium-high heat. Add sun-dried tomatoes and cook for about 2 minutes. Add spinach and garlic and cook 2 more minutes.

3. Add sauce to pan and cook 3 minutes until sauce begins to reduce. Add salt and pepper.

4. Place pizza crust on top of grill. Spread spinach mixture on top of crust. Sprinkle with cheese and grill 5–7 minutes or until cheese begins to melt.

Exchanges

3 Starch	2 Fat
1 Vegetable	

Calories	368
Calories from Fat	110
Total Fat	12 g
Saturated Fat	3 g
Cholesterol	6 mg
Sodium	754 mg
Total Carbohydrate	53 g
Dietary Fiber	3 g
Sugars	8 g
Protein	13 g

Chef's Tip: Grilled pizza isn't your traditional pizza, but it's delicious, with a crispy crust and smoky flavor.

Turkey Club

Makes: 4 servings   *Serving Size: 1 club*   *Prep Time: 5 minutes*

4 teaspoons light mayonnaise

8 slices whole-wheat bread, toasted

12 ounces thinly sliced deli turkey breast

8 slices turkey bacon, cooked

4 romaine lettuce leaves, torn into pieces

1 tomato, sliced in 8 thin slices

1. Spread 1 teaspoon mayonnaise on 1 slice of whole-wheat bread. Top with 3 ounces turkey breast, 2 slices turkey bacon, 1 lettuce leaf, and 2 slices tomato. Place 1 slice whole-wheat bread on top of sandwich.

2. Repeat process for remaining three sandwiches.

Exchanges

2 Starch	3 Lean Meat

Calories 314
  Calories from Fat 104
Total Fat . . . . 12 g
  Saturated Fat . . . . 4 g
Cholesterol . . . . 62 mg
Sodium . . . . 1399 mg
Total Carbohydrate . . . . . . 28 g
  Dietary Fiber . . . . 4 g
  Sugars . . . . 3 g
Protein . . . . 28 g

Dietitian's Tip: If your meal plan calls for more meat, you can add some extra lean deli ham to this sandwich.

Apple and Raisin-Stuffed Pork Chops

Makes: 4 servings   *Serving Size: 1 pork chop*   *Prep Time: 20 minutes*

4	4-ounce center-cut pork chops
1	teaspoon canola oil
1/4	cup finely diced red onion
1/2	cup peeled, finely diced apple
2	tablespoons raisins
1/2	teaspoon minced garlic
1 1/2	tablespoons brandy or apple cider vinegar
1/4	cup fat-free, reduced-sodium chicken broth
1/4	teaspoon each nutmeg, cinnamon, sage, salt, and ground black pepper

1. Prepare an indoor or outdoor grill. Prepare pork chops by slicing a 2-inch pocket in the side of each chop and set aside.

2. In a large sauté pan, heat oil over medium-high heat. Add onions and cook until they are caramelized (brown in color but not burned, about 7 minutes). Add apples and raisins and cook until the apples become soft.

3. Add garlic and cook for 30 seconds. Add brandy (or vinegar), chicken broth, and spices; cook until all of the moisture is reduced. Set aside to cool slightly.

4. Use a small spoon and gently stuff pork chops with apple mixture. Use only one to two spoonfuls of stuffing and do not overstuff chops.

5. Grill chops over medium-high heat for about 5–8 minutes per side or until done.

Exchanges

3 Lean Meat   1/2 Carbohydrate

Calories 182	
Calories from Fat 64	
Total Fat . . . . 7 g	
Saturated Fat . . . . 2 g	
Cholesterol . . . . 59 mg	
Sodium . . . . 222 mg	
Total Carbohydrate . . . . 7 g	
Dietary Fiber . . . . 1 g	
Sugars . . . . 5 g	
Protein . . . . 21 g	

Chef's Tip: Take care not to overstuff the pork chops in this recipe. If you do, the stuffing will burst out during cooking and create quite a mess!

Grilled Tomatoes

Makes: 4 servings   *Serving Size: 1 tomato*   *Prep Time: 5 minutes*

4 medium tomatoes, sliced into
1/2-inch-thick slices

1 tablespoon olive oil

1/2 teaspoon salt

1/4 teaspoon ground black pepper

1/4 teaspoon cayenne pepper

1. Prepare an indoor or outdoor grill. Brush each side of each tomato slice lightly with olive oil.

2. Sprinkle salt, pepper, and cayenne pepper on one side of each slice.

3. Grill tomatoes over medium heat for 2 minutes on each side.

Exchanges

1 Vegetable   1 Fat

Calories 62
  Calories from Fat 35
Total Fat . . . . 4 g
  Saturated Fat . . . . 0 g
Cholesterol . . . . 0 mg
Sodium . . . . 304 mg
Total Carbohydrate . . . . . . 7 g
  Dietary Fiber . . . . 2 g
  Sugars . . . . 4 g
Protein . . . . 1 g

Chef's Tip: Here's a great way to use those extra tomatoes from the garden. Grilling vegetables adds a unique flavor.

July ❖ Week 2

RECIPE LIST

DAY 1: Tangy Tarragon Turkey Burgers **228**
Red Potato Salad **229**

DAY 2: Beef and Broccoli **230**

DAY 3: Taco Salad with Black Beans **231**

DAY 4: Tuna Salad with Pasta **232**

DAY 5: Orange-Glazed Pork Loin
Medallions **233**
Mediterranean Couscous **234**

GROCERY LIST

Fresh Produce
Oranges – 2
Garlic – 1 head
Red new potatoes –
3 pounds
Red onion – 1 large
Onion – 1
Celery – small bag
Fresh dill – 1 small
bunch
Broccoli – 2 heads
Romaine lettuce –
1 large head
Tomatoes – 2 large

Meat/Poultry/Fish
Lean ground turkey –
1 pound
Turkey bacon –
1 package
Boneless beef sirloin –
1 pound

90% lean ground beef –
1 pound
Pork tenderloin –
1 pound

Grains/Bread/Pasta
Baked tortilla chips
Elbow macaroni – 1 box
10-ounce box
couscous – 1 box

Dairy and Cheese
Eggs
Shredded, reduced-fat
sharp cheddar cheese –
1 bag
Fat-free sour cream –
1 container

Canned Goods
and Sauces
Light mayonnaise –
1 jar

Lite soy sauce – small
bottle
14.5-ounce can reduced-
sodium, fat-free beef
broth – 1 can
Salsa – 1 jar
16-ounce can black
beans – 1 can
12-ounce can tuna
packed in water –
1 can
Dijon mustard – small
bottle

Staples/Seasonings/
Baking Needs
Salt/ground black pepper
Cooking spray
Dried tarragon
Dried sage
Sugar
Cornstarch
Rice wine vinegar
Sesame oil
Canola oil
Dried red chilies –
1 small bag
Hot pepper sauce

Miscellaneous
Orange juice – small
carton
Golden raisins – small
box
Pine nuts – small bag

Tangy Tarragon Turkey Burgers

Makes: 4 servings   *Serving Size: 1 burger*   *Prep Time: 15 minutes*

1 pound lean ground turkey
2 tablespoons dried tarragon
1/4 cup orange juice
1 teaspoon orange zest
1/4 teaspoon salt
1/4 teaspoon ground black pepper
1 garlic clove, minced
1/2 tablespoon hot pepper sauce

1. Prepare an indoor or outdoor grill. Combine all ingredients in a bowl. Divide turkey into 4 equal portions, shaping each into a 1/2-inch-thick patty.

2. Place patties on grill rack; grill 7 minutes on each side or until done. (Or coat a large nonstick skillet with cooking spray and cook patties over medium heat for 3–4 minutes per side, or until juices run clear.)

Exchanges

3 Lean Meat   1/2 Fat

Calories 205
  Calories from Fat 98
Total Fat . . . . 11 g
  Saturated Fat . . . . 3 g
Cholesterol . . . . 84 mg
Sodium . . . . 238 mg
Total Carbohydrate . . . . 3 g
  Dietary Fiber . . . . 0 g
  Sugars . . . . 2 g
Protein . . . . 23 g

Dietitian's Tip: Turkey burgers are traditionally lower in fat compared to beef burgers. However, this does not compromise any flavor in this recipe—the combination of orange, tarragon, and turkey makes for a mouthwatering burger.

Red Potato Salad

Makes: 10 servings　　　*Serving Size: 1 cup*　　　*Prep Time: 30 minutes*

3 pounds red new potatoes, quartered
1 cup finely diced red onion
1/2 cup finely diced celery
8 slices turkey bacon, cooked and cut into 1-inch strips
5 hard-boiled egg whites, sliced
1/2 cup light mayonnaise
1/2 cup fat-free sour cream
1/2 teaspoon salt
1/4 teaspoon ground black pepper
2 tablespoons fresh dill

1. Place potatoes in a large saucepan; cover with water. Bring to a boil; cook 12 minutes or longer until tender. Drain; cool.

2. In a large bowl, mix together remaining ingredients. Add potatoes and toss gently.

Exchanges

2 Starch　　　　　　　　1 Fat

Calories	203
Calories from Fat	56
Total Fat	6 g
Saturated Fat	2 g
Cholesterol	13 mg
Sodium	401 mg
Total Carbohydrate	31 g
Dietary Fiber	3 g
Sugars	4 g
Protein	6 g

Dietitian's Tip: Here's a twist on traditional potato salad, with a lot less fat but a unique, great taste.

Beef and Broccoli

Makes: 6 servings   *Serving Size: 1/6 recipe*   *Prep Time: 15 minutes*

2 teaspoons lite soy sauce
1/4 teaspoon sugar
1/4 teaspoon salt
1 pound boneless beef sirloin, cut across the grain into 1/4-inch-thick slices
1 tablespoon cornstarch
1 tablespoon lite soy sauce
1 tablespoon rice wine vinegar
1/4 cup reduced-sodium, fat-free beef broth or water
1 teaspoon sugar
1 teaspoon sesame oil
2 teaspoons canola oil
    Cooking spray
1 garlic clove, minced
2 dried whole red chilies or 1/2 teaspoon crushed red pepper flakes
4 cups broccoli florets
1/4 cup water

1. In a small bowl, whisk together soy sauce, sugar, and salt. Add beef and marinate for 20 minutes in the refrigerator.

2. Meanwhile, dissolve cornstarch in soy sauce and vinegar in a small bowl. Whisk in broth, sugar, and sesame oil and set aside.

3. Heat vegetable oil and a generous amount of cooking spray in a large non-stick skillet or wok over high heat. Stir-fry beef for 2 minutes and remove from pan. Coat pan again with cooking spray and add garlic and whole chilies or red pepper flakes. Stir-fry for 30 seconds, then add broccoli and stir-fry 2 more minutes.

4. Add water and steam broccoli, covered, for 1 1/2–2 minutes, or until it is tender-crisp. Stir sauce and add it to pan along with beef and bring to a boil.

5. Reduce heat and simmer for 2 minutes, or until sauce is thickened and beef is heated through. Remove whole chilies before serving.

Exchanges

2 Lean Meat	1 Vegetable

Calories	138
Calories from Fat	52
Total Fat	6 g
Saturated Fat	1 g
Cholesterol	43 mg
Sodium	329 mg
Total Carbohydrate	5 g
Dietary Fiber	1 g
Sugars	2 g
Protein	16 g

Dietitian's Tip: In traditional recipes, fat provided a lot of the flavor. If you add bold flavors instead, such as the garlic and red chilies in this recipe, you can enjoy great taste without extra calories.

Taco Salad with Black Beans

Makes: 7 servings   *Serving Size: about 1 3/4 cups*   *Prep Time: 20 minutes*

1 pound 90% lean ground beef
1 1/2 cups salsa
5 cups chopped romaine lettuce
1 cup canned black beans, rinsed and drained
3/4 cup shredded, reduced-fat, sharp cheddar cheese
2 large tomatoes, chopped
1 1/2 cups crumbled baked tortilla chips

1. In a large nonstick skillet, brown ground beef over high heat. Add salsa and bring to a boil. Set aside.

2. In a large salad bowl, add lettuce. Place cooked beef on top of lettuce in center. Top with black beans, cheese, tomatoes, and tortilla chips.

 Did you know there are great diabetes camps for kids in your state? Children and teenagers can meet friends, have fun, and learn something new about diabetes. Go to www.diabetes.org to find one near you.

Exchanges

1 Starch	1 Vegetable
2 Lean Meat	1/2 Fat

Calories 224
Calories from Fat 78
Total Fat . . . . 9 g
Saturated Fat . . . . 4 g
Cholesterol . . . . 48 mg
Sodium . . . . 391 mg
Total Carbohydrate . . . . . . 20 g
Dietary Fiber . . . . 4 g
Sugars . . . . 4 g
Protein . . . . 20 g

Chef's Tip: This recipe is just as tasty made with ground turkey or diced chicken breast.

Tuna Salad with Pasta

Makes: 7 servings   *Serving Size: about 1 cup*   *Prep Time: 15 minutes*

8 ounces elbow macaroni, uncooked (2 cups)

1/2 cup chopped onion

1 cup chopped celery

1/2 cup fat-free sour cream

1/4 cup light mayonnaise

1 12-ounce can tuna packed in water, drained

1/4 teaspoon salt

1/4 teaspoon ground black pepper

1. Cook pasta according to package directions, omitting salt. Drain and rinse under cold water.

2. In a salad bowl, add all ingredients and toss well. Refrigerate before serving.

Exchanges

2 Starch	2 Very Lean Meat

Calories 221
  Calories from Fat 33
Total Fat . . . . 4 g
  Saturated Fat . . . . 1 g
Cholesterol . . . . 16 mg
Sodium . . . . 338 mg
Total Carbohydrate . . . . . . 29 g
  Dietary Fiber . . . . 1 g
  Sugars . . . . 3 g
Protein . . . . 16 g

Dietitian's Tip: Tuna is a lean protein source that is healthy and quick to prepare. Just make sure to purchase tuna packed in water rather than oil.

Orange-Glazed Pork Loin Medallions

Makes: 4 servings   *Serving Size: 4 ounces*   *Prep Time: 15 minutes*

GLAZE

1 1/2 cups orange juice

  2 tablespoons Dijon mustard

  4 tablespoons rice wine vinegar

1/2 teaspoon dried sage

1/2 teaspoon sugar

PORK

  1 pound pork tenderloin, sliced into 1/2-inch-thick medallions
Cooking spray

1/4 teaspoon salt

1/4 teaspoon ground black pepper

1. In a small bowl, whisk together glaze ingredients.

2. Season tenderloin well with salt and pepper. Coat a medium sauté pan with cooking spray. Sear pork medallions over high heat on both sides for about 2 minutes. Remove meat from pan.

3. Add glaze mixture to pan and let it reduce by half or until it becomes thicker (a glaze consistency). Add meat back to pan for 30 seconds, cooking the meat in glaze on both sides.

Exchanges

3 Very Lean Meat   1 Carbohydrate

Calories 189
Calories from Fat 41
Total Fat . . . . 5 g
Saturated Fat . . . . 1 g
Cholesterol . . . . 65 mg
Sodium . . . . 373 mg
Total Carbohydrate . . . . . . 12 g
Dietary Fiber . . . . 0 g
Sugars . . . . 11 g
Protein . . . . 25 g

Chef's Tip: It is best to sear meat in a sauté pan that is not nonstick. That way the meat will turn a deep golden brown.

Mediterranean Couscous

Makes: 8 servings   *Serving Size: 1/2 cup*   *Prep Time: 5 minutes*

1 10-ounce box couscous
1/2 cup golden raisins
2 tablespoons pine nuts
1/4 teaspoon salt
1/4 teaspoon ground black pepper

1. Cook couscous according to package directions, omitting oil or butter. Fluff the cooked couscous with a fork.

2. Gently fold in raisins, pine nuts, salt, and pepper.

3. Serve warm.

Exchanges
2 Starch	1/2 Fruit

Calories	173
Calories from Fat	14
Total Fat	2 g
Saturated Fat	0 g
Cholesterol	0 mg
Sodium	78 mg
Total Carbohydrate	35 g
Dietary Fiber	2 g
Sugars	7 g
Protein	5 g

Chef's Tip: This quick and easy side dish can be a great accompaniment to many meals.

July ❖ Week 3

GROCERY LIST

Fresh Produce
Red onions – 2 large
Onion – 1 large
Fresh basil – 1 bunch
Fresh oregano – 1 bunch
Fresh tarragon – 1 bunch
Green bell peppers –
3 medium
Red bell peppers –
3 medium
Yellow or orange bell
peppers – 2 medium
Garlic – 1 head
Lemon – 1
Button mushrooms – 1
pint
Zucchini – 1 medium
Tomatoes – 2
Pears – 2 medium
Mixed field greens –
1 bag

Meat/Poultry/Fish
Flank steak – 4
(4-ounce) steaks
Orange roughy filets –
4 (4-ounce) filets
Boneless, skinless
chicken breasts –
1 pound

Grains/Bread/Pasta
Orzo pasta – 1 box
Gemelli pasta – 1 box
1-pound box lasagna
noodles – 1 box

Dairy and Cheese
Goat cheese – 1 package
Fat-free half-and-half –
1 pint
Fat-free ricotta cheese –
1 container
Grated Parmesan cheese
Eggs
Margarine

Canned Goods and Sauces
14.5-ounce can fat-free,
reduced-sodium
chicken broth – 1 can
16-ounce jar marinara
pasta sauce – 1 jar
Fat-free Italian dressing
– 1 small bottle

Staples/Seasonings/ Baking Needs
Salt/ground black pepper
Cooking spray
Olive oil
Balsamic vinegar
Garlic salt
Cornstarch
Dried parsley
Brown sugar
Honey

Miscellaneous
White wine – small
bottle
Toothpicks
Bamboo skewers
Pecans – 1 small
package

Grilled Flank Steak with Onion Rings

Makes: 4 servings   *Serving Size: 1 steak*   *Prep Time: 5 minutes*

4 4-ounce flank steaks
1/2 teaspoon salt
1/4 teaspoon ground black pepper
2 large red onions, cut into
    1/2-inch-thick rings
1 tablespoon olive oil

1. Prepare an indoor or outdoor grill. Season both sides of steaks with salt and pepper. Set aside.

2. In a large bowl, toss onion rings with oil to coat.

3. Place steaks and onions on grill over medium-high heat. Grill steaks for 5 minutes on each side. Grill onions for 6–7 minutes on each side.

Exchanges

3 Lean Meat	1/2 Fat
2 Vegetable	

Calories. 241
  Calories from Fat. 106
Total Fat . . . . 12 g
  Saturated Fat . . . . 4 g
Cholesterol . . . . 54 mg
Sodium . . . . 359 mg
Total Carbohydrate. . . . . . 10 g
  Dietary Fiber . . . . 2 g
  Sugars. . . . . 7 g
Protein. . . . . 23 g

Chef's Tip: Be sure to slice flank steak against the grain for maximum tenderness.

Orzo Salad

Makes: 4 servings   *Serving Size: 1/2 cup*   *Prep Time: 5 minutes*

2 cups cooked orzo pasta

1/4 cup fat-free, reduced-sodium chicken broth

1 tablespoon chopped fresh basil

1 tablespoon chopped fresh oregano

1 tablespoon chopped fresh tarragon

1/4 teaspoon salt

1/4 teaspoon ground black pepper

1. Toss all ingredients in a large bowl.

2. Refrigerate and serve cold.

Exchanges

1 1/2 Starch

Calories	108
Calories from Fat	5
Total Fat	1 g
Saturated Fat	0 g
Cholesterol	0 mg
Sodium	178 mg
Total Carbohydrate	22 g
Dietary Fiber	1 g
Sugars	3 g
Protein	4 g

Dietitian's Tip: Fresh herbs are a great way to add flavor to foods without adding extra fat or sodium. You may want to test your green thumb by growing your own small herb garden—it's easier than you may think!

Three-Pepper Pasta Salad with Goat Cheese

Makes: 10 servings　　　*Serving Size: 1 cup*　　　*Prep Time: 15 minutes*

DRESSING

1/2 cup balsamic vinegar
 2 tablespoons olive oil
1/2 teaspoon garlic salt
1/4 teaspoon ground black pepper
 2 tablespoons honey

SALAD

16 ounces gemelli pasta, uncooked
 2 medium green bell peppers, finely diced
 2 medium yellow or orange bell peppers, finely diced
 2 medium red bell peppers, finely diced
1/4 cup crumbled goat cheese
 2 tablespoons chopped fresh basil

1. In a small bowl, whisk together dressing ingredients.

2. Cook pasta according to package directions, omitting salt. Drain and rinse under cold water.

3. In a large salad bowl, toss cooled pasta with remaining salad ingredients. Drizzle dressing over pasta and toss to coat.

Exchanges

2 1/2 Starch	1/2 Fat
1 Vegetable	

Calories 246
　Calories from Fat 38
Total Fat . . . . 4 g
　Saturated Fat . . . . 1 g
Cholesterol . . . . 3 mg
Sodium . . . . 83 mg
Total Carbohydrate . . . . . . 46 g
　Dietary Fiber . . . . 3 g
　Sugars . . . . 8 g
Protein . . . . 7 g

Dietitian's Tip: Goat cheese is a fat source in this recipe, but you only need to use a small amount for a lot of flavor. If you don't like goat cheese, try substituting feta or Parmesan.

Orange Roughy with Citrus Cream Sauce

Makes: 4 servings   *Serving Size: 1 filet*   *Prep Time: 10 minutes*

Cooking spray
4 4-ounce orange roughy filets
1/4 teaspoon salt
1/4 teaspoon ground black pepper
1 pint fat-free half-and-half
2 tablespoons cornstarch
1 teaspoon olive oil plus
cooking spray
2 garlic cloves, minced
1/4 cup white wine
1/4 cup lemon juice (juice of
1 lemon)
1 tablespoon lemon zest
1/4 cup crumbled goat cheese

1. Preheat oven to 350 degrees. Coat a shallow baking dish with cooking spray. Season both sides of each orange roughy filet with salt and pepper.

2. Place filets in baking dish and bake for 15 minutes or until fish flakes with a fork.

3. Meanwhile, in a medium bowl, whisk together half-and-half and cornstarch to make a slurry. Set aside.

4. Heat oil and cooking spray in a medium nonstick skillet over medium-high heat. Sauté garlic for 30 seconds. Add wine, lemon juice, and lemon zest and let it reduce by half. Add slurry and bring to a boil. Reduce heat and simmer for 3 minutes.

5. Pour 1/4 cup sauce over each filet and top with 1 tablespoon goat cheese.

Exchanges

3 Very Lean Meat	1 Fat
1 Carbohydrate	

Calories	215
Calories from Fat	46
Total Fat	5 g
Saturated Fat	2 g
Cholesterol	38 mg
Sodium	429 mg
Total Carbohydrate	17 g
Dietary Fiber	0 g
Sugars	7 g
Protein	21 g

Dietitian's Tip: This fish is great served with a green vegetable, such as asparagus, broccoli, or Brussels sprouts.

Veggie Lasagna Roulades

Makes: 8 servings   *Serving Size: 2 roulades*   *Prep Time: 40 minutes*

1 pound lasagna noodles
  (16 noodles)
1 cup fat-free ricotta cheese
1/4 cup grated Parmesan cheese
1 tablespoon dried parsley
1 egg
  Cooking spray
1 cup mushrooms, finely diced
1 medium zucchini, finely diced
2 tomatoes, seeded and finely diced
3 garlic cloves, minced
1/4 teaspoon salt
1/4 teaspoon ground black pepper
1 16-ounce jar marinara pasta sauce

1. Preheat oven to 350 degrees. Cook lasagna noodles according to package directions, omitting salt. Drain. Lay out noodles on wax paper.

2. In a medium bowl, mix ricotta, Parmesan cheese, parsley, and egg. Set aside.

3. Coat a large nonstick skillet with cooking spray. Sauté mushrooms, zucchini, tomato, and garlic over high heat for 5–7 minutes. Remove from heat and let cool.

4. Fold vegetables into cheese mixture. Add salt and pepper. Heap 2 tablespoons cheese mixture at the end of each noodle.

5. Starting at the cheese mixture end, roll noodle to the other end. Secure with a toothpick. Repeat for remaining noodles.

6. Coat baking dish with cooking spray. Place roulades side by side in the dish. Pour sauce over roulades and bake for 20 minutes.

Exchanges

2 Starch   2 Vegetable
1 Lean Meat

Calories	254
Calories from Fat	25
Total Fat	3 g
Saturated Fat	1 g
Cholesterol	40 mg
Sodium	339 mg
Total Carbohydrate	44 g
Dietary Fiber	4 g
Sugars	9 g
Protein	14 g

See photo insert.

Chef's Tip: This recipe is a fun twist on regular lasagna.

Chicken Kabobs

Makes: 4 servings   *Serving Size: 2 skewers*   *Prep Time: 20 minutes*

1 pint button mushrooms

1 large onion, sliced into 1-inch chunks

1 red bell pepper, sliced into 1-inch chunks

1 green bell pepper, sliced into 1-inch chunks

1 pound boneless, skinless chicken breasts, cut into 1-inch cubes

8 bamboo skewers, soaked in warm water

1/2 cup fat-free Italian dressing

1. Prepare an indoor or outdoor grill.

2. Assemble kabobs by alternating mushrooms, onions, peppers, and chicken cubes on each skewer (making 8 skewers).

3. Brush all sides of kabobs with Italian dressing. Grill over medium heat for 10 minutes, turning occasionally.

Exchanges

3 Very Lean Meat	1/2 Fat
3 Vegetable	

Calories 200
  Calories from Fat 29
Total Fat . . . . 3 g
  Saturated Fat . . . . 1 g
Cholesterol . . . . 68 mg
Sodium . . . . 375 mg
Total Carbohydrate . . . . . . 15 g
  Dietary Fiber . . . . 3 g
  Sugars . . . . 9 g
Protein . . . . 27 g

Dietitian's Tip: Kabobs are a great way to work vegetables and protein into your meal plan. Serve over brown rice for a well-balanced meal.

Pear Pecan Salad

Makes: 8 servings   *Serving Size: 1/2 cup*   *Prep Time: 20 minutes*

2 teaspoons margarine
1 tablespoon brown sugar
1/4 cup chopped pecans
2 medium pears, diced
4 cups mixed field greens
2 tablespoons balsamic vinegar
2 teaspoons olive oil
1 teaspoon honey

1. Preheat oven to 350 degrees. Combine margarine and brown sugar in a small bowl and microwave for 30 seconds to melt margarine. Add pecans and toss to coat.

2. Spread pecan mixture in a small baking dish and bake for 15 minutes. Remove from oven and set aside to cool.

3. In a large salad bowl, toss together pears and greens.

4. In a small bowl, whisk together remaining ingredients. Drizzle dressing over salad and toss to coat. Serve with 1/2 tablespoon pecan mixture sprinkled on top of each serving.

Exchanges

1/2 Fruit	1 Fat

Calories 85
 Calories from Fat 45
Total Fat . . . . 5 g
 Saturated Fat . . . . 1 g
Cholesterol . . . . 0 mg
Sodium . . . . 15 mg
Total Carbohydrate . . . . . . 11 g
 Dietary Fiber . . . . 2 g
 Sugars . . . . 9 g
Protein . . . . 1 g

Chef's Tip: Nuts can be a great addition to any salad, offering different texture and flavor—transforming any recipe into a truly unique dish.

July ❖ Week 4

RECIPE LIST

DAY 1: Salmon Packet with Asparagus **244**

DAY 2: Chicken Caesar Wrap **245**

DAY 3: Pecan Chicken Salad **246**

DAY 4: BBQ Pork Cutlets **247**
Marinated Grilled Veggies **248**

DAY 5: Onion Burger **249**
Oriental Coleslaw **250**

DESSERT OF THE MONTH: Cherry
Tarts **251**

GROCERY LIST

Fresh Produce
Asparagus – 1 pound
Romaine lettuce –
2 heads
Tomato – 1
Carrots – small bag
Red onion – 1 small
Green bell peppers –
2 medium
Red bell peppers –
2 medium
Zucchini – 2 medium
Yellow squash –
2 medium
Onion – 1 large
Cabbage – 1 head
Scallions – 1 bunch

Meat/Poultry/Fish
Salmon – 4 (4-ounce)
filets
Boneless, skinless
chicken breasts – 8
(4-ounce) breasts
Boneless pork cutlets –
4 (3-ounce) cutlets
90% lean ground beef –
1 pound

Grains/Bread/Pasta
10-inch flour tortillas – 4
Cornflakes – small box
Bread crumbs
Whole-wheat hamburger
buns – 5

Dairy and Cheese
Fresh Parmesan cheese –
1 wedge
Eggs
8-ounce package light
cream cheese –
1 package
Fat-free cream cheese –
1 small package
Fat-free sour cream –
1 container

Canned Goods and Sauces
Reduced-fat Caesar
dressing – small bottle
Reduced-fat Ranch
dressing – small bottle
BBQ sauce – small bottle
Fat-free Italian dressing
– small bottle
16-ounce can crushed
pineapple in juice –
1 can

Staples/Seasonings/ Baking Needs
Salt/ground black pepper
Cooking spray
Dried thyme
Balsamic vinegar
Garlic salt
Onion salt
All-purpose flour
Sugar
Rice wine vinegar
Canola oil
Sesame oil
Vanilla extract
21-ounce can light cherry
pie topping – 1 can

Miscellaneous
Aluminum foil
Pecans – small package
1-ounce package onion
soup mix – 1 package
3-ounce package ramen-
style noodle soup
mix – 1 package
Sesame seeds
Sliced almonds –
1 package
Paper baking (muffin)
cups
Reduced-fat vanilla
wafers – 1 box

Salmon Packet with Asparagus

Makes: 4 servings   *Serving Size: 1 packet*   *Prep Time: 10 minutes*

4 12 × 19-inch sheets aluminum foil
Cooking spray
1 pound fresh asparagus, ends trimmed
4 4-ounce salmon filets
4 teaspoons dried thyme
6 tablespoons grated fresh Parmesan cheese
1/4 cup balsamic vinegar

1. Prepare an indoor or outdoor grill. Spray aluminum foil with cooking spray.

2. Place 1/4 pound asparagus on each sheet of foil. Place salmon filet on top of asparagus. Sprinkle 1 teaspoon thyme, 1 1/2 tablespoons Parmesan cheese, and 1 tablespoon balsamic vinegar over salmon.

3. Bring up sides of foil. Double-fold top and ends to seal packet (leave a little room in the packet for air circulation). Repeat for remaining 3 packets.

4. Place packets in covered outdoor grill over medium-high heat and cook for 12–14 minutes until salmon flakes with a fork.

Exchanges

4 Lean Meat	1 Vegetable

Calories 252
 Calories from Fat 113
Total Fat . . . . 13 g
 Saturated Fat . . . . 3 g
Cholesterol . . . . 78 mg
Sodium . . . . 127 mg
Total Carbohydrate . . . . 6 g
 Dietary Fiber . . . . 1 g
 Sugars . . . . 3 g
Protein . . . . 29 g

Chef's Tip: These packets can also be baked in the oven. Place packets on a baking sheet and bake at 450 degrees for 18–20 minutes. Cooking vegetables and fish this way can't get any easier!

Chicken Caesar Wrap

Makes: 4 servings   *Serving Size: 1 wrap*   *Prep Time: 20 minutes*

4 4-ounce boneless, skinless chicken breasts
1/4 teaspoon ground black pepper
4 cups chopped romaine lettuce
1 tomato, seeded and finely diced
1/4 cup grated fresh Parmesan cheese
1/4 cup reduced-fat Caesar dressing
4 10-inch flour tortillas

1. Prepare an indoor or outdoor grill. Season chicken breasts with pepper. Grill chicken for 4–6 minutes per side.

2. Remove chicken from grill and chop into 1-inch pieces.

3. In a large bowl, toss together lettuce, tomato, Parmesan cheese, and chicken. Drizzle with Caesar dressing and toss to coat.

4. Place 1 1/2 cups chicken mixture into 1 tortilla and wrap.

5. Repeat procedure for 3 remaining wraps.

Exchanges
2 1/2 Starch   1 Vegetable
4 Lean Meat

Calories 436
 Calories from Fat 114
Total Fat . . . . 13 g
 Saturated Fat . . . . 4 g
Cholesterol . . . . 74 mg
Sodium . . . . 603 mg
Total Carbohydrate . . . . . . 44 g
 Dietary Fiber . . . . 3 g
 Sugars . . . . 4 g
Protein . . . . 35 g

Dietitian's Tip: You can use whole-wheat tortillas for these wraps to increase dietary fiber.

Pecan Chicken Salad

Makes: 5 servings *Serving Size: 1 cup salad plus 3–4 chicken strips* *Prep Time: 15 minutes*

Cooking spray
- 1 cup cornflake crumbs
- 1/2 cup chopped pecans
- 1/2 teaspoon garlic salt
- 1/2 teaspoon onion salt
- 1 egg
- 2 egg whites
- 2 tablespoons all-purpose flour
- 4 4-ounce boneless, skinless chicken breasts
- 6 cups chopped romaine lettuce
- 1 cup shredded carrots
- 1/2 cup finely diced red onion
- 1/4 cup reduced-fat Ranch dressing

1. Preheat oven to 350 degrees. Coat a shallow baking pan with cooking spray.

2. In a medium bowl, combine cornflake crumbs, pecans, garlic salt, and onion salt.

3. In a separate bowl, lightly beat egg and egg whites.

4. Place flour in a separate bowl.

5. Dip each side of chicken breast in flour, then egg mixture, then cornflake and pecan mixture.

6. Place chicken breasts in baking pan. Spray chicken lightly with cooking spray and bake 30–35 minutes, until juices run clear.

7. In a large salad bowl, toss together lettuce, carrots, onion, and dressing. Remove chicken from pan and slice into 1-inch-thick strips.

8. Place a heaping cup of salad mixture on a plate and arrange 3–4 chicken strips on top. Repeat for remaining 4 salads.

Exchanges

1 Starch	1 Vegetable
3 Very Lean Meat	2 Fat

Calories	302
Calories from Fat	114
Total Fat	13 g
Saturated Fat	2 g
Cholesterol	87 mg
Sodium	531 mg
Total Carbohydrate	21 g
Dietary Fiber	3 g
Sugars	6 g
Protein	26 g

Dietitian's Tip: To reduce the fat content of this recipe, use fat-free Ranch dressing.

BBQ Pork Cutlets

Makes: 4 servings   *Serving Size: 1 cutlet*   *Prep Time: 5 minutes*

4 3-ounce boneless pork cutlets
1/2 cup bottled barbecue sauce
1 cup canned, crushed pineapple
   with juice
1/4 teaspoon ground black pepper
   Cooking spray

1. Preheat oven to 350 degrees.

2. Place one cutlet between two sheets of plastic wrap and, using a meat tenderizer or rolling pin, pound the cutlet to 1/4-inch thickness. Repeat for remaining 3 cutlets. Set aside.

3. In a medium bowl, combine barbecue sauce, pineapple, and pepper.

4. Coat a large, shallow baking dish with cooking spray. Line the bottom of the dish with the pork cutlets and cover with barbecue sauce mixture.

5. Bake for 20 minutes or until pork is done.

Exchanges
2 Medium-Fat Meat
1 Carbohydrate

Calories	220
Calories from Fat	94
Total Fat	10 g
Saturated Fat	4 g
Cholesterol	56 mg
Sodium	293 mg
Total Carbohydrate	12 g
Dietary Fiber	1 g
Sugars	10 g
Protein	19 g

Chef's Tip: Ask your butcher to prepare fresh cutlets for you. He can even pound them out for you, saving prep time.

Marinated Grilled Veggies

Makes: 8 servings   *Serving Size: 1/8 recipe*   *Prep Time: 30 minutes*

2 green bell peppers, seeded and sliced in fourths

2 red bell peppers, seeded and sliced in fourths

2 medium zucchini, sliced into 1/4-inch-thick slices length-wise

2 medium yellow squash, sliced into 1/4-inch-thick slices lengthwise

1 large onion, sliced into 1/4-inch-thick rings

1/2 cup fat-free Italian dressing

1. Prepare an indoor or outdoor grill.

2. Toss together all ingredients in a large bowl and marinate in the refrigerator for 20 minutes.

3. Place vegetables on grill over medium heat. Grill for 4 minutes on all sides.

Exchanges
2 Vegetable

Calories 53
  Calories from Fat 3
Total Fat . . . . 0 g
  Saturated Fat . . . . 0 g
Cholesterol . . . . 0 mg
Sodium . . . . 121 mg
Total Carbohydrate . . . . . . 12 g
  Dietary Fiber . . . . 3 g
  Sugars . . . . 7 g
Protein . . . . 2 g

Dietitian's Tip: Don't be afraid to grill these or your other favorite vegetables . . . they are delicious!

Onion Burger

Makes: 5 servings   *Serving Size: 1 burger*   *Prep Time: 5 minutes*

1 pound 90% lean ground beef
1 1-ounce package onion
  soup mix
1 egg
1/4 cup bread crumbs
5 whole-wheat hamburger buns

1. Prepare an indoor or outdoor grill.

2. Combine beef, soup mix, egg, and bread crumbs in a medium bowl and mix well to incorporate. Divide mixture into 5 equal portions and shape into 1/2-inch-thick patties.

3. Place burgers on grill over medium-high heat and grill 7 minutes on each side or until well done (meat should not be pink on the inside).

4. Serve each burger on a whole-wheat bun.

Exchanges

2 Starch   3 Lean Meat

Calories 329
  Calories from Fat 107
Total Fat . . . . 12 g
  Saturated Fat . . . . 4 g
Cholesterol . . . . 99 mg
Sodium . . . . 897 mg
Total Carbohydrate . . . . . . 30 g
  Dietary Fiber . . . . 3 g
  Sugars . . . . 6 g
Protein . . . . 25 g

Dietitian's Tip: Summer wouldn't be complete without a great grilled burger! Try ground turkey in this recipe instead of beef.

Oriental Coleslaw

Makes: 7 servings   *Serving Size: 1 cup*   *Prep Time: 10 minutes*

4 cups shredded cabbage

1 cup shredded carrots

4 scallions, sliced

1 3-ounce package ramen-style noodle soup mix, uncooked and crushed

2 tablespoons sesame seeds

3 tablespoons sliced almonds, toasted

1 Flavor packet from noodle soup mix

1 tablespoon sugar

3 tablespoons rice wine vinegar

1 tablespoon canola oil

1 teaspoon sesame oil

1. In a large bowl, toss cabbage, carrots, scallions, and crushed noodles together.

2. In a large nonstick skillet, sauté the sesame seeds and almonds over low-medium heat for 2 minutes or until toasted; set aside.

3. In a small bowl, whisk together remaining ingredients. Pour dressing over the salad and toss to coat. Sprinkle sesame seeds and almonds over top of salad.

Exchanges

1/2 Starch	1 1/2 Fat
1 Vegetable	

Calories 146
  Calories from Fat 76
Total Fat . . . . 8 g
  Saturated Fat . . . . 1 g
Cholesterol . . . . 0 mg
Sodium . . . . 226 mg
Total Carbohydrate . . . . . . 16 g
  Dietary Fiber . . . . 2 g
  Sugars . . . . 5 g
Protein . . . . 3 g

Chef's Tip: Buy packaged shredded cabbage at the store to save time.

Cherry Tarts

Makes: 15 servings   *Serving Size: 1 tart*   *Prep Time: 10 minutes*

8 ounces light cream cheese
4 ounces fat-free cream cheese
1/2 cup fat-free sour cream
1 egg
2 egg whites
1 tablespoon vanilla extract
15 reduced-fat vanilla wafers
1 21-ounce can light cherry pie topping
15 paper baking cups

> The ADA recommends eating only a small amount of saturated fat every day. This recipe is higher in saturated fat, so try to balance it by eating foods low in saturated fat at your other meals today.

1. Preheat oven to 350 degrees. Combine cream cheeses, sour cream, egg, egg whites, and vanilla extract and beat until smooth.

2. Line muffin pan with paper baking cups and place one vanilla water in the bottom of each cup.

3. Fill each muffin cup with approximately 1/4 cup cream cheese mixture.

4. Place muffin pan in oven and bake 40–45 minutes or until lightly golden brown.

5. Let cool and top each tart with 1 tablespoon cherry pie filling.

Exchanges

1 Fat   1 Carbohydrate

Calories	106
Calories from Fat	37
Total Fat	4 g
Saturated Fat	2 g
Cholesterol	26 mg
Sodium	139 mg
Total Carbohydrate	13 g
Dietary Fiber	1 g
Sugars	10 g
Protein	4 g

See photo insert.

Chef's Tip: These easy tarts look great on a holiday buffet table.

August

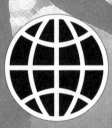

This month, try these easy and delicious recipes from different countries—without packing on vacation pounds! You'll add more variety to your meals, and discover that there are plenty of low-fat, healthy foods to enjoy from all over the world.

Embrace Ethnicity

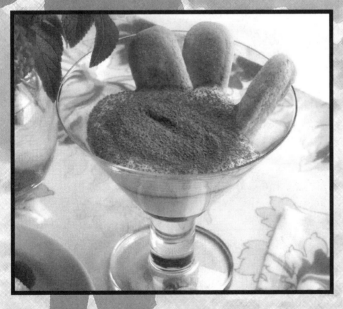

Tiramisu (page 287)
This version of the traditional Italian dessert is lighter,
but you can expect the same bold, rich flavors.

August ❖ Recipes

254

RECIPE LIST

DAY 1: Chicken Marsala **256**

DAY 2: Pork Chop Suey **257**
Fried Rice **258**

DAY 3: Crab Tostadas **259**

DAY 4: Curried Eggplant Couscous **260**

DAY 5: Spicy Szechwan Beef **261**
Spring Rolls **262**

GROCERY LIST

Fresh Produce
Mushrooms – 1 pint
Garlic – 1 head
Celery – small bag
Carrots – small bag
Scallions – 1 bunch
Lemon –1
Fresh cilantro – 1 bunch
Eggplant – 1
Sugar snap peas – 3 cups
Broccoli – 2 heads
Cucumbers – 2 medium
Bean sprouts – 1 cup
Napa (Chinese)
cabbage – 1 head
Avocado – 1 small

Meat/Poultry/Fish
Boneless, skinless
chicken breasts – 4
(4-ounce) breasts
Boneless pork chops –
1 pound
Imitation crabmeat –
1/2 pound
Beef tenderloin –
1 pound

Grains/Bread/Pasta
White rice
Corn tortillas – 5
10-ounce box
couscous – 1 box

Dairy and Cheese
Egg substitute – 1 carton
Fat-free sour cream –
1 container

Canned Goods
and Sauces
14.5-ounce can fat-free,
reduced-sodium
chicken broth – 5 cans
15-ounce can bean
sprouts – 1 can
8-ounce can water chest-
nuts – 1 can
Lite soy sauce – small
bottle
Salsa – 1 jar
8-ounce can bamboo
shoots – 2 cans
Light sugar-free apricot
preserves – 1 jar

Frozen Foods
10-ounce package peas –
1 package

Staples/Seasonings/
Baking Needs
Salt/ground black pepper
Cooking spray
All-purpose flour
Cornstarch
Rice wine vinegar
Sesame oil
Canola oil
Curry powder
Olive oil
Hot pepper sauce
Dried whole chilies –
1 package

Miscellaneous
Marsala wine – small
bottle
Golden raisins – small
box
Cashews – small
package
Rice paper spring roll
skins – 10

Chicken Marsala

Makes: 4 servings   *Serving Size: 1 chicken breast*   *Prep Time: 5 minutes*

Cooking spray

4 4-ounce boneless, skinless chicken breasts

4 cups sliced mushrooms

1 garlic clove, minced

1 tablespoon all-purpose flour

1/2 cup Marsala wine

1 14.5-ounce can fat-free, reduced-sodium chicken broth

1/4 teaspoon salt

1/4 teaspoon ground black pepper

1. Coat a large nonstick skillet with cooking spray. Over medium-high heat, sauté chicken breasts for 6 minutes on each side. Remove from pan and set aside.

2. Spray pan again with cooking spray and reduce heat to medium. Add mushrooms and garlic and sauté until all the liquid is evaporated. Add flour, stirring well to coat the mushrooms. Cook for 1 more minute. Add wine, stirring well to incorporate the flour. Add broth and turn heat to high. Let simmer for 5 minutes. Add salt and pepper.

3. Serve sauce over chicken breasts.

Exchanges

3 Very Lean Meat	1 Fat
1 Vegetable	

Calories 185
  Calories from Fat 29
Total Fat . . . . 3 g
  Saturated Fat . . . . 1 g
Cholesterol . . . . 68 mg
Sodium . . . . 459 mg
Total Carbohydrate . . . . 6 g
  Dietary Fiber . . . . 1 g
  Sugars . . . . 2 g
Protein . . . . 28 g

Chef's Tip: Serve over egg noodles, and save time by buying presliced mushrooms.

Pork Chop Suey

Makes: 4 servings   *Serving Size: 1 cup*   *Prep Time: 10 minutes*

Cooking spray

1 pound boneless pork chops, cut into 1-inch strips

2 stalks celery, thinly sliced

1 cup canned bean sprouts, rinsed and drained

1 cup canned water chestnuts, rinsed, drained, and sliced

1 14.5-ounce can fat-free, reduced-sodium chicken broth

1 tablespoon cornstarch

2 tablespoons lite soy sauce

1. Coat a large nonstick skillet or wok with cooking spray and stir-fry pork over high heat for 4 minutes. Remove pork from pan.

2. Spray pan again with cooking spray and reduce heat to medium. Stir-fry the celery, bean sprouts, and water chestnuts for about 5 minutes. Add pork back to pan.

3. In a small bowl, whisk together chicken broth and cornstarch. Pour over pork and vegetables in the pan and bring to a boil. Add soy sauce, reduce heat, and simmer for 3 minutes.

Exchanges

3 Lean Meat   1 Vegetable

Calories 201
  Calories from Fat 62
Total Fat . . . . 7 g
  Saturated Fat . . . . 3 g
Cholesterol . . . . 68 mg
Sodium . . . . 632 mg
Total Carbohydrate . . . . 7 g
  Dietary Fiber . . . . 1 g
  Sugars . . . . 2 g
Protein . . . . 26 g

Chef's Tip: You can use chicken breasts instead of pork in this recipe.

Fried Rice

Makes: 8 servings   *Serving Size: 1/2 cup*   *Prep Time: 10 minutes*

4 cups cooked white rice, chilled

2 tablespoons fat-free, reduced-sodium chicken broth

2 tablespoons rice wine vinegar

1 tablespoon lite soy sauce

1/2 teaspoon salt

1 teaspoon sesame oil

1/4 teaspoon ground black pepper
Cooking spray

1 tablespoon canola oil

1 cup egg substitute

1 bunch scallions, finely chopped (about 1 cup)

1 10-ounce package frozen peas, thawed

1. Spread rice in a shallow baking pan and separate grains with a fork.

2. In a small bowl, whisk together broth, vinegar, soy sauce, salt, sesame oil, and black pepper. Set aside.

3. Coat a large nonstick skillet or wok with cooking spray and heat canola oil over moderately high heat until hot. Stir-fry egg substitute until scrambled, about 30 seconds. Add scallions and stir-fry 1 minute.

4. Add peas and stir-fry until heated through. Add rice and stir-fry, stirring frequently, 2–3 minutes, or until heated through.

5. Stir liquid and add to fried rice, tossing to coat evenly.

Exchanges
2 Starch

Calories	168
Calories from Fat	23
Total Fat	3 g
Saturated Fat	0 g
Cholesterol	0 mg
Sodium	316 mg
Total Carbohydrate	29 g
Dietary Fiber	2 g
Sugars	3 g
Protein	7 g

Dietitian's Tip: This version of a classic favorite contains a lot less fat, but is just as delicious.

Crab Tostadas

Makes: 5 servings   *Serving Size: 1 tostada*   *Prep Time: 5 minutes*

5 corn tortillas

1 avocado, mashed

1/2 pound shredded imitation
    crabmeat

1 tablespoon lemon juice

1 tablespoon sliced scallions

1 teaspoon chopped cilantro

2 tablespoons fat-free sour
    cream

3 tablespoons salsa

1. Preheat oven to 400 degrees. Place corn tortillas on a baking sheet and bake for 5 minutes or until crisp.

2. In a medium bowl, combine remaining ingredients and mix well.

3. Spoon crab mixture on tortillas.

Exchanges

1 Starch	1/2 Carbohydrate
1 Very Lean Meat	1/2 Fat

Calories 166
    Calories from Fat 61
Total Fat . . . . 7 g
    Saturated Fat . . . . 1 g
Cholesterol . . . . 10 mg
Sodium . . . . 456 mg
Total Carbohydrate . . . . . . 20 g
    Dietary Fiber . . . . 3 g
    Sugars . . . . 6 g
Protein . . . . 8 g

Chef's Tip: Avocados are easy to ripen. Put them in a paper bag with an apple for 2–3 days at room temperature. When they turn dark purple or black and are soft to the touch, they're ready to eat! Garnish these tasty tostadas with shredded lettuce, chopped tomatoes, and a touch of hot salsa for an extra kick.

Curried Eggplant Couscous

Makes: 5 servings   *Serving Size: 1 cup*   *Prep Time: 5 minutes*

2 cups fat-free, reduced-sodium chicken broth, divided

1 cup uncooked couscous

1/2 teaspoon salt

1/4 teaspoon ground black pepper

2 tablespoons all-purpose flour

1 tablespoon curry powder

1 eggplant, cubed (about 4 cups)

2 teaspoons olive oil

1 cup shredded carrots

1/2 cup golden raisins

1. In a medium saucepan, bring 1 1/4 cups chicken broth to a boil; reserve remaining 3/4 cup. Add 1 cup uncooked couscous. Cover and remove from heat. Let stand for 5 minutes and fluff with fork.

2. In a large mixing bowl, combine salt, pepper, flour, and curry powder. Add eggplant and toss to coat.

3. Add oil to a large nonstick skillet over medium-high heat. Add eggplant and stir-fry for 5 minutes. Add remaining 3/4 cup chicken broth and stir well to incorporate the flour. Add carrots and raisins and cook 1 more minute. Stir in couscous and mix well.

Exchanges

2 Starch	1 Fruit
1 Vegetable	

Calories 236
 Calories from Fat 22
Total Fat . . . . 2 g
 Saturated Fat . . . . 0 g
Cholesterol . . . . 0 mg
Sodium . . . . 447 mg
Total Carbohydrate . . . . . . 48 g
 Dietary Fiber . . . . 5 g
 Sugars . . . . 14 g
Protein . . . . 7 g

Chef's Tip: This recipe is a great example of marrying different flavors—spicy curry, sweet raisins, and creamy eggplant—into a great palate-pleaser.

Spicy Szechwan Beef

Makes: 6 servings   *Serving Size: 1/6 recipe*   *Prep Time: 10 minutes*

Cooking spray
1 teaspoon sesame oil
1 pound beef tenderloin, sliced into 1-inch strips
1/4 cup cashews
3 cups sugar snap peas
4 cups broccoli florets (about 2 heads)
1 cup canned bamboo shoots, rinsed and drained
2 scallions, thinly sliced
1 14.5-ounce can fat-free, reduced-sodium chicken broth
3 tablespoons lite soy sauce
2 teaspoons hot pepper sauce
1 tablespoon cornstarch
3 dried whole red chilies

1. Coat a large nonstick skillet with cooking spray and heat oil over medium-high heat. Add beef and stir-fry for 3 minutes. Remove beef from pan.

2. Spray pan again with cooking spray; add cashews and stir-fry for 1 minute. Add sugar snap peas, broccoli, bamboo shoots, and scallions and stir-fry for 5 minutes over medium heat. Add beef back to pan.

3. In a small bowl, whisk together broth, soy sauce, hot pepper sauce, and cornstarch. Pour over meat and vegetables in pan. Add chilies. Bring to a boil, reduce heat, and simmer for 2 minutes.

4. Remove chilies before serving. Serve over brown rice.

Exchanges

2 Lean Meat	1/2 Fat
2 Vegetable	

Calories 194
Calories from Fat 77
Total Fat . . . . 9 g
Saturated Fat . . . . 3 g
Cholesterol . . . . 40 mg
Sodium . . . . 530 mg
Total Carbohydrate . . . . . . 11 g
Dietary Fiber . . . . 3 g
Sugars . . . . 4 g
Protein . . . . 18 g

Dietitian's Tip: Cashews are a good source of monounsaturated fat and vitamin E . . . plus they add great flavor and crunchiness to any dish.

Spring Rolls

Makes: 5 servings   *Serving Size: 2 rolls*   *Prep Time: 20 minutes*

SPRING ROLLS

1/2 cup canned bamboo shoots, rinsed, drained, and shredded
 2 medium carrots, cut into thin sticks
 2 medium cucumbers, seeded and cut into thin sticks
 1 cup fresh bean sprouts
 2 cups Napa cabbage, finely shredded
10 6-inch rice paper wrappers
   Medium bowl of warm water

DIPPING SAUCE

1/2 cup light sugar-free apricot preserves
 1 tablespoon lite soy sauce
1/2 teaspoon hot pepper sauce
1/4 teaspoon sesame oil

1. In a large bowl, toss bamboo shoots, carrots, cucumber, bean sprouts, and cabbage. Divide into 10 equal portions.

2. Soak one rice paper skin in warm water until softened, about 30 seconds. Lay rice paper on a clean, flat surface. Place one portion of the vegetable mixture in the center of the rice paper. Fold the left and right sides into the middle until almost touching. Roll paper from the bottom to form the roll. Repeat for remaining rice papers. Set aside.

3. Combine sauce ingredients in a small saucepan over high heat. Bring to a boil, stirring constantly. Boil for 2 minutes. Serve warm with cold spring rolls for dipping.

Exchanges

1 Starch	2 Vegetable

Calories 110
  Calories from Fat 6
Total Fat . . . . 1 g
  Saturated Fat . . . . 0 g
Cholesterol . . . . 0 mg
Sodium . . . . 164 mg
Total Carbohydrate . . . . . . 23 g
  Dietary Fiber . . . . 3 g
  Sugars . . . . 5 g
Protein . . . . 4 g

Chef's Tip: You can add anything you want to spring rolls to make them unique. Try adding finely diced chicken, stir-fried tofu cubes, chopped shrimp, or shredded pork to add protein.

August ❖ Week 2

GROCERY LIST

Fresh Produce
Garlic – 1 head
Mixed greens of choice
(collard, turnip,
mustard, or kale) –
2 pounds
Onions – 2
Lemons – 2
Red bell pepper –
1 medium
Carrots – small bag
Celery – small bag
Cucumber – 1 medium
Eggplant – 1
Portabello mushrooms –
2 large

Meat/Poultry/Fish
Boneless, skinless
chicken breasts –
1 pound plus 4
(4-ounce) breasts
Boneless pork chops –
1 1/4 pounds

Grains/Bread/Pasta
Penne pasta – 1 box
Cornflakes – small box
White rice
Brown rice
Whole-wheat pita
pockets – 5

Dairy and Cheese
Reduced-fat ricotta
cheese – 8 ounces
Eggs
Plain, fat-free yogurt –
8 ounces
Grated Parmesan cheese

Canned Goods and Sauces
15-ounce can crushed
tomatoes – 2 cans
14.5-ounce can fat-free,
reduced-sodium
chicken broth – 6 cans
Lite soy sauce – small
bottle
8-ounce can water
chestnuts – 1 can

Staples/Seasonings/Baking Needs
Salt/ground black pepper
Cooking spray
Olive oil
Dried oregano
Dried basil
Dried thyme
Garlic salt
Onion salt
Ground cinnamon
All-purpose flour
Cayenne pepper
Cornstarch
Rice wine vinegar
Hot pepper sauce
Brown sugar
Sesame oil

Miscellaneous
Liquid smoke
Peanuts – small package
Bamboo skewers

263

Penne with Ricotta and Tomato

Makes: 8 servings   *Serving Size: 1 cup*   *Prep Time: 15 minutes*

4 cups penne pasta, uncooked

1 teaspoon olive oil

3 garlic cloves, minced

1 15-ounce can crushed tomatoes

1 tablespoon dried oregano

1 tablespoon dried basil

8 ounces reduced-fat ricotta cheese

1. Cook pasta according to package directions, omitting salt. Drain.

2. Heat olive oil in a large nonstick skillet or wok over medium-high heat. Add garlic and sauté for 30 seconds. Add tomatoes, oregano, and basil and bring to a boil; reduce heat and simmer for about 10 minutes.

3. Add ricotta cheese to tomato mixture and stir well. Cook for 1–2 more minutes.

4. Toss sauce with pasta.

Exchanges

2 Starch	1/2 Fat
1 Vegetable	

Calories 215
  Calories from Fat 21
Total Fat . . . . 2 g
  Saturated Fat . . . . 1 g
Cholesterol . . . . 11 mg
Sodium . . . . 196 mg
Total Carbohydrate . . . . . . 37 g
  Dietary Fiber . . . . 3 g
  Sugars . . . . 5 g
Protein . . . . 12 g

Dietitian's Tip: Use whole-wheat pasta to boost the fiber content of this recipe.

Tasty "Fried" Chicken

Makes: 4 servings   Serving Size: 1 chicken breast   Prep Time: 15 minutes

Cooking spray
1 1/2 cups cornflake crumbs
1/2 teaspoon dried thyme
1/2 teaspoon garlic salt
1/2 teaspoon onion salt
1 egg
2 egg whites
1 teaspoon hot pepper sauce (optional)
2 tablespoons all-purpose flour
4 4-ounce boneless, skinless chicken breasts

1. Preheat oven to 350 degrees. Coat a shallow baking pan with cooking spray.

2. In a medium bowl, combine cornflake crumbs, thyme, garlic salt, and onion salt.

3. In a separate bowl, lightly beat egg and egg whites. Add hot pepper sauce and mix well.

4. Place flour in a separate bowl.

5. Dip each side of the chicken breast in flour, then egg mixture, then cornflake mixture.

6. Place chicken breasts in baking pan. Spray chicken lightly with cooking spray and bake 30–35 minutes, until juices run clear.

Exchanges

1 1/2 Starch   1/2 Fat
3 Very Lean Meat

Calories.	256
Calories from Fat.	34
Total Fat	4 g
Saturated Fat	1 g
Cholesterol	108 mg
Sodium	596 mg
Total Carbohydrate.	24 g
Dietary Fiber	1 g
Sugars.	3 g
Protein.	30 g

Chef's Tip: You will be amazed at how great this baked chicken tastes. The cornflakes retain their crunchiness, providing a fried-like texture and excellent flavor.

Spicy Greens

2 pounds mixed greens of choice (collard, turnip, mustard, or kale)

1 14.5-ounce can fat-free, reduced-sodium chicken broth

1 medium onion, chopped

2 garlic cloves, minced

1/4 teaspoon cayenne pepper

1/2 teaspoon ground black pepper

1 teaspoon liquid smoke

1. Wash greens thoroughly. Discard tough stems and cut greens into pieces.

2. Place greens in a large soup pot. Add chicken broth, onion, and garlic and simmer, covered, for 30–45 minutes or until tender. Season with cayenne pepper, black pepper, and liquid smoke.

Exchanges
2 Vegetable

Calories 57
   Calories from Fat 4
Total Fat . . . . 0 g
   Saturated Fat . . . . 0 g
Cholesterol . . . . 0 mg
Sodium . . . . 282 mg
Total Carbohydrate . . . . . . 12 g
   Dietary Fiber . . . . 5 g
   Sugars . . . . 3 g
Protein . . . . 3 g

Dietitian's Tip: Greens are a good source of folic acid. Folic acid may help protect against heart disease and helps lower the risk of birth defects, such as spina bifida.

Greek Lemon Rice Soup

Makes: 10 servings   *Serving Size: 1 cup*   *Prep Time: 5 minutes*

4 14.5-ounce cans fat-free, reduced-sodium chicken broth
1 cup rice, uncooked
1/4 cup lemon juice (juice of 1 lemon)
2 eggs
2 tablespoons cold water
2 tablespoons cornstarch
1/2 teaspoon salt
1/2 teaspoon ground black pepper

1. Bring chicken broth to a boil in a large soup pot. Add rice and reduce to a simmer for 20 minutes.

2. In a large bowl, whisk together lemon juice, eggs, water, and cornstarch.

3. Pour one ladle of the hot broth into the egg mixture, whisking constantly to temper the eggs. Repeat with two more ladles of soup.

4. Reduce heat to low. Add tempered egg mixture to soup, stirring constantly until fully incorporated. Remove from heat. Add salt and pepper.

Exchanges
1 Starch

Calories	102
Calories from Fat	10
Total Fat	1 g
Saturated Fat	0 g
Cholesterol	43 mg
Sodium	415 mg
Total Carbohydrate	18 g
Dietary Fiber	0 g
Sugars	1 g
Protein	4 g

Chef's Tip: A Greek salad made of lettuce, feta cheese, and olives would make a nice side dish for this meal.

Kung Pao Chicken

Makes: 4 servings   *Serving Size: 1 cup chicken*   *Prep Time: 10 minutes*
plus 1/2 cup rice

2 tablespoons cornstarch
1/2 cup fat-free, reduced-sodium chicken broth
2 tablespoons rice wine vinegar
2 tablespoons lite soy sauce
1/2 teaspoon hot pepper sauce
2 teaspoons brown sugar
2 teaspoons sesame oil, divided
1 garlic clove, minced
Cooking spray
1 pound boneless, skinless chicken breasts, cubed
1 medium red bell pepper, finely diced
1/2 cup finely diced carrots
1 8-ounce can water chestnuts, rinsed, drained, and chopped
1/4 cup chopped peanuts
2 cups brown rice, cooked

1. In a small bowl, combine cornstarch and chicken broth and whisk until cornstarch dissolves. Add vinegar, soy sauce, hot pepper sauce, brown sugar, 1 teaspoon sesame oil, and garlic; stir well and set aside.

2. In a large nonstick skillet or wok, heat cooking spray and 1 teaspoon sesame oil over medium-high heat. Add chicken breast and cook for 4 minutes. Remove from pan and set aside.

3. Add peppers, carrots, water chestnuts, and peanuts to pan. Stir-fry for 4 minutes. Add chicken broth mixture to skillet and bring to a boil. Add chicken back to pan and simmer for 3 minutes.

4. Serve over brown rice.

Exchanges

2 Starch	2 Vegetable
3 Very Lean Meat	1 1/2 Fat

Calories 376
  Calories from Fat 96
Total Fat . . . . 11 g
  Saturated Fat . . . . 2 g
Cholesterol . . . . 68 mg
Sodium . . . . 447 mg
Total Carbohydrate . . . . . . 38 g
  Dietary Fiber . . . . 4 g
  Sugars . . . . 7 g
Protein . . . . 31 g

Chef's Tip: No need to order out for Chinese food. Make your own low-fat version—you won't even taste the difference!

Souvlaki

Makes: 5 servings   *Serving Size: 1 stuffed pita*   *Prep Time: 20 minutes*

5 whole-wheat pita pockets
1 1/4 pounds boneless pork chops, cut into 1-inch cubes
1/2 cup lemon juice
2 garlic cloves, sliced
1 tablespoon dried oregano
1 cucumber, peeled, seeded, and shredded (about 1 1/2 cups)
8 ounces plain, fat-free yogurt
1 small garlic clove, minced
1/4 teaspoon salt
1/4 teaspoon ground black pepper
Bamboo skewers, soaked in warm water

1. Prepare an indoor or outdoor grill.

2. Slice one side of each pita to open pocket, but do not cut all the way through. Set aside.

1. In a medium bowl, combine pork cubes, lemon juice, garlic, and oregano. Marinate in refrigerator for 15 minutes.

2. In a medium bowl, mix cucumber, yogurt, garlic, salt, and pepper. Set aside.

3. Skewer 6–7 pork cubes on each bamboo skewer and grill over medium-high heat for 3 minutes on each side.

4. Toast pita bread and fill each pita with 1/2 cup pork and 1/2 cup sauce.

Exchanges

2 1/2 Starch   3 Lean Meat

Calories 335
 Calories from Fat 75
Total Fat . . . . 8 g
 Saturated Fat . . . . 3 g
Cholesterol . . . . 69 mg
Sodium . . . . 338 mg
Total Carbohydrate . . . . . . 36 g
 Dietary Fiber . . . . 3 g
 Sugars . . . . 7 g
Protein . . . . 32 g

Chef's Tip: These traditional Greek shishkabobs make an excellent light summer meal. They're great at a picnic.

Moussaka

Makes: 8 servings   *Serving Size: 1/8 recipe*   *Prep Time: 15 minutes*

1 large eggplant, unpeeled, cut into 1/4-inch-thick rounds
1 tablespoon olive oil
  Cooking spray
1 large onion, thinly sliced
1 cup finely chopped carrots
1 cup finely chopped celery
1 garlic clove, minced
2 large portabello mushrooms, cut into 1/2-inch pieces
1 teaspoon dried oregano
1/2 teaspoon ground cinnamon
1 15-ounce can crushed tomatoes
1/2 teaspoon salt
1/4 teaspoon ground black pepper
1/4 cup grated Parmesan cheese

1. Preheat oven to 425 degrees. Brush both sides of eggplant rounds with olive oil. Arrange in single layer on a baking sheet. Bake 10 minutes. Turn eggplant and continue baking until tender, about 15 minutes.

2. While eggplant is roasting, coat a large nonstick skillet with cooking spray. Over medium-high heat, add onion, carrots, and celery. Sauté until onion is clear, about 7 minutes.

3. Stir in garlic and mushrooms. Sauté until liquid evaporates, about 10 minutes. Add oregano, cinnamon, and tomatoes. Cook until mixture is thick, about 10 minutes. Add salt and pepper.

4. Reduce oven temperature to 350 degrees. Coat a shallow baking dish with cooking spray. Arrange half of eggplant rounds in single layer in dish. Spoon half of tomato mixture evenly over eggplant. Sprinkle with 2 tablespoons Parmesan cheese. Repeat layering with remaining eggplant, tomato mixture, and 2 tablespoons cheese, ending with cheese.

5. Bake until heated through and cheese is golden brown on top, about 20 minutes.

Chef's Tip: Traditional moussaka calls for a béchamel, or white cream sauce. We skipped that high-fat addition with an end result that's just as tasty.

Exchanges

3 Vegetable	1/2 Fat

Calories	95
Calories from Fat	29
Total Fat	3 g
Saturated Fat	1 g
Cholesterol	4 mg
Sodium	378 mg
Total Carbohydrate	14 g
Dietary Fiber	4 g
Sugars	8 g
Protein	4 g

August ❖ Week 3

RECIPE LIST

DAY 1: Spaghetti with Turkey Meatballs **272**

DAY 2: Meatball Sandwich **273**
Italian Green Beans **274**

DAY 3: Vegetable Paella **275**

DAY 4: Cajun Shrimp over Pasta **276**

DAY 5: Mediterranean Chicken **277**
Cucumber Tomato Salad **278**

GROCERY LIST

Fresh Produce
Garlic – 1 head
Italian (flat-leaf)
    parsley – 1 bunch
Onions – 4 medium
Red bell peppers –
    2 medium
Green bell peppers –
    2 medium
Green beans – 1 pound
    (if not using frozen)
Zucchini – 1 medium
Cucumbers – 2 large
Tomatoes – 2 medium

Meat/Poultry/Fish
Lean ground turkey –
    1 1/2 pounds
Shrimp – 1 pound
Boneless, skinless
    chicken breasts –
    3/4 pound

Grains/Bread/Pasta
Italian-style bread
    crumbs
Linguine – 2 boxes
French bread sandwich
    rolls – 4
Medium-grain white rice
Brown rice

Dairy and Cheese
Eggs
Grated Parmesan cheese
Shredded, reduced-fat
    mozzarella cheese –
    1 package

Canned Goods and Sauces
26-ounce jars marinara
    pasta sauce – 3 jars
15-ounce can no-salt-
    added diced
    tomatoes – 3 cans
14.5-ounce can fat-free,
    reduced-sodium
    chicken broth – 4 cans
15-ounce can cannellini
    beans – 1 can

Frozen Foods
Corn – 1 package
Italian green beans –
    1 pound (if not using
    fresh)

Staples/Seasonings/ Baking Needs
Salt/ground black pepper
Cooking spray
Olive oil
Dried minced onions
Dried basil
Dried oregano
Paprika
Onion salt
Cayenne pepper
Red wine vinegar

Miscellaneous
White wine – small
    bottle

271

Spaghetti with Turkey Meatballs

*Makes: 8 servings
(see Chef's Tip)*

*Serving Size: 3/4 cup pasta
with 1 cup meatball sauce
(about 2–3 meatballs)*

Prep Time: 15 minutes

1	teaspoon olive oil
4	garlic cloves, minced
3	26-ounce jars marinara pasta sauce
1 1/2	pounds lean ground turkey
1	egg
1/3	cup grated Parmesan cheese
1/4	cup chopped fresh Italian (flat-leaf) parsley
1/3	cup Italian-style bread crumbs
1 1/2	teaspoons dried minced onion
1/4	teaspoon ground black pepper
	12 ounces linguine, uncooked

1. In a large saucepan, heat oil and garlic over medium heat and sauté for 30 seconds. Add pasta sauce.

2. In a medium bowl, combine all remaining ingredients except linguine and mix well. Form meat into small balls (makes about 30 meatballs).

3. Add meatballs to sauce. Bring to a boil; reduce heat and simmer for about 1 hour; stirring occasionally.

4. Cook pasta according to package directions, omitting salt. Drain.

5. Serve meatball sauce over linguine.

Exchanges

2 1/2 Starch   3 Vegetable
2 Lean Meat

Calories 368	
Calories from Fat 67	
Total Fat . . . . 7 g	
Saturated Fat . . . . 2 g	
Cholesterol . . . . 57 mg	
Sodium . . . . 778 mg	
Total Carbohydrate . . . . . . 54 g	
Dietary Fiber . . . . 7 g	
Sugars . . . . 16 g	
Protein . . . . 23 g	

Chef's Tip: Reserve 2 cups sauce and 12 meatballs for tomorrow's Meatball Sandwich recipe.

Meatball Sandwich

Makes: 4 servings   *Serving Size: 1 sandwich*   *Prep Time: 5 minutes*

4 French bread sandwich rolls

2 cups spaghetti sauce (from recipe, page 272)

12 meatballs (from recipe, page 272)

1/4 cup shredded, part-skim mozzarella cheese

1. Preheat oven to 450 degrees.

2. Place French rolls on baking sheet. Spoon 1/2 cup sauce and about 3 meatballs onto each roll. Top each sandwich with 1 tablespoon mozzarella cheese.

3. Place in oven and bake for 10 minutes or until cheese is melted.

Exchanges

2 Starch	2 Vegetable
2 Lean Meat	1 Fat

Calories 367
  Calories from Fat 99
Total Fat . . . . 11 g
  Saturated Fat . . . . 4 g
Cholesterol . . . . 80 mg
Sodium . . . . 922 mg
Total Carbohydrate . . . . . . 42 g
  Dietary Fiber . . . . 5 g
  Sugars . . . . 13 g
Protein . . . . 26 g

Chef's Tip: This recipe is a great example of how to turn leftovers into a whole new meal.

Italian Green Beans

Makes: 6 servings   *Serving Size: 1/2 cup*   *Prep Time: 5 minutes*

1 pound frozen Italian green beans or fresh green beans, sliced

1 tablespoon olive oil

1 small onion, diced

2 garlic cloves, minced

1 15-ounce can no-salt-added diced tomatoes

1/4 teaspoon dried basil

1/4 teaspoon dried oregano

1. Steam green beans until tender-crisp. Set aside.

2. Heat olive oil in a medium non-stick skillet over medium-high heat. Sauté onions until clear. Add garlic; sauté 30 seconds. Add tomatoes, basil, and oregano and simmer for 15–20 minutes.

3. Pour tomato mixture over steamed green beans and mix well.

Exchanges

2 Vegetable   1/2 Fat

Calories 65
  Calories from Fat 24
Total Fat . . . . 3 g
  Saturated Fat . . . . 0 g
Cholesterol . . . . 0 mg
Sodium . . . . 33 mg
Total Carbohydrate . . . . . . 10 g
  Dietary Fiber . . . . 4 g
  Sugars . . . . 5 g
Protein . . . . 2 g

Chef's Tip: Italian green beans are wider and thicker than regular green beans. They're usually found in the frozen food aisle of your market.

Vegetable Paella

Makes: 6 servings   *Serving Size: 1 cup*   *Prep Time: 15 minutes*

1 tablespoon olive oil
1 red bell pepper, diced
1 onion, diced
2 large garlic cloves, minced
1/4 cup white wine
1 1/2 cups medium-grain white rice
2 14.5-ounce cans fat-free, reduced-sodium chicken broth
1 15-ounce can no-salt-added diced tomatoes, drained
1 1/2 teaspoons paprika
1/2 teaspoon salt
1/4 teaspoon ground black pepper
1 15-ounce can cannellini beans, rinsed and drained
1/2 cup frozen corn

1. Add oil to a large nonstick skillet over medium-high heat. Sauté bell pepper and onion for 3–4 minutes. Add garlic and sauté for 30 seconds.

2. Add wine and cook until liquid is reduced by half, about 3 minutes.

3. Stir in rice, broth, tomatoes, paprika, salt, and pepper. Bring to a boil. Reduce heat and simmer for 25 minutes.

4. Stir in beans and corn and simmer for 2 more minutes.

Exchanges

3 1/2 Starch	1 Vegetable

Calories 300
Calories from Fat 28
Total Fat . . . . 3 g
Saturated Fat . . . . 0 g
Cholesterol . . . . 0 mg
Sodium . . . . 597 mg
Total Carbohydrate . . . . . . 58 g
Dietary Fiber . . . . 6 g
Sugars . . . . 5 g
Protein . . . . 10 g

Chef's Tip: Cannellini beans are also called white kidney beans.

Cajun Shrimp over Pasta

Makes: 5 servings   *Serving Size: 1/5 recipe*   *Prep Time: 10 minutes*

10 ounces linguine, uncooked

2 teaspoons olive oil, divided

1 green bell pepper, thinly sliced

1 red bell pepper, thinly sliced

1 small onion, thinly sliced

1 garlic clove, minced

1 pound raw shrimp, peeled and deveined

1 14.5-ounce can fat-free, reduced-sodium chicken broth

1 teaspoon paprika

1 teaspoon onion salt

1/4 teaspoon cayenne pepper

1/2 teaspoon ground black pepper

1. Cook pasta according to package directions, omitting salt. Drain.

2. Add 1 teaspoon olive oil to a large nonstick skillet over medium-high heat. Add peppers and onion and stir-fry for 5 minutes. Remove from pan and set aside.

3. Add remaining teaspoon olive oil to pan and reduce heat to medium. Add garlic and shrimp and sauté for 1–2 minutes or until shrimp is done. Add peppers back to pan.

4. Pour chicken broth, paprika, onion salt, cayenne pepper, and black pepper in pan and bring to a simmer for 1 minute.

5. Serve shrimp and broth over pasta.

Exchanges

3 Starch	1 Vegetable
2 Very Lean Meat	

Calories 317
 Calories from Fat 33
Total Fat . . . . 4 g
 Saturated Fat . . . . 0 g
Cholesterol . . . . 116 mg
Sodium . . . . 593 mg
Total Carbohydrate . . . . . . 49 g
 Dietary Fiber . . . . 4 g
 Sugars . . . . 5 g
Protein . . . . 21 g

Chef's Tip: If you don't like shrimp, substitute chicken in this recipe by cooking it in step 3 for 7–9 minutes or until done.

Mediterranean Chicken

Makes: 5 servings   *Serving Size: about 1 1/3 cups*   *Prep Time: 13 minutes*

1 cup brown rice, uncooked
   Cooking spray
3/4 pound boneless, skinless
   chicken breasts, cubed
1/4 teaspoon ground black pepper
1 tablespoon olive oil
3 garlic cloves, minced
1 cup diced zucchini
1 green bell pepper, diced
1/2 cup diced onion
1 15-ounce can no-salt-added
   diced tomatoes with juice
1 cup fat-free, reduced-sodium
   chicken broth
1 tablespoon dried oregano
1/2 teaspoon salt

1. Cook rice according to package directions, omitting salt.

2. Coat a large nonstick skillet or wok with cooking spray. Season chicken with black pepper and sauté over medium-high heat for 3–4 minutes. Remove chicken from pan.

3. Add olive oil and garlic to skillet and sauté 30 seconds. Add zucchini, green pepper, and onion and sauté 3–4 minutes. Add chicken back to pan along with diced tomatoes, chicken broth, oregano, and salt.

4. Bring to a boil; reduce heat and simmer 6–7 minutes. Add cooked rice to pan and mix well.

Exchanges

2 Starch	1 Vegetable
2 Very Lean Meat	1/2 Fat

Calories 284
   Calories from Fat 53
Total Fat . . . . 6 g
   Saturated Fat . . . . 1 g
Cholesterol . . . . 41 mg
Sodium . . . . 407 mg
Total Carbohydrate . . . . . . 38 g
   Dietary Fiber . . . . 4 g
   Sugars . . . . 6 g
Protein . . . . 20 g

Chef's Tip: This dish is as tasty as it is beautiful. Garnish it with a few sprigs of fresh oregano for an extra flair.

Cucumber Tomato Salad

Makes: 5 servings   *Serving Size: 1/5 recipe*   *Prep Time: 10 minutes*

2 large cucumbers, peeled, seeded, and diced

2 medium tomatoes, seeded and diced

1 tablespoon olive oil

2 tablespoons red wine vinegar

1/2 teaspoon salt

Dash ground black pepper

1. In a medium bowl, toss cucumbers and tomatoes.

2. Drizzle oil and vinegar over vegetables and toss to coat. Season with salt and pepper.

 National Food Safety Month is in August. Always keep food safely stored in the refrigerator, and when in doubt, throw it out.

Exchanges

1 Vegetable	1/2 Fat

Calories 43
  Calories from Fat 26
Total Fat . . . . 3 g
  Saturated Fat . . . . 0 g
Cholesterol . . . . 0 mg
Sodium . . . . 237 mg
Total Carbohydrate . . . . 4 g
  Dietary Fiber . . . . 1 g
  Sugars . . . . 3 g
Protein . . . . 1 g

Chef's Tip: For added flavor, sprinkle some feta cheese on top of this salad.

August ❖ Week 4

RECIPE LIST

DAY 1: Greek Lemon Chicken and Rice **280**

DAY 2: Hungarian Goulash **281**

DAY 3: Cuban Black Beans and Rice **282**

DAY 4: Chicken Parmesan **283**
Ratatouille **284**

DAY 5: Moroccan Pork with Caramelized Radicchio **285**
Stuffed Tomatoes **286**

DESSERT OF THE MONTH: Tiramisu **287**

GROCERY LIST

Fresh Produce
Onions – 2 large
Green bell peppers –
2 large
Red bell pepper – 1 large
Garlic – 1 head
Lemon – 1
Fresh oregano – 1 bunch
Idaho potatoes –
2 medium
Eggplant – 1
Zucchini – 2 small
Radicchio – 1 head
Beefsteak tomatoes –
4 large
Lime – 1
Fresh cilantro – 1 bunch

Meat/Poultry/Fish
Boneless, skinless
chicken breasts –
3/4 pound plus 4
(4-ounce) breasts
Sirloin steak – 1 pound
Boneless pork chops –
4 (4-ounce) chops

Grains/Bread/Pasta
Brown rice
Egg noodles – 1 package
Italian-style bread
crumbs

Dairy and Cheese
Fat-free sour cream –
1 container
Eggs
Shredded, reduced-fat
mozzarella cheese –
1 package
Fresh Parmesan cheese –
1 wedge
Goat cheese – 1 package
Light cream cheese –
1 package

Canned Goods and Sauces
16-ounce can black
beans – 2 cans
14.5-ounce can fat-free,
reduced-sodium veg-
etable broth – 1 can
14.5-ounce can fat-free,
reduced-sodium
chicken broth – 2 cans
15-ounce can crushed
tomatoes – 1 can
Ketchup – small bottle
Worcestershire sauce –
small bottle
Marinara pasta sauce –
1 large jar

Frozen Foods
Corn – 1 package
Light whipped topping –
8 ounces

Staples/Seasonings/ Baking Needs
Salt/ground black pepper
Cooking spray
Canola oil
Olive oil
Cumin
Dried oregano
Apple cider vinegar
All-purpose flour
Dry mustard
Paprika
Cayenne pepper
Ground cinnamon
Sugar
1-ounce package sugar-
free vanilla instant
pudding – 1 package
Powdered sugar – small
bag
Unsweetened cocoa –
small package

Miscellaneous
Instant coffee granules –
small jar
Ladyfingers – 24

279

Greek Lemon Chicken and Rice

Makes: 4 servings   *Serving Size: 1 chicken breast and 1/2 cup brown rice*   *Prep Time: 35 minutes*

3 tablespoons fresh lemon juice
2 teaspoons olive oil
3 garlic cloves, minced
1 teaspoon chopped fresh oregano (or 1/4 teaspoon dried oregano)
4 4-ounce boneless, skinless chicken breasts
  Cooking spray
1/4 teaspoon salt
1/4 teaspoon ground black pepper
2 cups cooked brown rice

1. In a medium bowl, whisk together lemon juice, olive oil, garlic, and oregano. Add chicken breasts to marinade and turn to coat. Marinate chicken in refrigerator for 30 minutes.

2. Coat a large nonstick skillet with cooking spray. Remove chicken from marinade and season well with salt and pepper. Reserve marinade. Cook chicken over high heat for approximately 5–7 minutes on each side. Add reserved marinade to pan and bring to a boil for 1 minute.

3. Serve chicken breasts over brown rice.

Exchanges

1 1/2 Starch	1 Fat
3 Very Lean Meat	

Calories 268
  Calories from Fat 54
Total Fat . . . . 6 g
  Saturated Fat . . . . 1 g
Cholesterol . . . . 68 mg
Sodium . . . . 213 mg
Total Carbohydrate . . . . . . 24 g
  Dietary Fiber . . . . 2 g
  Sugars . . . . 2 g
Protein . . . . 28 g

Dietitian's Tip: Steamed broccoli and carrots would make a great side dish for this entrée.

Hungarian Goulash

Makes: 8 servings   *Serving Size: 1 cup*   *Prep Time: 15 minutes*

6 ounces egg noodles, uncooked
Cooking spray
1 pound sirloin steak, sliced into thin 1-inch pieces
1 medium onion, thinly sliced
2 medium Idaho potatoes, peeled and diced
2 tablespoons ketchup
1/2 teaspoon Worcestershire sauce
2 tablespoons all-purpose flour
2 14.5-ounce cans fat-free, reduced-sodium chicken broth
2 garlic cloves, minced
1 teaspoon dry mustard
1 tablespoon paprika
1/2 teaspoon salt
1/4 teaspoon ground black pepper
1/2 cup fat-free sour cream

1. Cook egg noodles according to package directions, omitting salt. Drain.

2. Coat a large nonstick skillet with cooking spray over high heat. Add sirloin and sauté for 3–4 minutes. Remove from pan and set aside.

3. Add onion to pan and sauté for 5–6 minutes or until onions begin to brown. Add potatoes and continue to sauté.

4. In a medium bowl, whisk together remaining ingredients except sour cream. Pour mixture over potatoes and onions and bring to a boil. Reduce heat and simmer for 20 minutes or until potatoes are soft.

5. Add steak back to pan and stir in sour cream.

Exchanges

2 Starch	1 Lean Meat

Calories	225
Calories from Fat	33
Total Fat	4 g
Saturated Fat	1 g
Cholesterol	53 mg
Sodium	494 mg
Total Carbohydrate	30 g
Dietary Fiber	2 g
Sugars	5 g
Protein	17 g

Chef's Tip: This version tastes just like your grandmother's! You can substitute fat-free sour cream for regular in any recipe and still achieve wonderful creaminess and flavor.

Cuban Black Beans and Rice

Makes: 4 servings   *Serving Size: 3/4 cup beans*   *Prep Time: 5 minutes*
and 1/2 cup rice

2 teaspoons canola oil

1 large onion, chopped

1 green bell pepper, cut into
1/2-inch strips

4 large garlic cloves, minced

1 teaspoon cumin

1/2 tablespoon dried oregano

2 16-ounce cans black beans,
rinsed and drained

1 cup canned fat-free, reduced-
sodium vegetable broth

1 tablespoon apple cider vinegar

1/2 teaspoon crushed red pepper
flakes (optional)

2 cups cooked brown rice

1. In a large saucepan, heat oil over medium heat. Add onion, green pepper, garlic, cumin, and oregano and sauté about 5 minutes.

2. Add black beans, vegetable broth, vinegar, and red pepper flakes to pan and simmer for 15 minutes.

3. Serve over brown rice.

Exchanges

4 Starch   1 Very Lean Meat

Calories 332
   Calories from Fat 38
Total Fat . . . . 4 g
   Saturated Fat . . . . 1 g
Cholesterol . . . . 0 mg
Sodium . . . . 406 mg
Total Carbohydrate . . . . . . 61 g
   Dietary Fiber . . . . 14 g
   Sugars . . . . 10 g
Protein . . . . 15 g

Dietitian's Tip: Beans and rice are a great combination, offering plenty of protein and fiber. Meatless meals don't have to be boring!

Chicken Parmesan

Makes: 4 servings   *Serving Size: 1/4 recipe*   *Prep Time: 10 minutes*

Cooking spray

3/4 pound boneless, skinless chicken breasts

1 cup Italian-style bread crumbs

4 egg whites

1/2 cup all-purpose flour

2 tablespoons olive oil

3 cups jarred marinara pasta sauce

1/3 cup shredded, reduced-fat mozzarella cheese

3 tablespoons grated fresh Parmesan cheese

Exchanges

1 1/2 Starch	3 Vegetable
3 Lean Meat	1/2 Fat

Calories 392
  Calories from Fat 114
Total Fat . . . . 13 g
  Saturated Fat . . . . 3 g
Cholesterol . . . . 60 mg
Sodium . . . . 1014 mg
Total Carbohydrate . . . . . . 37 g
  Dietary Fiber . . . . 5 g
  Sugars . . . . 13 g
Protein . . . . 34 g

1. Preheat oven to 350 degrees. Coat a shallow baking dish with cooking spray. Set aside.

2. Place one chicken breast in between two pieces of plastic wrap. Using a meat tenderizer or rolling pin, pound the chicken breast to 1/2-inch thickness. Repeat for remaining 3 breasts.

3. In three separate bowls, place the bread crumbs, egg whites, and flour. Dip each side of the chicken breast in flour, coating all sides, then egg whites, then bread crumbs, coating well. Repeat for remaining 3 breasts.

4. Add oil to a large nonstick skillet over medium-high heat. Place the chicken breasts in the pan and cook on each side for 2–3 minutes or just until lightly golden brown.

5. Line the baking dish with the chicken breasts. Cover with sauce and sprinkle both cheeses over the top. Bake for 25 minutes.

Chef's Tip: Serve this dish over pasta with some colorful steamed veggies.

Ratatouille

1 tablespoon olive oil
2 garlic cloves, minced
1 medium eggplant, cubed
2 small zucchini, sliced
1 green bell pepper, chopped
1 cup canned crushed tomatoes
1/2 teaspoon salt
1/4 teaspoon ground black pepper

1. Add oil to a large nonstick skillet over medium-high heat. Add garlic and sauté 30 seconds.

2. Add remaining ingredients and cook 10–15 minutes, stirring occasionally, until vegetables are tender.

Exchanges

2 Vegetable	1/2 Fat

Calories	65
Calories from Fat	23
Total Fat	3 g
Saturated Fat	0 g
Cholesterol	0 mg
Sodium	310 mg
Total Carbohydrate	10 g
Dietary Fiber	3 g
Sugars	6 g
Protein	2 g

Chef's Tip: This classic side dish is just as good served cold the next day.

Moroccan Pork with Caramelized Radicchio

Makes: 4 servings   *Serving Size: 1 pork chop*   *Prep Time: 10 minutes*

1 teaspoon cumin
1 teaspoon paprika
1/4 teaspoon cayenne pepper
1/4 teaspoon ground cinnamon
1/4 teaspoon dry mustard
4 4-ounce boneless pork chops
2 teaspoons olive oil
Cooking spray
1 head radicchio, chopped
1 teaspoon sugar
1/2 teaspoon salt
1/4 teaspoon ground black pepper

1. In a small bowl, combine the first 5 ingredients and mix well. Dredge one side of each pork chop in spice mixture.

2. Add oil and a generous amount of cooking spray to a large nonstick skillet over high heat. Place chops spice side down in the skillet. Cook for 6 minutes on each side. Remove from pan and set aside.

3. Spray skillet generously again and add radicchio to pan. Sauté radicchio for 2 minutes. Add sugar, salt, and pepper. Sauté 5–6 more minutes or until radicchio begins to caramelize. Serve radicchio on top of each pork chop.

Exchanges

3 Lean Meat	1 Vegetable

Calories	201
Calories from Fat	86
Total Fat	10 g
Saturated Fat	3 g
Cholesterol	68 mg
Sodium	352 mg
Total Carbohydrate	4 g
Dietary Fiber	1 g
Sugars	2 g
Protein	25 g

Dietitian's Tip: Most people just use radicchio in salads. You won't believe how good it tastes caramelized in this recipe. Try cooking other leafy salad greens ... they add fantastic texture and flavor to other dishes!

Stuffed Tomatoes

Makes: 8 servings   *Serving Size: 1/2 tomato*   *Prep Time: 15 minutes*

2 cups frozen corn, thawed

1 large red bell pepper, diced

4 large beefsteak tomatoes (each about 9–10 ounces)

1 tablespoon olive oil

2 tablespoons fresh lime juice

1 garlic clove, minced

2 tablespoons chopped fresh cilantro

1/2 teaspoon salt

1/4 teaspoon ground black pepper

1/2 cup crumbled goat cheese

1. Toss corn and bell pepper in a medium bowl and set aside.

2. Cut tomatoes horizontally in half. Using a small spoon, scoop center of tomatoes into small bowl, leaving a shell. Discard tomato seeds and juices and chop tomato meat; add to corn mixture.

3. In a small bowl, whisk together oil, lime juice, garlic, cilantro, salt, and pepper. Drizzle over corn mixture. Spoon corn salad into tomato shells.

4. Sprinkle each tomato with 1 tablespoon goat cheese and serve cold.

Exchanges

1/2 Starch	1/2 Fat
1 Vegetable	

Calories 99
 Calories from Fat 35
Total Fat . . . . 4 g
 Saturated Fat . . . . 1 g
Cholesterol . . . . 8 mg
Sodium . . . . 194 mg
Total Carbohydrate . . . . . . 15 g
 Dietary Fiber . . . . 3 g
 Sugars . . . . 5 g
Protein . . . . 4 g

Dietitian's Tip: Tomatoes offer great nutritional value. Not only are they a good source of vitamins A and C, but they also contain a pigment called lycopene, which may slow the development of some cancers.

Tiramisu

Makes: 16 servings   *Serving Size: 1/2 cup*   *Prep Time: 35 minutes*

1 cup cold water

1 1-ounce package sugar-free vanilla instant pudding mix

1/2 cup powdered sugar

12 ounces light cream cheese

8 ounces fat-free whipped topping

1 cup hot water

2 tablespoons instant coffee granules

24 ladyfingers

3 tablespoons unsweetened cocoa, divided

The ADA recommends eating only a small amount of saturated fat every day. This recipe is higher in saturated fat, so try to balance it by eating foods low in saturated fat at your other meals today.

1. In a medium bowl, combine cold water, vanilla pudding mix, and powdered sugar and stir with whisk. Chill 20 minutes.

2. Add cream cheese to pudding mixture and beat with a mixer at medium speed until well blended. Fold in whipped topping.

3. In a small bowl or mug, mix hot water and coffee granules.

4. Split lady fingers in half lengthwise. Arrange 16 ladyfingers halves flat side down in a trifle or large glass bowl. Drizzle ladyfingers with coffee. Spread 1/3 of the pudding mixture over the ladyfingers and sprinkle with 1 tablespoon cocoa. Repeat layers, ending with cocoa.

5. Cover and chill 4 hours or longer.

See photo insert.

Dietitian's Tip: You can still enjoy any dessert if you have diabetes . . . just enjoy it in moderation! This one is beautiful served in a trifle bowl.

Exchanges

1 Fat	1 Carbohydrate

Calories. 136
Calories from Fat. 46
Total Fat . . . . .5 g
Saturated Fat . . . . 3 g
Cholesterol . . . . 24 mg
Sodium . . . . 193 mg
Total Carbohydrate. . . . . . 19 g
Dietary Fiber . . . . 0 g
Sugars. . . . . 11 g
Protein. . . . . 3 g

September

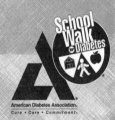

The School Walk for Diabetes®
is a school-based ADA
fundraising event great for
enhancing team spirit and
community fun! Walkers of all
age levels learn about diabetes
and raise money for their
schools at the same time.
For more info, call
1-888-diabetes.

Super Salad Meals

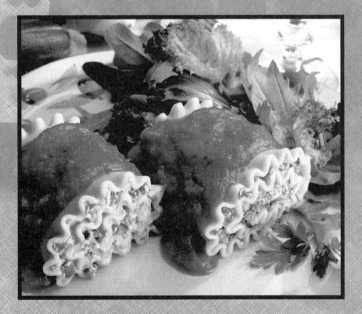

Veggie Lasagna Roulades (page 240)
Green Salad with Raspberry Vinaigrette (page 428)
What's better together than great lasagna, a crisp salad, and warm French bread? You'll like this rolled pasta dish—it looks impressive, but is so easy to make!

September ❖ Recipes

September ❖ Week 1

RECIPE LIST

DAY 1: Chicken Caesar Salad **292**

DAY 2: Shrimp Fajitas **293**
Corn Fritters **294**

DAY 3: Beef Tips with Mushroom
Gravy **295**
Texas Toast **296**

DAY 4: Black-Eyed Pea Soup **297**

DAY 5: Chicken Couscous Salad **298**

GROCERY LIST

Fresh Produce
Garlic – 1 head
Lemons – 2
10-ounce bag romaine
lettuce – 1 bag
Red bell pepper –
1 medium
Green bell pepper –
1 medium
Onions – 2 medium
Sliced mushrooms –
1 pint
Carrots – small bag
Mixed field greens –
4 cups

Meat/Poultry/Fish
Boneless, skinless
chicken breasts –
2 pounds
Shrimp – 1 pound

Beef tenderloin tips –
1 pound
Turkey bacon –
1 package

Grains/Bread/Pasta
6-inch corn or flour
tortillas – 8
Thickly sliced white
bread – 4 slices
Couscous – 1 package

Dairy and Cheese
Fat-free sour cream –
1 container
Fat-free milk
Grated Parmesan cheese
Eggs
Margarine

Canned Goods and Sauces
Light mayonnaise – 1 jar
15.5-ounce can black-
eyed peas – 2 cans
14.5-ounce can fat-free,
reduced-sodium
chicken broth – 3 cans
14.5-ounce can fat-free,
reduced-sodium beef
broth – 1 can

Frozen Foods
Corn – 1 package
Chopped spinach –
1 small package

Staples/Seasonings/Baking Needs
Salt/ground black pepper
Cooking spray
Canola oil
Olive oil
Dry mustard
Chili powder
Cumin
Cayenne pepper
Crushed red pepper
flakes
All-purpose flour
Cornstarch

Miscellaneous
Honey
Golden raisins – 1 box
Raisins – 1 box
Walnuts – small package

Chicken Caesar Salad

Makes: 6 servings   *Serving Size: 1/6 recipe*   *Prep Time: 10 minutes*

DRESSING

  2 tablespoons light mayonnaise

1/4 cup fat-free sour cream

1/4 cup fat-free milk

  2 tablespoons lemon juice

1/2 teaspoon dry mustard

  3 tablespoons grated Parmesan cheese

1/4 teaspoon salt

    Dash ground black pepper

SALAD

  1 pound boneless, skinless chicken breasts

  1 10-ounce bag romaine lettuce

  2 tablespoons grated Parmesan cheese

1. Prepare an indoor or outdoor grill. In a medium bowl, whisk together dressing ingredients. Reserve 1/2 cup of dressing.

2. Add chicken breasts to remaining dressing and marinate in the refrigerator for 15 minutes.

3. Remove chicken breasts from marinade and grill over medium-high heat for 5–6 minutes on each side or until done. Slice grilled chicken into strips.

4. In a large bowl, toss together salad ingredients. Drizzle with reserved dressing and toss well to coat.

5. Divide salad among 6 plates and top with sliced chicken breast.

Exchanges

2 Very Lean Meat	1 Fat
1 Vegetable	

Calories 145	
Calories from Fat 46	
Total Fat . . . . 5 g	
Saturated Fat . . . . 2 g	
Cholesterol . . . . 53 mg	
Sodium . . . . 265 mg	
Total Carbohydrate . . . . 4 g	
Dietary Fiber . . . . 0 g	
Sugars . . . . 2 g	
Protein . . . . 21 g	

Dietitian's Tip: Caesar salad dressing is typically very high in fat, but we've solved that problem by using light mayo, fat-free sour cream, and fat-free milk.

Shrimp Fajitas

Makes: 4 servings   *Serving Size: 2 fajitas*   *Prep Time: 10 minutes*

Cooking spray

2 teaspoons canola oil

1 medium red bell pepper, cut into 1/4-inch strips

1 medium green bell pepper, cut into 1/4-inch strips

1 medium onion, cut into 1/4-inch strips

1 pound uncooked shrimp, peeled and deveined

2 tablespoons water

1 teaspoon chili powder

1/2 teaspoon cumin

1/4 teaspoon cayenne pepper

1/2 teaspoon salt

1/4 teaspoon ground black pepper

8 6-inch flour or corn tortillas, warmed

1. Coat a large nonstick skillet with cooking spray and add oil; heat over medium-high heat. Sauté peppers for 10 minutes. Add remaining ingredients except tortillas and cook for another 5 minutes or until shrimp is done.

2. Fill each tortilla with 1/8 of shrimp and pepper mixture.

Exchanges

2 Starch	2 Vegetable
2 Very Lean Meat	1 Fat

Calories 327
  Calories from Fat 69
Total Fat . . . . 8 g
  Saturated Fat . . . . 1 g
Cholesterol . . . . 145 mg
Sodium . . . . 754 mg
Total Carbohydrate . . . . . . 42 g
  Dietary Fiber . . . . 4 g
  Sugars . . . . 5 g
Protein . . . . 22 g

Chef's Tip: Bell peppers come in a variety of colors—try orange and yellow peppers in this dish for a colorful and tasty meal.

Corn Fritters

Makes: 8 servings   *Serving Size: 2 fritters*   *Prep Time: 10 minutes*

2 cups frozen corn, thawed
1 egg
1/3 cup fat-free milk
1/2 cup all-purpose flour
1 teaspoon salt
Dash of ground black pepper
Cooking spray

1. In a large bowl, combine all ingredients and mix well. Coat a mini-muffin pan with cooking spray.

2. Fill 16 muffin cups with 1 tablespoon corn mixture. Bake for 15–18 minutes or until golden brown. Remove from oven and let sit for 5 minutes before removing from muffin pan.

Exchanges

1 Starch

Calories 74
Calories from Fat 8
Total Fat . . . . 1 g
Saturated Fat . . . . 0 g
Cholesterol . . . . 27 mg
Sodium . . . . 306 mg
Total Carbohydrate . . . . . . 15 g
Dietary Fiber . . . . 1 g
Sugars . . . . 1 g
Protein . . . . 3 g

Chef's Tip: If you don't have a mini-muffin pan, drop tablespoonfuls of batter onto a cookie sheet coated with cooking spray and bake for 15 minutes.

Beef Tips with Mushroom Gravy

Makes: 4 servings   *Serving Size: 1/4 recipe*   *Prep Time: 10 minutes*

Cooking spray
1 pound beef tenderloin tips
1 pint sliced mushrooms
1 cup fat-free, reduced-sodium beef broth
1 tablespoon cornstarch
1/2 teaspoon salt
1/4 teaspoon ground black pepper

1. Coat a large nonstick skillet with cooking spray over high heat. Add beef tips to skillet and sauté for 5–6 minutes or until browned well. Remove beef from pan and set aside. Cover beef.

2. Add mushrooms to pan and sauté for 4–5 minutes.

3. In a small bowl, whisk together broth and cornstarch. Pour over mushrooms and bring to a boil, scraping brown bits up from the bottom of the pan. Reduce heat and simmer for 2 minutes.

4. Stir in salt and pepper. Return beef tips and any juice and stir into gravy.

Exchanges

3 Lean Meat	1 Vegetable

Calories 169
   Calories from Fat 64
Total Fat . . . . 7 g
   Saturated Fat . . . . 3 g
Cholesterol . . . . 60 mg
Sodium . . . . 447 mg
Total Carbohydrate . . . . 4 g
   Dietary Fiber . . . . 0 g
   Sugars . . . . 1 g
Protein . . . . 21 g

Chef's Tip: Serve this homestyle favorite over Texas Toast (see page 296).

Texas Toast

1 tablespoon margarine
  Cooking spray
1 garlic clove, minced
1/4 teaspoon salt
4 slices white bread, thickly
  sliced (6 ounces total)

1. Preheat broiler.

2. Coat a small nonstick skillet with cooking spray. Add margarine and melt over medium heat. Add garlic and salt and sauté for 30 seconds. Remove from heat.

3. Place bread on baking sheet. Brush garlic butter on one side of each slice of bread. Place in broiler for 3 minutes to toast.

Exchanges

1 1/2 Starch	1/2 Fat

Calories	140
Calories from Fat	39
Total Fat	4 g
Saturated Fat	1 g
Cholesterol	0 mg
Sodium	407 mg
Total Carbohydrate	21 g
Dietary Fiber	1 g
Sugars	2 g
Protein	4 g

Chef's Tip: Serve this easy toast with any meat dish and a side salad.

Black-Eyed Pea Soup

Makes: 8 servings   *Serving Size: 1 cup*   *Prep Time: 10 minutes*

2 teaspoons olive oil

5 strips turkey bacon, chopped

1 small onion, finely diced

1 cup shredded carrots

1/4 cup frozen chopped spinach, thawed and drained

2 15.5-ounce cans black-eyed peas, rinsed and drained

3 14.5-ounce cans fat-free, reduced-sodium chicken broth

1/2 teaspoon salt (optional)

1/4 teaspoon ground black pepper

1/4 teaspoon crushed red pepper flakes

1. Add oil to a large soup pot over high heat. Add bacon and sauté for 3 minutes or until bacon is crispy. Add onion and sauté 4 minutes or until clear. Add carrots and spinach. Sauté 3–4 minutes.

2. Add remaining ingredients and bring to a boil. Reduce heat and simmer for 20 minutes.

Exchanges

1 Starch   1 Vegetable
1 Very Lean Meat

Calories 140
  Calories from Fat 28
Total Fat . . . . 3 g
  Saturated Fat . . . . 1 g
Cholesterol . . . . 7 mg
Sodium . . . . 613 mg
Total Carbohydrate . . . . . . 19 g
  Dietary Fiber . . . . 6 g
  Sugars . . . . 5 g
Protein . . . . 9 g

Dietitian's Tip: Soups can be a great way to incorporate more legumes and beans into your diet. Beans and legumes, such as lentils, pinto beans, red beans, and navy beans, are low in fat and a great source of fiber.

Chicken Couscous Salad

Makes: 6 servings   *Serving Size: 1/6 recipe*   *Prep Time: 15 minutes*

DRESSING

1/4 cup lemon juice
  2 tablespoons honey
  2 tablespoons olive oil
1/4 teaspoon salt
    Dash of ground black pepper

SALAD

  4 cups couscous, cooked and
    cooled
  2 cups cooked, chopped chicken
    breast meat
1/4 cup golden raisins
1/4 cup raisins
1/4 cup chopped walnuts, toasted
  4 cups mixed field greens

1. In a medium bowl, whisk together dressing ingredients and set aside.

2. In another medium bowl, toss couscous, chicken, raisins, and walnuts. Drizzle dressing over couscous and toss to coat.

3. Arrange field greens on a plate and mound 1 cup of couscous salad in center. Repeat for remaining 5 plates.

Exchanges

1 1/2 Starch	1 Fruit
2 Very Lean Meat	1 1/2 Fat

Calories 325
  Calories from Fat 83
Total Fat . . . . 9 g
  Saturated Fat . . . . 1 g
Cholesterol . . . . 36 mg
Sodium . . . . 141 mg
Total Carbohydrate . . . . . . 42 g
  Dietary Fiber . . . . 3 g
  Sugars . . . . 15 g
Protein . . . . 19 g

Chef's Tip: This recipe shows you how to mix different textures and flavors for a unique and outstanding meal.

September ❖ Week 2

GROCERY LIST

Fresh Produce
Lime – 1
Fresh mint – 1 bunch
Cucumbers – 2 medium
Carrots – small bag
Scallions – 1 bunch
Romaine lettuce –
1 head
Green beans – 4 cups
Red new potatoes –
1 pound
Tomatoes – 2
Red cabbage – 1 head
Granny Smith apples –
2 small

Meat/Poultry/Fish
Top sirloin steak –
1 pound
Boneless, skinless
chicken breasts –
1 pound
Boneless veal chops –
4 (4-ounce) chops
Lean ground beef –
1 pound

Grains/Bread/Pasta
Soba noodles or linguine
pasta – 1 box
Crispy rice cereal –
small box
Grits – small box
Prepackaged 12-inch
pizza crust

Dairy and Cheese
Eggs
Shredded, reduced-fat
cheddar cheese –
1 package
Shredded, reduced-fat
Mexican-style cheese
– 1 package

Canned Goods and Sauces
Lite soy sauce – small
bottle
6-ounce can tuna packed
in water – 2 cans
Light Italian dressing –
small bottle
14.5-ounce can fat-free,
reduced-sodium
chicken broth – 1 can
Salsa – 1 jar

Staples/Seasonings/ Baking Needs
Salt/ground black pepper
Cooking spray
Sesame oil
Olive oil
Cayenne pepper
Rice wine vinegar
Red wine vinegar
Apple cider vinegar
All-purpose flour
Dijon mustard
Allspice
Cumin
Chili powder
Cayenne pepper
Onion salt
Hot pepper sauce
Honey

Miscellaneous
Smooth peanut butter –
small jar
Roasted, salted peanuts
– small package
Sesame seeds

Asian Beef Noodle Salad

Makes: 6 servings   *Serving Size: 1/6 recipe*   *Prep Time: 15 minutes*

DRESSING

2 tablespoons smooth peanut butter
2 tablespoons lite soy sauce
1 tablespoon fresh lime juice
1/4 teaspoon cayenne pepper
1/2 cup chopped fresh mint

SALAD

1 pound soba noodles or linguine, uncooked
2 tablespoons lite soy sauce
2 tablespoons rice wine vinegar
1 pound top sirloin steak, cut into 3-inch strips
2 teaspoons sesame oil
   Cooking spray
2 medium cucumbers, peeled, seeded, and sliced into thin sticks

2 medium carrots, shredded
4 scallions, cut diagonally
1/4 cup roasted salted peanuts, coarsely chopped
2 tablespoons sesame seeds, toasted

1. In a medium bowl, whisk together dressing ingredients. Set aside.

2. Cook noodles according to package directions, omitting salt; drain and rinse under cold water to cool.

3. In a medium bowl, whisk together soy sauce and rice wine vinegar. Add beef and toss to coat.

4. Add the sesame oil and a generous amount of cooking spray to a large sauté pan or wok over high heat. Stir-fry beef in batches; set aside to cool slightly.

5. In a large salad bowl, toss remaining ingredients, except sesame seeds, with cooled noodles. Drizzle the dressing over the salad and toss to coat.

6. Arrange 6 portions of the salad on salad plates and top with a portion of beef. Garnish with toasted sesame seeds.

Exchanges

3 1/2 Starch	1 Vegetable
2 Medium-Fat Meat	1/2 Fat

Calories	476
Calories from Fat	122
Total Fat	14 g
Saturated Fat	3 g
Cholesterol	43 mg
Sodium	1177 mg
Total Carbohydrate	59 g
Dietary Fiber	7 g
Sugars	8 g
Protein	30 g

Chef's Tip: This is a great luncheon dish . . . easy and impressive!

Chicken Fingers

Makes: 5 servings   *Serving Size: 3 chicken strips*   *Prep Time: 15 minutes*

Cooking spray
1/2 cup all-purpose flour
1/2 teaspoon salt
1/4 teaspoon ground black pepper
1 egg
2 egg whites
1/2 teaspoon hot pepper sauce
2 cups crispy rice cereal, crushed
1 pound boneless, skinless chicken breasts, cut into strips (about 15 strips)

1. Preheat oven to 350 degrees. Coat a large baking dish with cooking spray.

2. Combine flour, salt, and pepper and spread out on a plate. In a medium bowl, whisk together egg, egg whites, and hot pepper sauce. Spread crushed cereal out on a plate.

3. Dredge each strip in flour, dip in egg mixture, then roll in cereal, coating completely.

4. Line strips in the bottom of the baking dish and spray generously with cooking spray. Bake for 25 minutes.

✔ *Children's Eye Health and Safety Month is in September. Teach your kids how to keep their eyes safe and well!*

Exchanges

1 Starch	3 Very Lean Meat

Calories 205
  Calories from Fat 32
Total Fat . . . . 4 g
  Saturated Fat . . . . 1 g
Cholesterol . . . . 97 mg
Sodium . . . . 364 mg
Total Carbohydrate . . . . . . 17 g
  Dietary Fiber . . . . 0 g
  Sugars . . . . 1 g
Protein . . . . 24 g

Chef's Tip: Use heated barbecue sauce or low-fat Ranch dressing as dipping sauces for these crispy chicken fingers.

Savory Grits

Makes: 7 servings   *Serving Size: 1/2 cup*   *Prep Time: 10 minutes*

3 1/2 cups water
3/4 cup grits
1/2 teaspoon salt
3 ounces shredded, reduced-fat cheddar cheese
1/4 cup chopped scallions

1. In a medium saucepan, bring water to a boil. Stir in grits and salt, stirring vigorously. Reduce heat and simmer covered for 15–20 minutes, stirring occasionally.

2. Stir in cheese and scallions until cheese melts.

Exchanges
1 Starch

Calories 82
Calories from Fat 25
Total Fat . . . . 3 g
Saturated Fat . . . . 2 g
Cholesterol . . . . 9 mg
Sodium . . . . 270 mg
Total Carbohydrate . . . . . . 13 g
Dietary Fiber . . . . 1 g
Sugars . . . . 0 g
Protein . . . . 4 g

Dietitian's Tip: This tasty recipe is a healthy version of the old Southern favorite.

Salad Niçoise

Makes: 4 servings   *Serving Size: 1/4 recipe*   *Prep Time: 20 minutes*

DRESSING

1/4 cup red wine vinegar

2 tablespoons Dijon mustard

2 tablespoons olive oil

SALAD

4 cups chopped romaine lettuce

2 6-ounce cans tuna packed in water, drained

4 cups green beans, steamed to tender-crisp and cooled

1 pound red new potatoes, boiled and quartered

4 hard-boiled egg whites, quartered

2 cups tomatoes, diced

1. In a small bowl, whisk together dressing ingredients; set aside.

2. Place 1 cup romaine lettuce on a plate and top with 1/4 of the tuna, 1 cup green beans, 8 potato quarters, 4 egg white slices, and 1/4 of the tomatoes.

3. Drizzle 1/4 of the dressing over salad. Repeat procedure for remaining 3 salads.

Exchanges

2 Starch	3 Vegetable
3 Lean Meat	1/2 Fat

Calories 419

Calories from Fat 121

Total Fat . . . . 13 g

Saturated Fat . . . . 3 g

Cholesterol . . . . 234 mg

Sodium . . . . 522 mg

Total Carbohydrate . . . . . . 44 g

Dietary Fiber . . . . 7 g

Sugars . . . . 9 g

Protein . . . . 33 g

Chef's Tip: This French classic is easy and delicious.

Grilled Veal Chops

Makes: 4 servings   *Serving Size: 1 veal chop*   *Prep Time: 5 minutes*

4 4-ounce boneless veal chops
2 tablespoons light Italian dressing
1/2 teaspoon salt
1/4 teaspoon ground black pepper

1. Prepare an indoor or outdoor grill. Trim any visible fat from chops. Brush each side with dressing. Season well with salt and pepper.

2. Grill for 4–6 minutes on each side over medium heat.

Exchanges
3 Lean Meat

Calories 175	
Calories from Fat 67	
Total Fat . . . . 7 g	
Saturated Fat . . . . 2 g	
Cholesterol . . . . 91 mg	
Sodium . . . . 420 mg	
Total Carbohydrate . . . . 1 g	
Dietary Fiber . . . . 0 g	
Sugars . . . . 1 g	
Protein . . . . 25 g	

Chef's Tip: You can use pork instead of veal if you wish.

Braised Red Cabbage

Makes: 4 servings   *Serving Size: 1/2 cup*   *Prep Time: 10 minutes*

1 14.5-ounce can fat-free, reduced-sodium chicken broth

1/2 cup apple cider vinegar

2 tablespoons red wine vinegar

1 tablespoon honey

1/2 teaspoon allspice

1/4 teaspoon salt

4 cups shredded red cabbage

2 small Granny Smith apples, grated

1. In a large saucepan, bring broth, vinegars, honey, allspice, and salt to a boil.

2. Add cabbage and apples. Reduce heat and simmer uncovered for 30 minutes.

Exchanges

1 Vegetable	1 Fruit

Calories	78
Calories from Fat	4
Total Fat	0 g
Saturated Fat	0 g
Cholesterol	0 mg
Sodium	403 mg
Total Carbohydrate	19 g
Dietary Fiber	3 g
Sugars	15 g
Protein	2 g

Chef's Tip: Use the large holes on your cheese grater to grate the apples for this recipe.

Taco Pizza

Makes: 8 servings   *Serving Size: 1 slice*   *Prep Time: 15 minutes*

1/2 pound lean ground beef
1/3 cup water
1/2 teaspoon cumin
1/2 tablespoon chili powder
1/8 teaspoon cayenne pepper
1/2 teaspoon onion salt
1 12-inch prepackaged pizza crust
1 1/2 cups salsa
1 1/4 cups shredded, reduced-fat Mexican-style cheese

1. Preheat oven to 450 degrees.

2. Brown beef in a large nonstick skillet over medium-high heat until thoroughly cooked and no longer pink. Drain fat. Add water, cumin, chili powder, cayenne pepper, and onion salt and simmer 2–4 minutes.

3. Place pizza crust on baking sheet. Spread salsa over pizza crust.

4. Spoon taco meat over pizza crust and distribute evenly. Top with cheese. Bake 10 minutes or until pizza crust is crisp and cheese is melted.

Exchanges

1 1/2 Starch	1/2 Fat
2 Lean Meat	

Calories 248
Calories from Fat 88
Total Fat . . . . 10 g
Saturated Fat . . . . 4 g
Cholesterol . . . . 30 mg
Sodium . . . . 634 mg
Total Carbohydrate . . . . . . 25 g
Dietary Fiber . . . . 1 g
Sugars . . . . 2 g
Protein . . . . 16 g

Chef's Tip: You can top this pizza with lettuce, tomato, and fat-free sour cream after baking if you like.

September ❖ Week 3

GROCERY LIST

Fresh Produce
Garlic – 1 head
Oranges – 2
10-ounce bag romaine
lettuce – 2 bags
Onions – 2 small
Tomato – 1 large
Broccoli – 2 heads
Russet potatoes –
4 medium

Meat/Poultry/Fish
Boneless, skinless
chicken breasts –
3/4 pound
Perch filets – 4
(4-ounce) filets
Lean ground turkey –
3/4 pound
Ham steaks – 4
(4-ounce) steaks
Whole roaster chicken –
5–6 pounds

Grains/Bread/Pasta
Long-grain white rice

Dairy and Cheese
Shredded, reduced-fat
cheddar cheese –
1 package
Fat-free milk

Canned Goods and Sauces
Lite soy sauce – small
bottle
11-ounce can Mandarin
oranges in juice –
2 cans
Fat-free Italian dressing
– small bottle
15-ounce can crushed
tomatoes – 1 can
14.5-ounce can fat-free,
reduced-sodium
chicken broth – 1 can
12-ounce can evaporated
fat-free milk – 1 can
16-ounce can black
beans – 1 can
15-ounce can chickpeas
(garbanzo beans)–
1 can
Light sugar-free apricot
preserves – small jar
Ketchup – small bottle
10 3/4-ounce can
reduced-fat condensed
cream of celery soup –
1 can

Staples/Seasonings/ Baking Needs
Salt/ground black pepper
Cooking spray
Canola oil
Sesame oil
Chili powder
Cumin
Dried oregano
Dried basil
Curry powder
Ground nutmeg
Cayenne pepper
Ground cinnamon

Miscellaneous
Coconut flakes – small
bag

Mandarin Orange Chicken Salad

Makes: 4 servings   *Serving Size: 1/4 recipe*   *Prep Time: 35 minutes*

SALAD

1/2 cup orange juice
  1 teaspoon canola oil
  1 tablespoon lite soy sauce
  1 garlic clove, sliced
3/4 pound boneless, skinless
    chicken breasts
    Cooking spray
  1 10-ounce bag romaine lettuce
  2 11-ounce cans mandarin
    oranges packed in juice,
    drained (reserve 1/4 cup juice)

DRESSING

1/2 cup fat-free Italian dressing
1/4 cup reserved mandarin orange
    juice

1. Preheat boiler. Combine orange juice, canola oil, soy sauce, and garlic in a large mixing bowl. Place chicken in bowl and marinate in the refrigerator for 15 minutes.

2. Coat broiler with cooking spray and place chicken on broiler rack. Broil 3 inches away from heat until lightly brown (approximately 4 minutes on each side).

3. Cut cooked chicken into cubes. In a large salad bowl, toss lettuce, chicken, and mandarin oranges.

4. In a small bowl, whisk together Italian dressing and mandarin orange juice.

5. Drizzle dressing over salad and toss well to coat.

Exchanges

3 Very Lean Meat	1/2 Fruit
1 Vegetable	1/2 Fat

Calories 177	
Calories from Fat 26	
Total Fat . . . . 3 g	
Saturated Fat . . . . 1 g	
Cholesterol . . . . 51 mg	
Sodium . . . . 441 mg	
Total Carbohydrate . . . . . . 16 g	
Dietary Fiber . . . . 1 g	
Sugars . . . . 13 g	
Protein . . . . 21 g	

Chef's Tip: Instead of broiling the chicken, you can also grill it on an indoor or outdoor grill.

Baked Perch

Makes: 4 servings   *Serving Size: 1 filet*   *Prep Time: 10 minutes*

Cooking spray
4 4-ounce perch filets
1 15-ounce can crushed tomatoes
2 garlic cloves, minced
2 teaspoons chili powder
1/2 teaspoon cumin
1 teaspoon dried oregano
1/2 teaspoon salt (optional)

1. Preheat oven to 350 degrees.

2. Coat a shallow baking dish with cooking spray. Arrange perch filets in bottom of dish.

3. In a small bowl, mix remaining ingredients and pour over fish filets. Bake for 15–20 minutes or until fish flakes easily.

Exchanges

3 Very Lean Meat   2 Vegetable

Calories 155
  Calories from Fat 14
Total Fat . . . . 2 g
  Saturated Fat . . . . 0 g
Cholesterol . . . . 102 mg
Sodium . . . . 379 mg
Total Carbohydrate . . . . . . 10 g
  Dietary Fiber . . . . 3 g
  Sugars . . . . 6 g
Protein . . . . 24 g

Dietitian's Tip: Fish is always a great protein choice. Just remember that baked or broiled fish is much healthier than fried.

Spiced Rice

Makes: 6 servings   *Serving Size: 1/2 cup*   *Prep Time: 15 minutes*

1 tablespoon canola oil

1 small onion, minced

2 garlic cloves, minced

1 1/2 cups long-grain white rice, uncooked

1 teaspoon curry powder

1/2 teaspoon ground nutmeg

1/4 teaspoon cayenne pepper

1/2 teaspoon ground cinnamon

1 1/2 cups fat-free, reduced-sodium chicken broth

1 12-ounce can evaporated fat-free milk

1/4 cup coconut flakes, toasted

1. Add oil to a medium saucepan over medium heat. Add onion and garlic and sauté 3–4 minutes until onion turns clear.

2. Add rice and spices (curry powder through cinnamon), stirring constantly for 1 minute. Add remaining ingredients and bring to a boil. Reduce heat and simmer, covered, for 20 minutes or until all liquid is absorbed.

Exchanges

2 1/2 Starch	1/2 Fat
1/2 Fat-Free Milk	

Calories 268
  Calories from Fat 35
Total Fat . . . . 4 g
  Saturated Fat . . . . 1 g
Cholesterol . . . . 0 mg
Sodium . . . . 216 mg
Total Carbohydrate . . . . . . 48 g
  Dietary Fiber . . . . 1 g
  Sugars . . . . 9 g
Protein . . . . 9 g

Chef's Tip: There are a lot of ways to liven up everyday rice. This recipe is just one way to turn a plain side dish into an exciting accompaniment.

Southwest Salad

1 small onion, diced
3/4 pound lean ground turkey
2 teaspoons chili powder
1/2 teaspoon cumin
1/4 teaspoon cayenne pepper
1 16-ounce can black beans, rinsed and drained
1 15-ounce can chickpeas, rinsed and drained
1 large tomato, seeded and diced
4 cups chopped romaine lettuce
1/3 cup shredded, reduced-fat cheddar cheese

1. Add onion and ground turkey to a large nonstick skillet over medium-high heat. Cook about 8–10 minutes or until turkey is cooked through (no longer pink).

2. Add chili powder, cumin, and cayenne pepper and cook 2 more minutes. Gently stir in beans, chickpeas, and tomatoes and cook an additional 2 minutes. Set aside to cool slightly.

3. Toss meat mixture with lettuce in a large bowl. Sprinkle with cheese.

Exchanges

2 Starch	1 Vegetable
3 Lean Meat	1/2 Fat

Calories 376
 Calories from Fat 113
Total Fat . . . . 13 g
 Saturated Fat . . . . 4 g
Cholesterol . . . . 70 mg
Sodium . . . . 350 mg
Total Carbohydrate . . . . . . 37 g
 Dietary Fiber . . . . 11 g
 Sugars . . . . 9 g
Protein . . . . 32 g

Chef's Tip: Chickpeas are also known as garbanzo beans.

Glazed Ham Steaks

Makes: 4 servings   *Serving Size: 1 ham steak*   *Prep Time: 10 minutes*

1/2 cup light sugar-free apricot preserves
1 tablespoon lite soy sauce
1 tablespoon ketchup
Cooking spray
4 4-ounce ham steaks

1. Preheat oven to 375 degrees.

2. In a small saucepan, bring the preserves, soy sauce, and ketchup to a boil. Reduce heat and simmer for 4–5 minutes.

3. Coat a shallow baking dish with cooking spray. Arrange ham steaks in the bottom of the dish. Brush glaze on top and sides of ham steaks. Bake for 15–20 minutes.

Exchanges

3 Lean Meat   1/2 Carbohydrate

Calories 164
Calories from Fat 44
Total Fat . . . . 5 g
Saturated Fat . . . . 2 g
Cholesterol . . . . 51 mg
Sodium . . . . 1635 mg
Total Carbohydrate . . . . 6 g
Dietary Fiber . . . . 0 g
Sugars . . . . 1 g
Protein . . . . 22 g

Chef's Tip: Fruits such as apricots, prunes, pears, and apples go well with pork dishes.

Broccoli Casserole

Makes: 8 servings   *Serving Size: 1/2 cup*   *Prep Time: 10 minutes*

4 cups broccoli florets, steamed
10 3/4-ounce can reduced-fat condensed cream of celery soup

1/2 cup fat-free milk

1/2 cup shredded, reduced-fat cheddar cheese

1/8 teaspoon ground black pepper

1. Preheat oven to 350 degrees.

2. In a large bowl, combine all ingredients. Pour into a medium casserole dish and bake for 30 minutes.

Exchanges

1/2 Fat   1/2 Carbohydrate

Calories	54
Calories from Fat	25
Total Fat	3 g
Saturated Fat	2 g
Cholesterol	7 mg
Sodium	350 mg
Total Carbohydrate	6 g
Dietary Fiber	1 g
Sugars	2 g
Protein	4 g

Dietitian's Tip: Broccoli is a cruciferous vegetable, like cauliflower and Brussels sprouts, and may help protect you against some cancers. Broccoli also has plenty of vitamins A and C, folic acid, and lots of fiber!

Thai-Spiced Roasted Chicken with Potatoes

Makes: 8 servings   *Serving Size: 3 ounces chicken*   *Prep Time: 15 minutes*
plus 4 potato wedges

1 5 1/2-pound whole
  roaster chicken
1 teaspoon salt, divided
1 teaspoon ground black pepper,
  divided
1 tablespoon sesame oil
1 tablespoon curry powder
1 tablespoon dried basil
  Cooking spray
4 medium russet potatoes, cut into
  eighths

> **Chef's Tip:** To make this chicken Italian-style, substitute olive oil for sesame oil and dried oregano for the curry powder.

Exchanges (without skin)

1 Starch	1 Fat
4 Lean Meat	

Calories. 277	
Calories from Fat. 87	
Total Fat . . . . 10 g	
Saturated Fat . . . . 2 g	
Cholesterol . . . . 88 mg	
Sodium . . . . 382 mg	
Total Carbohydrate. . . . . . 15 g	
Dietary Fiber . . . . 2 g	
Sugars. . . . . 1 g	
Protein. . . . . 31 g	

1. Preheat oven to 450 degrees. Remove and discard giblet and neck from chicken cavity. Trim excess fat around neck and cavity opening. Rinse chicken with cold water and pat dry.

2. Season inside of cavity with 1/2 teaspoon salt and 1/2 teaspoon pepper. Starting at the neck, loosen skin around breast using your finger. Rub entire chicken (including breast meat under the skin) with sesame oil.

3. In a small bowl, mix curry and basil together. Rub half of mixture onto the breasts under the skin and rub the entire chicken with remaining mixture.

4. Place chicken breast side up into a roasting pan coated with cooking spray. Place potatoes around the chicken. Sprinkle entire chicken and potatoes with remaining 1/2 teaspoon salt and 1/2 teaspoon pepper.

5. Bake in oven for 30 minutes. After 30 minutes, reduce heat to 350 degrees and bake chicken an additional 45 minutes.

September ❖ Week 4

GROCERY LIST

Fresh Produce
Lemons – 2
Fresh tarragon – 1 bunch
Red bell peppers –
2 medium
Green bell pepper –
1 medium
Carrots – medium bag
Broccoli – 2 heads
Mushrooms – 1/2 pint
10-ounce bag fresh
spinach – 1 bag
Plum (Roma)
tomatoes – 4
Italian (flat-leaf)
parsley – 1 bunch

Meat/Poultry/Fish
Imitation crabmeat –
1 pound
Ground pork tenderloin –
1 pound
Turkey bacon –
1 package
Boneless, skinless
chicken breasts –
3/4 pound
Top sirloin steak –
1 pound

Grains/Bread/Pasta
Medium pasta shells –
1 box
Penne pasta – 1 box
Brown rice
Saltine crackers – small
box
Crispy rice cereal –
small box

Dairy and Cheese
Eggs
Fresh mozzarella cheese,
packed in water –
6 ounces

Canned Goods and Sauces
Light mayonnaise – 1 jar
14.5-ounce can fat-free,
reduced-sodium
chicken broth – 1 can
14.5-ounce can fat-free,
reduced-sodium beef
broth – 1 can
Lite soy sauce – small
bottle
15.5-ounce can pink
salmon – 2 cans
Dijon mustard – small
bottle

Frozen Foods
Light or fat-free cookies
and cream ice cream –
1 quart

Staples/Seasonings/Baking Needs
Salt/ground black pepper
Whole black peppercorns
Cooking spray
Olive oil
Cornstarch
Dijon mustard
Garlic salt
Dried minced onion
Dried tarragon
Apple cider vinegar
Balsamic vinegar
Sugar
Light chocolate syrup –
small bottle
Semi-sweet chocolate
chips – small bag
Honey

Crab Pasta Salad

Makes: 6 servings　　　　*Serving Size: 1/6 recipe*　　　　*Prep Time: 15 minutes*

DRESSING

1/4 cup light mayonnaise
　1 tablespoon lemon juice
　2 tablespoons chopped fresh
　　tarragon
1/4 teaspoon salt
　　Dash ground black pepper

SALAD

　1 pound medium pasta shells,
　　uncooked
　1 pound chopped imitation
　　crabmeat
　1 medium red bell pepper, diced
　1 medium green bell pepper,
　　diced
　1 large carrot, diced

1. In a small bowl, whisk together dressing ingredients; set aside.

2. Cook pasta according to package directions, omitting salt; drain and rinse under cold water until cooled.

3. In a large bowl, toss together cooled pasta with remaining salad ingredients. Drizzle dressing over salad and toss well to coat.

Exchanges

2 Starch	1 Vegetable
1 Very Lean Meat	1/2 Fat

Calories 239
　Calories from Fat 46
Total Fat . . . . 5 g
　Saturated Fat . . . . 1 g
Cholesterol . . . . 19 mg
Sodium . . . . 820 mg
Total Carbohydrate . . . . . . 35 g
　Dietary Fiber . . . . 2 g
　Sugars . . . . 11 g
Protein . . . . 13 g

Chef's Tip: Imitation crabmeat is also known as surimi. It has an excellent flavor and is much lower in cost than crab or lobster meat. Look for it in the fresh or frozen seafood section of your market.

Pork Stir-Fry

Makes: 4 servings   *Serving Size: 1/4 recipe*   *Prep Time: 15 minutes*

1 pound ground pork tenderloin
Cooking spray
2 cups broccoli florets
1 medium red bell pepper, thinly sliced
1/2 pint sliced mushrooms
1/2 cup fat-free, reduced-sodium chicken broth
2 teaspoons cornstarch
2 tablespoons lite soy sauce
1/2 teaspoon garlic salt
2 cups brown rice, cooked

1. Cook pork in a large nonstick skillet or wok over medium-high heat for 5–7 minutes or until no longer pink. Drain any excess fat and remove from pan.

2. Coat the pan with cooking spray. Add broccoli, bell pepper, and mushrooms and sauté for 5–6 minutes. Add pork back to pan.

3. In a small bowl, whisk broth, cornstarch, soy sauce, and garlic salt. Pour over mixture and bring to a boil. Reduce heat and simmer 2–3 minutes. Serve over brown rice.

Exchanges

1 1/2 Starch	1 Vegetable
3 Very Lean Meat	1/2 Fat

Calories 282
Calories from Fat 47
Total Fat . . . . 5 g
Saturated Fat . . . . 2 g
Cholesterol . . . . 66 mg
Sodium . . . . 570 mg
Total Carbohydrate . . . . . . 29 g
Dietary Fiber . . . . 4 g
Sugars . . . . 4 g
Protein . . . . 29 g

Dietitian's Tip: Tired of chicken stir-fry? Try this dish for a nice change.

Salmon Loaf

Makes: 6 servings   *Serving Size: 1 slice*   *Prep Time: 10 minutes*

Cooking spray

1 egg

2 egg whites

2 tablespoons water

2 15.5-ounce cans pink salmon with liquid

2 cups coarse cracker crumbs

1 tablespoon dried minced onion

1 teaspoon dried tarragon

1/2 teaspoon salt (optional)

1/4 teaspoon ground black pepper

1. Preheat oven to 350 degrees. Coat a 9-inch loaf pan with cooking spray.

2. In a large bowl, beat eggs and water. Add remaining ingredients and mix well to incorporate.

3. Gently spread into loaf pan and bake for 60 minutes.

Exchanges

1 Starch   4 Lean Meat

Calories 325
　Calories from Fat 112
Total Fat . . . . 12 g
　Saturated Fat . . . . 1 g
Cholesterol . . . . 118 mg
Sodium . . . . 1145 mg
Total Carbohydrate . . . . . . 18 g
　Dietary Fiber . . . . 1 g
　Sugars . . . . 1 g
Protein . . . . 33 g

Chef's Tip: Be sure to pick through the meat carefully and remove any bones from canned salmon—the spinal bones are often still intact.

Spinach Salad with Warm Bacon Dressing

Makes: 8 servings   *Serving Size: 1/2 cup*   *Prep Time: 5 minutes*

Cooking spray

6 strips turkey bacon, diced

1/2 cup apple cider vinegar

1 tablespoon olive oil

2 tablespoons honey

1/4 teaspoon salt

1 10-ounce bag fresh spinach leaves, torn

1. Coat a small sauté pan with cooking spray and heat over medium-high heat. Add bacon and sauté 3 minutes or until bacon is crispy. Add remaining ingredients except spinach and bring to a boil. Boil for 5–7 minutes or until slightly thickened.

2. Place spinach in a large bowl. Drizzle hot dressing over spinach and toss to coat.

✔ *September is National Cholesterol Education Month . . . high fat intake can cause too much cholesterol to build up in your bloodstream! Watch your fat intake every day.*

Exchanges

1/2 Fat	1/2 Carbohydrate

Calories 63
  Calories from Fat 33
Total Fat . . . . 4 g
  Saturated Fat . . . . 1 g
Cholesterol . . . . 8 mg
Sodium . . . . 229 mg
Total Carbohydrate . . . . 6 g
  Dietary Fiber . . . . 1 g
  Sugars . . . . 5 g
Protein . . . . 3 g

Chef's Tip: Turkey bacon is an excellent, healthier substitute for real bacon. Use it in any recipe— you won't be able to tell the difference!

Chicken Pasta Salad with Fresh Mozzarella

Makes: 9 servings   *Serving Size: 1 cup*   *Prep Time: 15 minutes*

DRESSING

- **5** tablespoons balsamic vinegar
- **2** tablespoons olive oil
- **1/2** teaspoon Dijon mustard

SALAD

- **8** ounces penne pasta, uncooked
- **3/4** pound boneless, skinless chicken breasts, cooked and cubed
- **4** ripe plum (Roma) tomatoes, diced
- **1/4** cup chopped flat-leaf parsley
- **6** ounces fresh Mozzarella cheese, cubed

1. In a small bowl, whisk together dressing ingredients; set aside.

2. Cook pasta according to package directions, omitting salt. Drain pasta and run under cold water until pasta is cooled. In a large bowl, toss cooled pasta with remaining salad ingredients.

3. Drizzle dressing over salad and toss well to coat.

Exchanges

1 1/2 Starch	2 Lean Meat

Calories	224
Calories from Fat	71
Total Fat	8 g
Saturated Fat	3 g
Cholesterol	29 mg
Sodium	132 mg
Total Carbohydrate	22 g
Dietary Fiber	1 g
Sugars	3 g
Protein	16 g

Chef's Tip: This is a refreshing and beautiful dish that is easy to prepare.

Steak au Poivre

Makes: 4 servings   *Serving Size: 1/4 recipe*   *Prep Time: 5 minutes*

1 pound boneless top sirloin steak
1/2 teaspoon salt
1/2 teaspoon ground black pepper
    Cooking spray
1 teaspoon black peppercorns, crushed
1/2 cup fat-free, reduced-sodium beef broth

1. Trim any visible fat from sirloin. Season both sides with salt and pepper.

2. Coat a medium oven-safe skillet with cooking spray over high heat. Sear both sides of steak for 3–4 minutes or until brown. Place skillet in oven and bake for 10 minutes. Remove from oven.

3. Remove steak from pan and set aside. Cover steak. Place skillet back on stove over high heat. Add remaining ingredients to skillet and bring to a boil for 5–7 minutes or until sauce is reduced by one-fourth. Pour sauce over steak.

Exchanges
3 Lean Meat

Calories 141
  Calories from Fat 44
Total Fat . . . . 5 g
  Saturated Fat . . . . 2 g
Cholesterol . . . . 64 mg
Sodium . . . . 395 mg
Total Carbohydrate . . . . 0 g
  Dietary Fiber . . . . 0 g
  Sugars . . . . 0 g
Protein . . . . 22 g

Chef's Tip: Find whole black peppercorns in the spice aisle of your market.

Carrot Salad

1 1/2 tablespoons lemon juice

1 tablespoon olive oil

2 tablespoons finely chopped fresh parsley

1/2 teaspoon salt

1/2 teaspoon sugar

6 large carrots, peeled and grated

1. In a medium bowl, whisk together all ingredients except carrots.

2. Add carrots and toss well to coat.

Exchanges

2 Vegetable	1/2 Fat

Calories 79
Calories from Fat 26
Total Fat . . . . 3 g
Saturated Fat . . . . 0 g
Cholesterol . . . . 0 mg
Sodium . . . . 277 mg
Total Carbohydrate . . . . . . 13 g
Dietary Fiber . . . . 4 g
Sugars . . . . 8 g
Protein . . . . 1 g

Dietitian's Tip: Many people think carrots are in the starch exchange group, but they're not. They're in the vegetable group, which means you can eat more of them without your blood sugar going up!

Cookie Ice Cream Pie

Makes: 8 servings   *Serving Size: 1/8 pie*   *Prep Time: 25 minutes*

Cooking spray
1/2 cup light chocolate syrup
2 tablespoons semi-sweet
  chocolate chips
2 cups crispy rice cereal
4 cups light or fat-free cookies
  and cream ice cream, softened

1. Coat an 8-inch pie plate with cooking spray.

2. In a small microwave-safe bowl, combine chocolate syrup and chocolate chips. Microwave on high for 45–60 seconds. Stir until smooth. Reserve 1/4 cup of chocolate mixture.

3. In a medium bowl, combine remaining chocolate mixture and cereal and stir gently to coat.

4. Press mixture into pie plate, covering bottom and sides of plate. Freeze until firm, about 15 minutes.

5. Spread half the ice cream (2 cups) into the pie plate. Drizzle with half the chocolate sauce mixture. Top with remaining ice cream and drizzle with remaining chocolate mixture.

6. Freeze pie, covered, about 1 hour or until firm.

Exchanges

2 1/2 Carbohydrate

Calories 185
  Calories from Fat 27
Total Fat . . . . 3 g
  Saturated Fat . . . . 2 g
Cholesterol . . . . 5 mg
Sodium . . . . 172 mg
Total Carbohydrate . . . . . . 36 g
  Dietary Fiber . . . . 1 g
  Sugars . . . . 23 g
Protein . . . . 4 g

Chef's Tip: You can top this dessert with 4 crushed Oreo cookies right before serving.

October

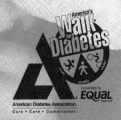

America's Walk for Diabetes®
is the ADA's signature walk
fundraising event. Each mile
you walk and event dollar
you raise helps in the fight to
prevent and cure diabetes and
improve the lives of all
people affected by diabetes.
Call 1-888-diabetes
to register today!

Great Veggie Fare

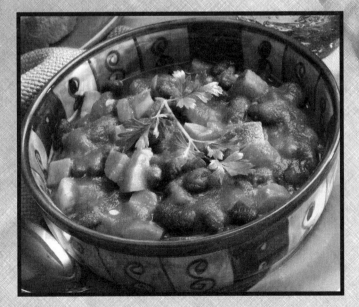

Veggie Chili (page 350)
If you're looking for a great vegetarian chili recipe,
this is it. You won't miss the meat at all! Serve it
with a crunchy salad and warm muffins or bread.

October ❖ Recipes

October ❖ Week 1

GROCERY LIST

Fresh Produce
Garlic – 1 head
Celery – small bag
Onions – 3 medium
Green bell pepper – 1
Fresh cilantro – 1 bunch
Fresh tarragon – 1 bunch
Mushrooms – 1 1/2 pints
Zucchini – 2 medium
Carrots – small bag
Idaho potatoes –
2 medium

Meat/Poultry/Fish
95% fat-free turkey kiel-
basa – 1 pound
Boneless, skinless
chicken breasts –
1 pound

Grains/Bread/Pasta
Farfalle pasta – 1 box
Cornmeal – 1 box
Whole-wheat bread –
10 slices

Dairy and Cheese
Low-fat buttermilk –
small carton
Fat-free milk – small
carton
Fat-free half-and-half –
1 pint
Eggs
Shredded, reduced-fat
cheddar cheese –
1 package
Light cream cheese –
7 ounces
Bleu cheese – 1 package
Fresh Parmesan cheese –
1 wedge
Plain, fat-free yogurt –
small carton

Canned Goods and Sauces
15-ounce can black
beans – 3 cans
14.5-ounce can no-salt-
added diced
tomatoes – 2 cans
4-ounce can chopped
green chilies – 1 can
15-ounce can pumpkin –
1 can
15-ounce can chickpeas
(garbanzo beans) –
1 can
14.5-ounce can fat-free,
reduced-sodium
chicken broth – 3 cans
Light mayonnaise – 1 jar

Frozen Foods
10-ounce package
spinach – 1 package

Staples/Seasonings/ Baking Needs
Salt/ground black pepper
Cooking spray
Olive oil
Canola oil
Cumin
Dried oregano
Bay leaf
Cayenne pepper
Dried sage
Paprika
Onion salt
Ground nutmeg
Dried thyme
Reduced-fat baking mix
Cornstarch

Miscellaneous
White wine – small
bottle
Slivered almonds –
small package

Black Bean Soup

Makes: 10 servings   *Serving Size: 1 cup*   *Prep Time: 15 minutes*

1 teaspoon olive oil

1 pound 95% fat-free turkey kielbasa, chopped

3 medium onions, coarsely chopped

2 medium celery stalks, diced

3 garlic cloves, minced

3 16-ounce cans black beans, rinsed and drained

4 cups water

1 15-ounce can no-salt-added diced tomatoes

1 4-ounce can chopped green chilies

1 teaspoon ground cumin

2 teaspoons dried oregano

1 bay leaf

1 green bell pepper, diced

1/2 teaspoon salt (optional)

1/4 teaspoon ground black pepper

1 tablespoon chopped fresh cilantro

1. Add oil to a large soup pot over high heat. Add kielbasa and sauté for 4–5 minutes or until beginning to brown.

2. Stir in onions, celery, and garlic. Sauté an additional 5 minutes or until onions turn clear.

3. Stir in remaining ingredients except cilantro and bring to a boil. Reduce heat and simmer 15 minutes.

4. Remove bay leaf and stir in cilantro.

Exchanges

1 1/2 Starch   2 Vegetable
1 Very Lean Meat

Calories 199
  Calories from Fat 36
Total Fat . . . . 4 g
  Saturated Fat . . . . 1 g
Cholesterol . . . . 21 mg
Sodium . . . . 555 mg
Total Carbohydrate . . . . . . 30 g
  Dietary Fiber . . . . 9 g
  Sugars . . . . 8 g
Protein . . . . 13 g

Chef's Tip: Serve a dollop of fat-free sour cream and a sprig of fresh cilantro on each serving of soup.

Cheese Muffins

Makes: 12 servings   *Serving Size: 1 muffin*   *Prep Time: 5 minutes*

Cooking spray
2 cups reduced-fat baking mix
2/3 cup low-fat buttermilk
1 tablespoon canola oil
1 egg
3/4 cup shredded, reduced-fat cheddar cheese
1/4 teaspoon ground black pepper

1. Preheat oven to 400 degrees. Coat a muffin pan with cooking spray.

2. In a medium bowl, mix together baking mix, buttermilk, oil, and egg with a fork. Stir vigorously.

3. Fold in remaining ingredients. Divide batter evenly among tins. Bake for 20 minutes until golden brown.

✔ *National Family Health Month is in October . . . serve delicious, nutritious meals every day!*

Exchanges

1 Starch   1/2 Fat

Calories 106
  Calories from Fat 42
Total Fat . . . . 5 g
  Saturated Fat . . . . 1 g
Cholesterol . . . . 23 mg
Sodium . . . . 330 mg
Total Carbohydrate . . . . . . 14 g
  Dietary Fiber . . . . 1 g
  Sugars . . . . 2 g
Protein . . . . 4 g

Chef's Tip: To add some color to these muffins, stir in 1 tablespoon chopped fresh parsley when you add the cheese.

Pumpkin Pasta

Makes: 10 servings   *Serving Size: 1 cup*   *Prep Time: 15 minutes*

16 ounces farfalle pasta, uncooked

1 teaspoon olive oil

7 ounces light cream cheese, cubed

1/4 cup grated fresh Parmesan cheese

1/2 cup fat-free milk

1 15-ounce can pumpkin

1/2 teaspoon cayenne pepper

1/4 teaspoon salt

1/4 teaspoon ground black pepper

1/4 teaspoon dried sage

Pinch ground nutmeg

1. Cook pasta according to package directions, omitting salt. Drain.

2. In a large saucepan, heat olive oil, cream cheese, Parmesan cheese, and milk over low heat until cream cheese is melted, stirring frequently. Add remaining ingredients and cook until thoroughly heated.

3. Add cooked pasta to pan and toss gently to coat.

Exchanges

2 1/2 Starch	1 Fat

Calories 251
  Calories from Fat 56
Total Fat . . . . 6 g
  Saturated Fat . . . . 3 g
Cholesterol . . . . 16 mg
Sodium . . . . 171 mg
Total Carbohydrate . . . . . . 39 g
  Dietary Fiber . . . . 3 g
  Sugars . . . . 5 g
Protein . . . . 10 g

Dietitian's Tip: This rare combination of flavors will have your guests coming back for more. This recipe is not only great in flavor, but an excellent source of vitamin A.

Mushroom and Bleu Cheese Polenta

Makes: 6 servings   *Serving Size: 1 cup*   *Prep Time: 10 minutes*

2 cups cornmeal

6 cups water

1 teaspoon olive oil

6 cups mushrooms, finely chopped

2 garlic cloves, minced

1/2 teaspoon dried thyme

1/2 cup white wine

1/2 cup fat-free half-and-half

1/2 teaspoon salt

1/4 teaspoon ground black pepper

1/4 cup bleu cheese

3 tablespoons grated Parmesan cheese

1. In a large saucepan, combine cornmeal and water. While whisking, bring to a boil. Reduce to a simmer, whisking occasionally. Cook 20 minutes.

2. While polenta is cooking, heat oil in a medium nonstick skillet. Add mushrooms to skillet and sauté until all the liquid is evaporated (about 6–7 minutes). Add garlic and thyme and sauté for 30 seconds. Add wine and cook until liquid is evaporated.

3. Fold half-and-half into cooked polenta. Fold in salt, pepper, bleu and Parmesan cheeses, and mushrooms until well mixed.

Exchanges

2 1/2 Starch   1/2 Fat

1 Vegetable

Calories	245
Calories from Fat	41
Total Fat	5 g
Saturated Fat	2 g
Cholesterol	9 mg
Sodium	358 mg
Total Carbohydrate	42 g
Dietary Fiber	4 g
Sugars	3 g
Protein	9 g

Chef's Tip: Polenta is an Italian-style cornmeal that is served in different ways. This is a creamy version, but you can also cool it, slice it, and pan-fry it with a little cooking spray, salt, pepper, and Parmesan cheese.

Creamed Spinach

Makes: 5 servings   *Serving Size: 1/4 cup*   *Prep Time: 10 minutes*

2 teaspoons olive oil
1 10-ounce package frozen
   spinach, thawed and drained
1 garlic clove, minced
1 tablespoon cornstarch
1 cup fat-free half-and-half
1/2 teaspoon salt
1/4 teaspoon ground black pepper

1. Add oil to a medium nonstick skillet over medium heat. Add spinach and cook 5–6 minutes or until liquid is evaporated. Stir in garlic and sauté an additional 30 seconds.

2. In a small bowl, whisk together remaining ingredients until all the cornstarch is dissolved. Pour over spinach, stirring constantly. Bring to a boil, then reduce to a simmer for 5 minutes.

 October is Breast Cancer Awareness Month. Please do self-checks every week and get a yearly mammogram!

Exchanges

1/2 Fat   1/2 Carbohydrate

Calories	68
Calories from Fat	23
Total Fat	3 g
Saturated Fat	1 g
Cholesterol	3 mg
Sodium	340 mg
Total Carbohydrate	9 g
Dietary Fiber	1 g
Sugars	3 g
Protein	3 g

Dietitian's Tip: Although spinach is a nutritious food, creamed spinach is usually loaded with fat. We fixed that problem with some fat-free half-and-half.

Toasted Almond Chicken Salad Sandwich

Makes: 5 servings   *Serving Size: 1 sandwich*   *Prep Time: 20 minutes*

1 pound boneless, skinless chicken breasts

2 14.5-ounce cans fat-free, reduced-sodium chicken broth

1 tablespoon fresh tarragon, chopped

1/4 cup almond slivers, toasted

1/3 cup light mayonnaise

2 tablespoons plain, fat-free yogurt

1/2 teaspoon salt
   Dash ground black pepper

10 slices whole-wheat bread, toasted

1. Place chicken breasts in a large saucepan over medium heat. Pour chicken broth over the chicken breasts and bring to a low simmer for 20 minutes or until done. Shred chicken meat and set aside to cool.

2. In a medium bowl, combine remaining ingredients, except bread, and mix well.

3. Add chicken to mixture and toss well to coat. Divide the chicken salad into 5 equal portions. Top one slice of toasted wheat bread with one portion of chicken salad. Top with another slice of bread. Repeat for remaining 4 sandwiches.

Exchanges

2 Starch	2 Fat
3 Very Lean Meat	

Calories	338
Calories from Fat	118
Total Fat	13 g
Saturated Fat	2 g
Cholesterol	59 mg
Sodium	731 mg
Total Carbohydrate	29 g
Dietary Fiber	5 g
Sugars	3 g
Protein	27 g

Chef's Tip: How to make the ordinary more special: add a gourmet touch with fresh tarragon and toasted almonds.

Vegetarian Stew

Makes: 7 servings   *Serving Size: 1 cup*   *Prep Time: 15 minutes*

1/4 cup fat-free, reduced-sodium chicken broth

2 medium zucchini, diced

2 medium carrots, diced

2 celery stalks, diced

2 medium Idaho potatoes, peeled and finely diced

1 14.5-ounce can no-salt-added diced tomatoes

1 teaspoon paprika

1 1/2 teaspoons cumin

1 teaspoon onion salt

1 15-ounce can chickpeas (garbanzo beans)

1/4 teaspoon salt

1/4 teaspoon ground black pepper

1. In a large soup pot, add chicken broth, zucchini, carrots, celery, and potatoes over medium-high heat. Simmer for 5–6 minutes or until vegetables just begin to soften.

2. Add remaining ingredients and bring to a boil. Reduce heat and simmer, covered, for 30 minutes.

✔ *October is Vegetarian Awareness Month. Try a meatless meal today!*

Exchanges

1 1/2 Starch	1 Vegetable

Calories 143
Calories from Fat 10
Total Fat . . . . 1 g
Saturated Fat . . . . 0 g
Cholesterol . . . . 0 mg
Sodium . . . . 512 mg
Total Carbohydrate . . . . . . 30 g
Dietary Fiber . . . . 6 g
Sugars . . . . 8 g
Protein . . . . 5 g

Dietitian's Tip: This recipe is an excellent twist on a traditional stew—and packs in a lot of flavorful vegetables!

October ❖ Week 2

GROCERY LIST

Fresh Produce
Garlic – 1 head
Red onion – 1 medium
Tomato – 1 large
Cucumber – 1 medium
Acorn squash – 2 large
Butternut squash –
1 large or 2 medium
Carrots – small bag
Celery – small bag
Onion – 1 medium
Romaine lettuce – small
head

Meat/Poultry/Fish
Lean turkey Italian
sausage links – 5
(3-ounce) sausages
Tuna steaks – 4
(4-ounce) steaks

Grains/Bread/Pasta
Whole-wheat pita
pockets – 4
Mostaccioli pasta –
1 box
Farfalle pasta – 1 box

Dairy and Cheese
2 1/4 ounces reduced-fat
Swiss cheese
Hummus – 1 package
Shredded, part-skim
mozzarella cheese –
2 packages
Fat-free ricotta cheese –
1 container
Grated Parmesan cheese
Fat-free half-and-half –
1/2 pint
Low-fat buttermilk –
small carton
Eggs

Canned Goods and Sauces
Light mayonnaise – 1 jar
45-ounce jar marinara
pasta sauce – 1 jar
26-ounce jar marinara
pasta sauce – 1 jar
14.5-ounce can fat-free,
reduced-sodium
chicken broth – 3 cans
15-ounce can pumpkin –
1 can

Frozen Foods
10-ounce package
veggie burgers –
1 package

Staples/Seasonings/ Baking Needs
Salt/ground black pepper
Cooking spray
Olive oil
Canola oil
Garlic salt
Dried basil
Dried parsley
Paprika
Dried thyme
Chili powder
Cayenne pepper
All-purpose flour
Sugar
Baking powder –
1 package
Baking soda – 1 box
Ground cinnamon
Ground nutmeg

Miscellaneous
Sunflower seeds – small
package

Cheese and Veggie Pitas

Makes: 4 servings　　　*Serving Size: 1 pita*　　　*Prep Time: 15 minutes*

4 whole-wheat pita pockets

2 tablespoons light mayonnaise

1/2 teaspoon garlic salt

2 1/4 ounces reduced-fat Swiss cheese

1 cup hummus

1/4 cup sunflower seeds

4 romaine lettuce leaves

1 medium red onion, thinly sliced

1 large tomato, cut into 4 equal slices

1 medium cucumber, thinly sliced

1. Slice one side of each pita to open pocket, but do not cut all the way through. Set aside.

2. In a small bowl, whisk together mayonnaise and garlic salt. Spread 1 tablespoon of mayonnaise in each pita.

3. Slice Swiss cheese into 4 even slices. Spread 1/4 cup of hummus on each cheese slice and sprinkle 2 teaspoons sunflower seeds on top.

4. Layer lettuce leaf, onion slices, tomato slices, and cucumber slices on top of hummus.

5. Stuff each pita with sandwich filling.

Exchanges

2 1/2 Starch	2 Vegetable
1 Medium-Fat Meat	2 Fat

Calories 404
　Calories from Fat 152
Total Fat . . . . 17 g
　Saturated Fat . . . . 3 g
Cholesterol . . . . 10 mg
Sodium . . . . 693 mg
Total Carbohydrate . . . . . . 49 g
　Dietary Fiber . . . . 8 g
　Sugars . . . . 11 g
Protein . . . . 20 g

Chef's Tip: You can often find different flavors of hummus at your grocery store. Experiment with roasted red pepper hummus, garlic hummus, or chili pepper hummus.

Mostaccioli with Italian Sausage

Makes: 10 servings   *Serving Size: 1 cup*   *Prep Time: 10 minutes*

16 ounces mostaccioli, uncooked
5 lean turkey Italian sausage links, sliced into 1/2-inch pieces (about 14–15 ounces)
3 garlic cloves, minced
1 45-ounce jar marinara pasta sauce
1/2 tablespoon dried basil
1/2 cup shredded, part-skim mozzarella cheese

1. Cook pasta according to package directions, omitting salt. Drain.

2. In a large saucepan, cook sausage over medium-high heat about 8 minutes or until sausage is no longer pink. Drain fat.

3. Add garlic and sauté 30 seconds. Add pasta sauce and basil. Bring to a boil; reduce heat and simmer about 10 minutes.

4. Add cooked pasta and mozzarella cheese to sauce and mix well.

Sign up today for the ADA's America's Walk for Diabetes®. You can make a difference by joining thousands of walkers across the nation and helping us find the cure we need! Go to www. diabetes.org to sign up.

Exchanges

2 1/2 Starch	2 Vegetable
1 Medium-Fat Meat	

Calories	311
Calories from Fat	56
Total Fat	6 g
Saturated Fat	2 g
Cholesterol	33 mg
Sodium	640 mg
Total Carbohydrate	46 g
Dietary Fiber	5 g
Sugars	10 g
Protein	18 g

Chef's Tip: The turkey Italian sausage in this recipe is a great substitute for regular sausage. The taste is superb without the added fat.

Blackened Tuna Steaks

Makes: 4 servings   *Serving Size: 1 steak*   *Prep Time: 10 minutes*

1 tablespoon paprika
1 teaspoon dried thyme
1/2 teaspoon ground black pepper
1/2 teaspoon garlic salt
1/2 teaspoon chili powder
1/4 teaspoon cayenne pepper
4 4-ounce tuna steaks
Cooking spray

1. In a small bowl, combine first 6 ingredients and mix well to incorporate.

2. Dredge one side of each tuna steak in blackening spice.

3. Coat a large nonstick skillet with cooking spray. Add tuna steaks spice side down to pan over medium-high heat. Cook on both sides for 4–5 minutes or until done.

Exchanges

4 Very Lean Meat	1/2 Fat

Calories 163
Calories from Fat 51
Total Fat . . . . 6 g
Saturated Fat . . . . 0 g
Cholesterol . . . . 42 mg
Sodium . . . . 206 mg
Total Carbohydrate . . . . 1 g
Dietary Fiber . . . . 1 g
Sugars . . . . 1 g
Protein . . . . 26 g

Chef's Tip: Blackened meat or seafood dishes have great, bold flavor without added fat.

Roasted Acorn Squash

Makes: 8 servings   *Serving Size: 1/8 recipe*   *Prep Time: 5 minutes*

2 large acorn squash (4 pounds total)

Cooking spray

1/2 teaspoon salt

1/4 teaspoon ground black pepper

2 teaspoons olive oil

1. Preheat oven to 400 degrees.

2. Cut stem off of each squash and cut in half lengthwise. Scoop out seeds; rinse and dry each squash half. Spray all sides of squash halves with cooking spray. Season inside of each half with salt and pepper. Place cut side down on a nonstick or cooking spray-coated baking sheet. Bake for 45 minutes.

3. Scoop squash meat out into a medium bowl; discard skins. Add olive oil and beat with a sturdy whisk until fluffy.

✔ *National Health Education Week is in October . . . read something today about staying healthy with diabetes.*

Exchanges

1 Starch

Calories	80
Calories from Fat	12
Total Fat	1 g
Saturated Fat	0 g
Cholesterol	0 mg
Sodium	150 mg
Total Carbohydrate	18 g
Dietary Fiber	6 g
Sugars	5 g
Protein	1 g

Dietitian's Tip: Acorn squash is an excellent source of fiber, with about 8 grams per cup. Some people are unsure how to prepare squash, but this recipe proves it couldn't be easier.

Roasted Butternut Squash Soup

Makes: 12 servings   *Serving Size: 1 cup*   *Prep Time: 45 minutes*

1 large (or 2 medium) butternut squash (2 pounds total)
1 teaspoon olive oil
Cooking spray
3 medium carrots, finely diced
3 celery stalks, finely diced
1 medium onion, finely diced
3 14.5-ounce cans fat-free, reduced-sodium chicken broth
1 teaspoon dried thyme
1/2 teaspoon salt
1/4 teaspoon ground black pepper
1 cup fat-free half-and-half, heated

Exchanges
1 Carbohydrate

Calories 61
Calories from Fat 7
Total Fat . . . . 1 g
Saturated Fat . . . . 0 g
Cholesterol . . . . 1 mg
Sodium . . . . 394 mg
Total Carbohydrate . . . . . . 12 g
Dietary Fiber . . . . 2 g
Sugars . . . . 5 g
Protein . . . . 3 g

1. Preheat oven to 400 degrees.

2. Cut ends off of each squash and cut in half lengthwise. Scoop out seeds; rinse and dry each squash half. Spray all sides of squash halves with cooking spray. Place cut side down on a non-stick or cooking spray-coated baking sheet. Bake for 45 minutes.

3. While squash is roasting, add oil and a generous amount of cooking spray to a large soup pot. Sauté carrots, celery, and onion over medium-high heat for 5–6 minutes or until onion is clear.

4. Add chicken broth, thyme, salt, and pepper and bring to a boil. Reduce heat and simmer for 15 minutes.

5. Remove squash from oven and scoop out squash meat into soup pot; discard skins. Simmer for an additional 15 minutes, stirring occasionally.

6. Stir in heated half-and-half. Working in batches, purée soup in a blender until smooth. (You can also use an immersion blender right in the soup pot to purée soup.)

Chef's Tip: Serve this delicious fall soup with Pumpkin Bread (see page 341) and a green salad.

Pumpkin Bread

Makes: 12 servings   *Serving Size: 1 slice*   *Prep Time: 12 minutes*

Cooking spray
1 15-ounce can pumpkin
1/3 cup low-fat buttermilk
1/4 cup canola oil
1 egg
2 egg whites
2 cups all-purpose flour
1/2 cup sugar
2 teaspoons baking powder
1 teaspoon baking soda
1/2 teaspoon salt
1 1/2 teaspoons ground cinnamon
1/4 teaspoon ground nutmeg

1. Preheat oven to 350 degrees. Coat a 9-inch loaf pan with cooking spray.

2. In a medium bowl, combine the pumpkin, buttermilk, oil, egg, and egg whites and mix well. Set aside.

3. In a large bowl, sift together the remaining ingredients.

4. Make a well in the center of the dry ingredients. Add pumpkin mixture all at once. Mix well.

5. Pour batter into loaf pan. Bake 50–60 minutes or until toothpick inserted in center comes out clean.

Exchanges

1/2 Fat	2 Carbohydrate

Calories	172
Calories from Fat	48
Total Fat	5 g
Saturated Fat	1 g
Cholesterol	18 mg
Sodium	286 mg
Total Carbohydrate	28 g
Dietary Fiber	2 g
Sugars	10 g
Protein	4 g

Dietitian's Tip: Pumpkin is a source of vitamin A, which helps your body's immune system and general repair and renewal.

Meatless Skillet Lasagna

Makes: 9 servings   *Serving Size: 1 cup*   *Prep Time: 5 minutes*

10 ounces farfalle pasta, uncooked

1 10-ounce package veggie burgers (4 burgers), crumbled

1 26-ounce jar marinara pasta sauce

1 cup fat-free ricotta cheese

1 cup shredded, part-skim mozzarella cheese

1/4 cup grated Parmesan cheese

1 tablespoon dried parsley

1. Cook pasta according to package directions, omitting salt; drain.

2. In a deep nonstick skillet or wok, cook veggie meat for 3–4 minutes until done. Add pasta sauce and heat.

3. In a medium bowl, combine remaining ingredients and mix well. Add cheese mixture to sauce and mix well until thoroughly heated.

4. Add cooked pasta to sauce and toss to coat.

✔ *Mental Health Awareness Week is in October. Be aware how your attitudes and beliefs are affecting your health.*

Exchanges

2 Starch	2 Vegetable
1 Lean Meat	

Calories 273
  Calories from Fat 44
Total Fat . . . . 5 g
  Saturated Fat . . . . 3 g
Cholesterol . . . . 26 mg
Sodium . . . . 503 mg
Total Carbohydrate . . . . . . 41 g
  Dietary Fiber . . . . 5 g
  Sugars . . . . 8 g
Protein . . . . 17 g

Chef's Tip: Look for veggie burgers in interesting flavors, such as Italian-style or spicy.

October ❖ Week 3

GROCERY LIST

Fresh Produce
Garlic – 1 head
Shallot – 1
Zucchini – 2 medium
Yellow squash –
1 medium
Portabello mushrooms –
3 small
Fresh basil – 1 bunch
Fresh oregano – 1 bunch
Beets – 3 large
Broccoli – 2 heads
Onion – 1 medium
Carrots – small bag
Green bell pepper –
1 medium

Meat/Poultry/Fish
Scallops – 1 pound
Shrimp – 1 pound
Lean ground beef –
1 pound
Cod filets – 4 (4-ounce)
filets

Grains/Bread/Pasta
Arborio rice (risotto,
pearl, or other small-
grain rice) – 1 box
Hearty Italian bread –
10 slices
Bread crumbs
Cornflakes – small box

Dairy and Cheese
Grated Parmesan cheese
Eggs
Shredded, reduced-fat,
sharp cheddar cheese
– 1 package

Canned Goods and Sauces
14.5-ounce can fat-free,
reduced-sodium
chicken broth – 2 cans
Light mayonnaise – 1 jar
16-ounce can kidney
beans – 1 can
16-ounce can black
beans – 1 can
15-ounce can tomato
sauce – 1 can
14.5-ounce can no-salt-
added diced tomatoes
– 2 cans

Staples/Seasonings/Baking Needs
Salt/ground black pepper
Cooking spray
Olive oil
Canola oil
Dried oregano
Garlic salt
Onion salt
Dried parsley
Chili powder
All-purpose flour
Hot pepper sauce

Miscellaneous
White wine – small
bottle

Seafood Risotto

Makes: 9 servings   *Serving Size: 1 cup*   *Prep Time: 15 minutes*

Cooking spray
1 shallot, minced
2 1/2 cups Arborio rice
2 14.5-ounce cans fat-free, reduced-sodium chicken broth
3 1/2 cups water
2 teaspoons olive oil
1 pound fresh scallops
1 pound uncooked shrimp, peeled and deveined
1/2 cup white wine
1/2 teaspoon salt
1/4 teaspoon ground black pepper
1/4 cup grated Parmesan cheese

1. Coat a large soup pot generously with cooking spray. Over medium-high heat, sauté shallots for 3–4 minutes or until they turn clear. Stir in Arborio rice and sauté for 1 more minute.

2. Stir in chicken broth and water and bring to a boil. Reduce heat to a simmer and stir constantly with a large wooden spoon for 20 minutes. Cover and remove from heat.

3. Add oil to a large nonstick skillet over medium-high heat. Add scallops and shrimp and sauté for 2 minutes. Add wine and cook until wine is reduced by half.

4. Fold seafood, salt, pepper, and cheese gently into risotto.

Exchanges

2 1/2 Starch   2 Very Lean Meat

Calories 274
Calories from Fat 34
Total Fat . . . . 4 g
Saturated Fat . . . . 1 g
Cholesterol . . . . 80 mg
Sodium . . . . 552 mg
Total Carbohydrate . . . . . . 39 g
Dietary Fiber . . . . 2 g
Sugars . . . . 1 g
Protein . . . . 19 g

Chef's Tip: If you can't find Arborio rice, try pearl rice or any other small-grain rice in this recipe.

Roasted Veggie Panini

Makes: 5 servings   *Serving Size: 1 sandwich*   *Prep Time: 40 minutes*

1 medium zucchini
1 medium yellow squash
3 small portabello mushrooms
2 teaspoons olive oil
1 teaspoon garlic salt
2 teaspoons dried oregano
1/2 cup basil leaves, washed and dried
5 tablespoons light mayonnaise
Cooking spray
10 slices hearty Italian bread

1. Preheat oven to 400 degrees and prepare an indoor or outdoor grill.

2. Slice the zucchini and squash thinly lengthwise and then in half to make 3-inch strips. Pull the stem out of the portabella mushrooms and scrape out the scales with a spoon. Slice the mushrooms into 1-inch strips.

3. In a large bowl, combine the zucchini, squash, and mushrooms. Drizzle the olive oil over the vegetables and toss to coat. Sprinkle the garlic salt and oregano over the top and toss again to distribute.

4. Place the vegetable mixture in a 13 × 9-inch baking dish and roast in the oven for 30 minutes.

5. While the vegetables are roasting, finely chop basil leaves. In a small bowl, combine basil leaves with mayonnaise. Set aside in the refrigerator.

6. To assemble sandwiches, spread 1/2 tablespoon mayo on 5 slices of bread. Place 1/2 cup of the vegetable mixture on top of 1 slice of bread and top with other slice of bread. Repeat this process for remaining 4 sandwiches. Spray sandwiches with cooking spray and grill sandwiches on an indoor or outdoor grill over medium heat for 4 minutes on each side.

Exchanges

2 Starch	1 1/2 Fat
1 Vegetable	

Calories 252
Calories from Fat 83
Total Fat . . . . 9 g
Saturated Fat . . . . 2 g
Cholesterol . . . . 5 mg
Sodium . . . . 729 mg
Total Carbohydrate . . . . . . 36 g
Dietary Fiber . . . . 4 g
Sugars . . . . 4 g
Protein . . . . 7 g

Chef's Tip: This sandwich can also be grilled in a nonstick skillet coated with cooking spray—cook for 4 minutes on each side over medium-high heat.

Herbed Meatloaf

Makes: 6 servings   *Serving Size: 1 piece*   *Prep Time: 10 minutes*

Cooking spray
1 pound lean ground beef
4 garlic cloves, minced
1/4 cup finely chopped fresh basil leaves
1/4 cup finely chopped fresh oregano leaves
1 tablespoon dried parsley
1 egg, slightly beaten
1/4 cup bread crumbs
1/2 teaspoon salt
1/4 teaspoon ground black pepper

1. Preheat oven to 400 degrees.

2. Coat a 5 × 9-inch loaf pan generously with cooking spray. In a medium bowl, combine all ingredients. Mix well.

3. Spread mixture evenly into loaf pan. Bake for 50–60 minutes or until no longer pink.

Exchanges

1/2 Starch	2 Lean Meat

Calories 153
Calories from Fat 65
Total Fat . . . . 7 g
Saturated Fat . . . . 3 g
Cholesterol . . . . 81 mg
Sodium . . . . 289 mg
Total Carbohydrate . . . . . . 4 g
Dietary Fiber . . . . 0 g
Sugars . . . . 1 g
Protein . . . . 17 g

Chef's Tip: This recipe is a great example of what herbs can do for a meal! Ordinary meatloaf is transformed into a mouthwatering delight. Make meatloaf sandwiches with leftovers for lunch the next day.

Roasted Beets

Makes: 6 servings   *Serving Size: 1/6 recipe*   *Prep Time: 5 minutes*

Cooking spray
3 large fresh beets (18 ounces total)
1 teaspoon olive oil
2 teaspoons chopped fresh basil
1/2 teaspoon salt

1. Preheat oven to 400 degrees.

2. Coat a 13 × 9-inch glass baking dish with cooking spray. Wash and dry beets; slice in half lengthwise. Place beets cut side down in the dish. Spray the beets generously with cooking spray. Roast in oven for 40 minutes. Remove beets from baking dish and let cool for 5 minutes.

3. Peel the skin off the roasted beets and slice into 1/4-inch-thick half moons. On a medium plate, arrange slices of beets in layers. Drizzle with olive oil and sprinkle with basil and salt. Serve hot.

Exchanges

1 Vegetable

Calories	27
Calories from Fat	8
Total Fat	1 g
Saturated Fat	0 g
Cholesterol	0 mg
Sodium	228 mg
Total Carbohydrate	5 g
Dietary Fiber	1 g
Sugars	3 g
Protein	1 g

Dietitian's Tip: Beets are low in carbohydrate and calories but high in nutrition.

Crispy Cod

Makes: 4 servings   *Serving Size: 1 filet*   *Prep Time: 10 minutes*

Cooking spray
1 1/2 cups cornflake crumbs
1/2 teaspoon garlic salt
1/2 teaspoon onion salt
1 egg
2 egg whites
1 teaspoon hot pepper sauce (optional)
2 tablespoons all-purpose flour
4 4-ounce cod filets

1. Preheat oven to 350 degrees. Coat a shallow baking pan with cooking spray.

2. In a medium bowl, combine cornflake crumbs, garlic salt, and onion salt.

3. In a separate bowl, lightly beat egg and egg whites. Add hot pepper sauce and mix well.

4. Place flour in a separate bowl.

5. Dip each cod filet in flour, then egg mixture, then cornflake mixture, coating well.

6. Place filets in baking pan. Spray filets lightly with cooking spray and bake 18–20 minutes.

Exchanges

1 1/2 Starch   3 Very Lean Meat

Calories	216
Calories from Fat	14
Total Fat	2 g
Saturated Fat	0 g
Cholesterol	90 mg
Sodium	606 mg
Total Carbohydrate	24 g
Dietary Fiber	1 g
Sugars	3 g
Protein	25 g

Dietitian's Tip: This is a great-tasting replacement for traditional high-fat fried fish.

Broccoli with Cheddar Cheese

Makes: 8 servings   *Serving Size: 1/2 cup*   *Prep Time: 10 minutes*

4 cups broccoli florets
1/2 teaspoon salt
1/4 teaspoon ground black pepper
3 ounces shredded, reduced-fat, sharp cheddar cheese

1. Steam broccoli until tender-crisp.

2. Sprinkle hot broccoli with salt, pepper, and cheese.

✔ *October is Healthy Lung Month. Stop smoking—now!*

Exchanges
1/2 Fat	1 Vegetable

Calories	32
Calories from Fat	22
Total Fat	2 g
Saturated Fat	1 g
Cholesterol	7 mg
Sodium	245 mg
Total Carbohydrate	2 g
Dietary Fiber	1 g
Sugars	1 g
Protein	4 g

Dietitian's Tip: Steaming vegetables in a small amount of water helps them retain their nutrients.

Veggie Chili

1 tablespoon canola oil

1 medium onion, chopped

4 carrots, sliced

1 green bell pepper, chopped

1 zucchini, chopped

2 garlic cloves, minced

1 tablespoon chili powder

1 16-ounce can kidney beans, rinsed and drained

1 16-ounce can black beans, rinsed and drained

1 15-ounce can tomato sauce

2 14.5-ounce cans no-salt-added diced tomatoes with juice

1. Heat oil in a large soup pot over medium-high heat.

2. Add onion and carrots and sauté 5 minutes. Add green pepper and zucchini and sauté another 2 minutes.

3. Add garlic and sauté 30 seconds. Add chili powder and all remaining ingredients; bring to a boil.

4. Cover, reduce heat, and simmer 30–35 minutes or until the vegetables are tender.

Exchanges

1 Starch	1/2 Fat
3 Vegetable	

Calories 179
  Calories from Fat 24
Total Fat . . . . 3 g
  Saturated Fat . . . . 0 g
Cholesterol . . . . 0 mg
Sodium . . . . 492 mg
Total Carbohydrate . . . . . . 33 g
  Dietary Fiber . . . . 10 g
  Sugars . . . . 12 g
Protein . . . . 9 g

See photo insert.

Dietitian's Tip: The beans and veggies in this dish make it a great source of fiber, with 10 grams per serving. You should aim to get 20–35 grams of dietary fiber daily.

October ❖ Week 4

RECIPE LIST

DAY 1: Pasta Primavera **352**

DAY 2: Shrimp Jambalaya **353**

DAY 3: Eggplant Parmesan **354**

DAY 4: Pork Chops with Cranberry Glaze **355**
Roasted Butternut Squash with Pecans **356**

DAY 5: Veggie Omelet **357**
Banana-Oat Pancakes **358**

DESSERT OF THE MONTH: Apple Crisp **359**

GROCERY LIST

Fresh Produce
Garlic – 1 head
Green bell pepper – 1 large
Broccoli – 2 heads
Plum tomatoes – 2
Onion – 1 medium
Celery – small bag
Eggplant – 1 medium
Red onion – 1 large
Butternut squash – 1 large
Zucchini – 1 small
Red bell pepper – 1 medium
Mushrooms – 1/2 pint
Red apples – 5 medium
Bananas – 2 large or 3 medium

Meat/Poultry/Fish
Medium shrimp – 1 pound
Bone-in, center-cut pork chops – 4 (4-ounce) chops

Grains/Bread/Pasta
Penne pasta – 1 box
White rice
Bread crumbs
Old-fashioned oats – 1 box

Dairy and Cheese
Grated Parmesan cheese
Eggs
Shredded, part-skim mozzarella cheese – 1 package
Shredded, reduced-fat cheddar cheese – 1 package
Margarine
Egg substitute – 1 pint
Low-fat buttermilk – small carton

Canned Goods and Sauces
4-ounce can tomato paste – 1
14.5-ounce can no-salt-added chopped tomatoes – 2
26-ounce jar marinara pasta sauce – 1 jar

Staples/Seasonings/Baking Needs
Salt/ground black pepper
Cooking spray
Olive oil
Garlic salt
Dried basil
Ground nutmeg
Ground cinnamon
Cajun seasoning
Cumin
All-purpose flour
Balsamic vinegar
Brown sugar
Crushed red pepper flakes
Cayenne pepper
Vanilla extract
Reduced-fat baking mix
Honey

Miscellaneous
Dried cranberries – 1 package
Pecans – 1 package

Pasta Primavera

Makes: 5 servings   *Serving Size: 2 cups*   *Prep Time: 15 minutes*

12 ounces penne pasta, uncooked
  Cooking spray
 2 tablespoons olive oil
 1 large green bell pepper, cut into 2-inch strips
 4 cups broccoli florets
1/4 teaspoon garlic salt
1/2 teaspoon ground black pepper
 3 garlic cloves, minced
 2 plum (Roma) tomatoes, cut into 1-inch chunks
 3 tablespoons grated Parmesan cheese

1. Cook pasta according to package directions, omitting salt. Drain.

2. Coat a large nonstick skillet with cooking spray and add olive oil over medium-high heat. Sauté green peppers for 5 minutes. Add broccoli, garlic salt, and pepper and cook another 5–7 minutes; add garlic and sauté 30 seconds.

3. Add tomatoes and cook 2 more minutes.

4. In a large bowl, toss together the pasta and vegetable mixture. Sprinkle with Parmesan cheese and serve immediately.

National Dental Hygiene Month is in October . . . did you know you should brush your teeth for at least one minute twice a day? Count the seconds as you brush . . . you'd be surprised how long one minute is!

Exchanges

3 1/2 Starch	1 Fat
1 Vegetable	

Calories	354
Calories from Fat	75
Total Fat	8 g
Saturated Fat	2 g
Cholesterol	5 mg
Sodium	164 mg
Total Carbohydrate	58 g
Dietary Fiber	5 g
Sugars	6 g
Protein	13 g

Dietitian's Tip: The vegetables in this dish add great flavor, plus lots of fiber to fill you up.

Shrimp Jambalaya

Makes: 8 servings   *Serving Size: 1 cup*   *Prep Time: 15 minutes*

1 1/2 teaspoons olive oil
1 medium onion, chopped
2 celery stalks, chopped
2 tablespoons tomato paste
1 teaspoon dried basil
1 tablespoon Cajun seasoning
    Dash cayenne pepper
    (optional)
3 garlic cloves, minced
1/4 teaspoon cumin
2 14.5-ounce cans no-salt-added chopped tomatoes with juice
1 pound uncooked medium shrimp, peeled and deveined
3 cups white rice, cooked

1. Add oil to a large, deep nonstick skillet or wok over medium-high heat. Add onions and celery and sauté for 5–7 minutes or until vegetables begin to caramelize. Stir in tomato paste and seasonings. Sauté for 1 minute.

2. Stir in tomatoes and bring to a simmer for 10 minutes.

3. Add shrimp and cook for 4 minutes or until shrimp is done. Fold in cooked rice.

Exchanges

1 Starch	2 Vegetable
1 Very Lean Meat	

Calories	156
Calories from Fat	15
Total Fat	2 g
Saturated Fat	0 g
Cholesterol	73 mg
Sodium	527 mg
Total Carbohydrate	25 g
Dietary Fiber	3 g
Sugars	5 g
Protein	11 g

Chef's Tip: Spice up this dish even more with a dash of Cajun hot sauce.

Eggplant Parmesan

Makes: 8 servings   *Serving Size: 1 slice eggplant*   *Prep Time: 15 minutes*

1/2 cup all-purpose flour
1/2 teaspoon salt
1/4 teaspoon ground black pepper
 1 cup bread crumbs
1/4 cup grated Parmesan cheese
 2 eggs, beaten
 1 medium eggplant, sliced into
    8 1/2-inch-thick round slices
    (1 pound)
 2 teaspoons olive oil
    Cooking spray
 1 26-ounce jar marinara pasta
    sauce
1/4 cup shredded, part-skim
    mozzarella cheese

1. Preheat oven to 375 degrees.

2. In a medium bowl, combine flour, salt, and pepper. In another medium bowl, add bread crumbs and Parmesan cheese. In a third medium bowl, add eggs.

3. Dredge both sides of the eggplant slices in flour, then eggs, then bread crumbs, coating well. Set aside.

4. Add oil and a generous amount of cooking spray to a large nonstick skillet over medium-high heat. Cook eggplant in batches, recoating pan with cooking spray as necessary, for 2 minutes each side.

5. In a 13 × 9-inch baking dish, layer the eggplant slices along the bottom. Pour entire jar of sauce over the eggplant so all the slices are covered. Sprinkle mozzarella over the top and bake for 30 minutes.

Exchanges

1 Starch	1/2 Fat
2 Vegetable	

Calories	158
Calories from Fat	40
Total Fat	4 g
Saturated Fat	2 g
Cholesterol	58 mg
Sodium	541 mg
Total Carbohydrate	23 g
Dietary Fiber	4 g
Sugars	8 g
Protein	8 g

Chef's Tip: This dish can be served alone or over pasta.

Pork Chops with Cranberry Glaze

Makes: 4 servings   *Serving Size: 1 pork chop*   *Prep Time: 10 minutes*

4 bone-in, center-cut pork chops
(20 ounces total)
1/4 teaspoon garlic salt
1/2 teaspoon ground black pepper
1 teaspoon olive oil
Cooking spray
1 large red onion, thinly sliced
and separated into rings
1 tablespoon honey
1/2 cup balsamic vinegar
1/3 cup water
1/3 cup dried cranberries

1. Season pork chops well with garlic salt and pepper.

2. Add oil to a large nonstick skillet over medium-high heat. Sauté chops for 6–8 minutes or until browned, turning once. Remove from pan and keep chops warm.

3. Spray pan with cooking spray. Add onions and cook for 5–6 minutes or until they begin to caramelize. Stir in honey, balsamic vinegar, water, and cranberries and simmer for 5–7 minutes or until cranberries are soft and sauce takes on a glaze consistency.

4. Pour cranberry sauce over pork chops.

Exchanges

2 Lean Meat   1 1/2 Carbohydrate
1/2 Fat

Calories 240
Calories from Fat 66
Total Fat . . . . 7 g
Saturated Fat . . . . 2 g
Cholesterol . . . . 59 mg
Sodium . . . . 126 mg
Total Carbohydrate . . . . . . 23 g
Dietary Fiber . . . . 2 g
Sugars . . . . 19 g
Protein . . . . 21 g

Dietitian's Tip: Dried fruit contains more carbohydrate than fresh fruit, but adding just a few raisins, prunes, or cranberries is a great way to liven up a dish.

Roasted Butternut Squash with Pecans

Makes: 6 servings   *Serving Size: 1/2 cup*   *Prep Time: 5 minutes*

1 large butternut squash, cut in half lengthwise, seeds discarded (2 pounds)
Cooking spray
2 teaspoons margarine, divided
1 tablespoon brown sugar, divided
1/4 cup chopped pecans

 National Youth Health Awareness Day is October 22 . . . help the young person in your life eat less fast food and more fresh fruits and veggies!

1. Preheat oven to 400 degrees.

2. Spray both sides of squash with cooking spray and place face down in a glass baking dish. Bake for 45 minutes.

3. In a small bowl, mix 1 teaspoon margarine and 1 1/2 teaspoons brown sugar and microwave for 30 seconds to melt margarine. Add pecans and mix well. Spread mixture on a small baking sheet and bake for 3 minutes to toast nuts.

4. Remove squash from oven. Scoop squash meat into a large bowl; discard skins. Add remaining margarine and brown sugar and whip with a whisk until smooth. Fold in pecans.

Exchanges

1 Starch   1/2 Fat

Calories	98
Calories from Fat	45
Total Fat	5 g
Saturated Fat	1 g
Cholesterol	0 mg
Sodium	20 mg
Total Carbohydrate	14 g
Dietary Fiber	2 g
Sugars	5 g
Protein	1 g

Chef's Tip: Roasting vegetables really intensifies their flavors, as this dish shows. The brown sugar and pecans add sweet crunchiness.

Veggie Omelet

Makes: 4 servings   *Serving Size: 1 omelet*   *Prep Time: 10 minutes*

Cooking spray
1/2 cup shredded zucchini
1/2 small red bell pepper, finely diced
1/2 cup sliced mushrooms
2 cups egg substitute
1/2 teaspoon salt
1/4 teaspoon ground black pepper
1/4 teaspoon crushed red pepper flakes
1/2 cup shredded, reduced-fat cheddar cheese

1. Add cooking spray to a large non-stick skillet over medium-high heat. Add zucchini, bell pepper, and mushrooms to pan and sauté for 5–6 minutes or until vegetables are soft.

2. Add cooking spray to a small non-stick pan (omelet pan) over medium heat. Pour 1/2 cup egg substitute in hot pan. Sprinkle with salt, pepper, and red pepper flakes.

3. Once eggs set up and are still a little runny in the center, spread 1/4 cup of vegetable mixture on one side of eggs. Sprinkle the vegetable mixture with 2 tablespoons cheese.

4. Fold the other half of the eggs over the vegetables and gently flip the omelet using a wide spatula.

5. Repeat process for remaining three omelets.

Exchanges

2 Very Lean Meat	1/2 Fat
1 Vegetable	

Calories 108
  Calories from Fat 28
Total Fat . . . . 3 g
  Saturated Fat . . . . 2 g
Cholesterol . . . . 10 mg
Sodium . . . . 642 mg
Total Carbohydrate . . . . 4 g
  Dietary Fiber . . . . 1 g
  Sugars. . . . . 2 g
Protein . . . . 16 g

Chef's Tip: Spoon a little salsa over each omelet for added flavor.

Banana-Oat Pancakes

Makes: 9 servings   *Serving Size: 1 pancake*   *Prep Time: 7 minutes*

1/2 cup old-fashioned oats
1 1/4 cups low-fat buttermilk
1 cup mashed bananas (about 2–3 bananas)
2 large eggs, beaten
1 teaspoon vanilla extract
1 1/2 cups reduced-fat baking mix
    Cooking spray

1. In a large bowl, combine oats and buttermilk. Let stand until oats soften. Mix in mashed bananas, eggs, and vanilla extract. Gradually stir in baking mix.

2. Coat a griddle or nonstick skillet with cooking spray. Use 1/4 cup batter for each pancake and cook pancake until brown on bottom and some bubbles begin to break around edges. Turn pancake over. Cook until brown on bottom and firm to touch in center.

3. Repeat procedure until all batter is gone. Serve pancakes with sugar-free syrup.

Exchanges

1 Starch	1/2 Fat
1/2 Fruit	

Calories 142
  Calories from Fat 30
Total Fat . . . . 3 g
  Saturated Fat . . . . 1 g
Cholesterol . . . . 49 mg
Sodium . . . . 300 mg
Total Carbohydrate . . . . . . 24 g
  Dietary Fiber . . . . 2 g
  Sugars . . . . 7 g
Protein . . . . 5 g

Chef's Tip: If you like, serve sliced bananas on top of these pancakes.

Apple Crisp

Makes: 7 servings   *Serving Size: 1/2 cup*   *Prep Time: 15 minutes*

Cooking spray

1/4 cup packed brown sugar

1/4 cup all-purpose flour

1/2 cup old-fashioned oats

2 tablespoons margarine, softened

1 teaspoon ground cinnamon

1/2 teaspoon ground nutmeg

1 teaspoon vanilla extract

5 cups peeled, sliced red apples (about 5 apples)

1. Preheat oven to 375 degrees. Coat a 13 × 9-inch pan with cooking spray.

2. In a small bowl, combine brown sugar, flour, oats, margarine, cinnamon, nutmeg, and vanilla. Blend with a fork until moistened (mixture should be crumbly).

3. Layer apples in pan and sprinkle brown sugar mixture evenly over top. Bake 30 minutes.

 World Food Day is in October . . . sponsor a hungry child today.

Exchanges

2 Carbohydrate

Calories	145
Calories from Fat	36
Total Fat	4 g
Saturated Fat	1 g
Cholesterol	0 mg
Sodium	41 mg
Total Carbohydrate	27 g
Dietary Fiber	2 g
Sugars	18 g
Protein	2 g

Chef's Tip: Top with light vanilla ice cream or frozen yogurt.

November

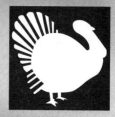

Having diabetes doesn't mean
the end of the world, food-wise.
You can still eat a lot of your old
favorites—just healthier versions
of them, in moderation.
Celebrate this month with
delicious, low-fat,
heart-healthy recipes.

American Diabetes Month

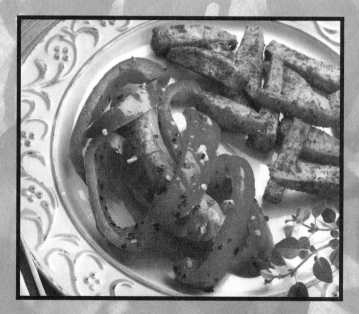

Italian Sausage with Pepper Medley (page 389)
Spicy Sweet Potato Fries (page 158)
When the days grow shorter, you'll enjoy these hearty, slightly
spicy foods! Sweet potato fries are a great alternative to the usual
fries. Try them with this sausage medley or a tasty turkey burger.

November ❖ Recipes

November ❖ Week 1

RECIPE LIST

DAY 1: Barbeque Shrimp over
Wild Rice **364**

DAY 2: Baked Potato Soup **365**

DAY 3: Pesto Chicken Pita **366**
Brussels Sprouts with Citrus
Butter **367**

DAY 4: Ten-Minute Tostadas **368**
Tomato Salad with Cilantro
Vinaigrette **369**

DAY 5: Beef Stew **370**

GROCERY LIST

Fresh Produce
Onions – 2 medium
Russet potatoes –
8 medium
Scallions – 1 bunch
Fresh basil – 1 bunch
Lemon – 1
Iceberg lettuce – 1 small
head
Tomatoes – 6 medium
Fresh cilantro – 1 bunch
Shallot – 1
Carrots – small bag
Celery – small bag
Garlic – 1 head

Meat/Poultry/Fish
Shrimp – 1 pound
Turkey bacon –
1 package

Boneless, skinless
chicken breasts –
1 pound
Beef round roast –
1 pound

Grains/Bread/Pasta
Long-grain and wild rice
mix – 1 package
Whole-wheat pocket
pitas – 4
Tostada shells – 4

Dairy and Cheese
Margarine
Fat-free half-and-half –
1/2 pint
Shredded, reduced-fat
cheddar cheese –
2 packages
Grated Parmesan cheese

Canned Goods and Sauces
Ketchup – small bottle
Worcestershire sauce –
small bottle
14.5-ounce can fat-free,
reduced-sodium
chicken broth – 3 cans
Light mayonnaise – 1 jar
16-ounce can fat-free
refried beans with
green chilies – 1 can
Salsa – 1 jar
14.5-ounce can fat-free,
reduced-sodium beef
broth – 2 cans

Frozen Foods
1-pound bag Brussels
sprouts – 1 bag

Staples/Seasonings/ Baking Needs
Salt/ground black pepper
Cooking spray
Olive oil
Dried oregano
Dried thyme
Dried parsley
Paprika
Cayenne pepper
Brown sugar
Bay leaf
White wine vinegar
All-purpose flour
Hot pepper sauce

Miscellaneous
Pine nuts – small bag

Barbeque Shrimp over Wild Rice

Makes: 4 servings   *Serving Size: 3/4 cup shrimp*   *Prep Time: 5 minutes*
and 1/2 cup rice

1 6-ounce package long-grain and wild rice mix (discard seasoning packet)

1/2 cup ketchup

1/4 cup Worcestershire sauce

1 tablespoon margarine

1/4 cup water

1 teaspoon dried oregano

1/2 teaspoon dried thyme

1 teaspoon paprika

1 tablespoon brown sugar

1/8 teaspoon cayenne pepper

1/4 teaspoon ground black pepper

3 garlic cloves, minced

1 pound uncooked shrimp, peeled and deveined

1. Cook rice according to package directions, omitting salt.

2. In a large nonstick skillet, add all ingredients except shrimp and bring to a boil. Reduce heat and simmer; add shrimp. Cook 4–6 minutes or until shrimp is done.

3. Serve shrimp over cooked rice.

Exchanges

2 Starch	1/2 Fat
2 Very Lean Meat	1 Carbohydrate

Calories 318
    Calories from Fat 40
Total Fat . . . . 4 g
    Saturated Fat . . . . 1 g
Cholesterol . . . . 145 mg
Sodium . . . . 756 mg
Total Carbohydrate . . . . . . 48 g
    Dietary Fiber . . . . 3 g
    Sugars . . . . 12 g
Protein . . . . 23 g

Chef's Tip: If you like things a little spicier, double the cayenne pepper in this recipe.

Baked Potato Soup

Makes: 9 servings   *Serving Size: 1 cup*   *Prep Time: 15 minutes*

Cooking spray

1 medium onion, finely diced

5 strips turkey bacon, finely diced

6 medium russet potatoes, peeled and diced

3 14.5-ounce cans fat-free, reduced-sodium chicken broth

1 bay leaf

1/2 teaspoon salt (optional)

1/4 teaspoon ground black pepper

1 cup fat-free half-and-half

1/2 cup scallions, chopped

1/2 cup shredded, reduced-fat cheddar cheese

1. Coat a large soup pot with cooking spray. Sauté onion for 3 minutes over medium heat. Add bacon and sauté for 3 minutes. Add potatoes, chicken broth, bay leaf, salt, and pepper. Turn heat to high and bring to a boil; then reduce heat to a low boil for 20 minutes.

2. Remove bay leaf.

3. Remove 4 cups of soup and purée in a blender or with a handheld immersion blender. Pour puréed soup back into pot and add half-and-half.

4. Garnish with scallions and cheddar cheese.

Exchanges

1 1/2 Starch	1/2 Fat

Calories 139
 Calories from Fat 29
Total Fat . . . . 3 g
 Saturated Fat . . . . 2 g
Cholesterol . . . . 12 mg
Sodium . . . . 525 mg
Total Carbohydrate . . . . . . 21 g
 Dietary Fiber . . . . 2 g
 Sugars . . . . 5 g
Protein . . . . 7 g

Chef's Tip: The immersion blender is a must-have kitchen tool for puréeing soups, sauces, smoothies, and desserts. It's easy to use and cleans up quickly!

Pesto Chicken Pita

Makes: 4 servings   *Serving Size: 1 pita*   *Prep Time: 10 minutes*

4 whole-wheat pita pockets
1/2 cup whole basil leaves
2 tablespoons pine nuts
2 tablespoons grated Parmesan cheese
1/4 cup light mayonnaise
1/4 cup fat-free half-and-half
1 pound boneless, skinless chicken breasts

1. Slice one side of each pita to open pocket, but do not cut all the way through. Set aside.

2. In a blender or food processor, purée basil leaves, pine nuts, Parmesan cheese, and mayonnaise until a paste forms, about 2 minutes.

3. In a medium bowl, add basil mixture and half-and-half and whisk together. Reserve 4 tablespoons of basil sauce for later use.

4. Place each chicken breast between two pieces of plastic wrap and pound with a meat tenderizer or rolling pin until breasts are about 1/4 inch thick.

5. Place chicken breasts in a shallow dish and pour basil sauce over chicken.

6. Cook chicken breasts on an indoor or outdoor grill for 4 minutes on each side.

7. Toast pita pockets. Slice breast into strips and stuff inside pita. Add 1 tablespoon reserved basil sauce to each pita. Repeat procedure for remaining 3 pitas.

Exchanges

2 Starch	2 Fat
4 Very Lean Meat	

Calories 377
  Calories from Fat 118
Total Fat . . . . 13 g
  Saturated Fat . . . . 3 g
Cholesterol . . . . 78 mg
Sodium . . . . 395 mg
Total Carbohydrate . . . . . . 34 g
  Dietary Fiber . . . . 2 g
  Sugars . . . . 3 g
Protein . . . . 34 g

Chef's Tip: You can also bake the chicken breasts in a 350-degree oven for 20 minutes or until done instead of grilling them.

Brussels Sprouts with Citrus Butter

Makes: 5 servings   *Serving Size: 1/5 recipe*   *Prep Time: 8 minutes*

1 1-pound bag frozen Brussels
sprouts
2 tablespoons margarine
1 tablespoon lemon juice
1/4 teaspoon salt

1. Cook Brussels sprouts according to package directions.

2. Add remaining ingredients to a medium nonstick skillet over medium heat. Cook until margarine melts.

3. Add cooked Brussels sprouts and toss to coat.

Exchanges

1 Vegetable   1 Fat

Calories 79
Calories from Fat 44
Total Fat . . . . 5 g
Saturated Fat . . . . 1 g
Cholesterol . . . . 0 mg
Sodium . . . . 190 mg
Total Carbohydrate . . . . . . 8 g
Dietary Fiber . . . . 4 g
Sugars . . . . 2 g
Protein . . . . 3 g

Dietitian's Tip: Brussels sprouts are also good topped with chopped, toasted nuts.

Ten-Minute Tostadas

Makes: 4 servings   *Serving Size: 1 tostada*   *Prep Time: 5 minutes*

4 tostada shells
1 16-ounce can fat-free refried beans with green chilies
3/4 cup shredded, reduced-fat cheddar cheese
1 cup shredded lettuce
1 cup tomatoes, seeded and chopped
  Salsa and hot pepper sauce to taste

1. Preheat oven to 350 degrees.

2. Place tostada shells on a baking sheet. Spread 1/2 cup refried beans evenly on each tostada. Top each tostada with cheese. Bake in oven for 8–10 minutes or until cheese is melted.

3. Top with 1/4 cup lettuce and 1/4 cup tomatoes. Add salsa and hot pepper sauce as desired.

Exchanges

1 1/2 Starch   1 Vegetable
1 Medium-Fat Meat

Calories	196
Calories from Fat	63
Total Fat	7 g
Saturated Fat	3 g
Cholesterol	15 mg
Sodium	668 mg
Total Carbohydrate	26 g
Dietary Fiber	7 g
Sugars	3 g
Protein	12 g

Dietitian's Tip: This tasty recipe works great when you're crunched for time. It's nutritious, with carbohydrate and fiber from the beans and protein and calcium from the cheese—all in minutes!

Tomato Salad with Cilantro Vinaigrette

Makes: 8 servings   *Serving Size: 1/2 cup salad*   *Prep Time: 10 minutes*

2 tablespoons white wine vinegar

2 tablespoons olive oil

1 tablespoon chopped fresh cilantro

1 small shallot, minced

1/4 teaspoon salt

Dash ground black pepper

5 medium tomatoes, seeded and chopped

1. In a medium bowl, whisk together all ingredients except tomatoes.

2. Add tomatoes to bowl and toss gently to coat.

Exchanges

1 Vegetable	1/2 Fat

Calories 49

Calories from Fat 33

Total Fat . . . . 4 g

Saturated Fat . . . . 0 g

Cholesterol . . . . 0 mg

Sodium . . . . 80 mg

Total Carbohydrate . . . . 4 g

Dietary Fiber . . . . 1 g

Sugars . . . . 2 g

Protein . . . . 1 g

Chef's Tip: You can add some chopped cucumber to this salad if you like.

Beef Stew

- **2** teaspoons olive oil
- **1** pound beef round roast, cut into 1/2-inch cubes
- **2** 14.5-ounce cans fat-free, reduced-sodium beef broth
- **1/4** teaspoon ground black pepper
- **2** medium carrots, chopped
- **2** medium russet potatoes, peeled and chopped
- **2** medium celery stalks, chopped
- **1** medium onion, unevenly chopped
- **1** bay leaf
- **2** teaspoons dried parsley
- **1/4** cup cold water
- **2** tablespoons all-purpose flour

1. Add oil to a large soup pot over high heat. Add beef and cook for 15 minutes or until beef begins to brown. Add broth and pepper and bring to a boil. Reduce heat to a simmer, cover, and cook for 1 1/2 hours.

2. Add remaining ingredients except water and flour. Cover again and simmer 30 more minutes.

3. In a small bowl, whisk flour into cold water. Gradually stir the flour and water into the stew. Bring to a boil, stirring constantly, for 5 more minutes.

Exchanges

1 Starch	1 Vegetable
2 Lean Meat	

Calories	222
Calories from Fat	54
Total Fat	6 g
Saturated Fat	2 g
Cholesterol	54 mg
Sodium	391 mg
Total Carbohydrate	19 g
Dietary Fiber	3 g
Sugars	5 g
Protein	23 g

Chef's Tip: This recipe takes a little longer to prepare, but is well worth it—especially for the great-tasting leftovers.

November ❖ Week 2

GROCERY LIST

Fresh Produce
Onion – 1 medium
Russet potatoes –
2 medium
Fresh dill – 1 bunch
Mushrooms – 1 pint
Spinach – 1 (6-ounce)
bag
Strawberries – 1 pint
Blueberries – 1/2 pint
Green grapes – small
bag
Lemon – 1

Meat/Poultry/Fish
Turkey bacon –
1 package
Boneless, skinless
chicken breasts –
4 (4-ounce) breasts
90% lean ground beef –
1 pound
Deli ham, extra lean,
thinly sliced – 8
ounces

Grains/Bread/Pasta
Brown rice
Rotini pasta – 1 box
Whole-wheat bread –
8 slices
Farfalle pasta – 1 box

Dairy and Cheese
Fat-free milk
Fat-free half-and-half –
1/2 pint
Plain, fat-free yogurt –
small container
Margarine
Shredded, reduced-fat
cheddar cheese –
2 packages
1-ounce slices reduced-
fat Swiss cheese –
4 slices

Canned Goods
and Sauces
10-ounce can chopped
clams – 2 cans
Teriyaki sauce – small
bottle
6-ounce can pineapple
juice – 1 can
14.5-ounce can crushed
tomatoes – 1 can
8-ounce can tomato
sauce – 1 can
Light mayonnaise – 1 jar
Dijon mustard – small
bottle
10 3/4-ounce can low-fat
cream of mushroom
condensed soup –
1 can
6-ounce can tuna packed
in water – 2 cans

Frozen Foods
1-pound bag stir-fry veg-
etables – 1 bag
1-pound bag green
beans – 1 bag

Staples/Seasonings/
Baking Needs
Salt/ground black pepper
Cooking spray
Chili powder
Cayenne pepper
Garlic powder
Sugar
Vanilla extract
Honey

Miscellaneous
Sesame seeds
Slivered almonds –
small package

New England Clam Chowder

Makes: 5 servings   *Serving Size: 1 cup*   *Prep Time: 10 minutes*

Cooking spray
- **4** strips turkey bacon, chopped
- **1** medium onion, finely diced
- **2** 10-ounce cans chopped clams with juice
- **1/2** cup water
- **2** medium russet potatoes, finely diced
- **1** cup fat-free milk
- **1** cup fat-free half-and-half
- **1/2** teaspoon salt (optional)
- **1/4** teaspoon ground black pepper

1. Coat a medium soup pot with cooking spray. Add bacon and cook over medium-high heat for 4 minutes or until beginning to brown. Add onion and continue to cook another 3 minutes or until onion is clear.

2. Add clams with juice, water, and potatoes. Increase heat to high and bring to a boil. Boil for 20 minutes or until potatoes are soft.

3. Reduce heat to low and add milk and half-and-half. Simmer for 1 minute. Do not boil. Add salt and pepper.

Exchanges
2 Lean Meat   1 1/2 Carbohydrate

Calories	213
Calories from Fat	35
Total Fat	4 g
Saturated Fat	1 g
Cholesterol	49 mg
Sodium	425 mg
Total Carbohydrate	24 g
Dietary Fiber	2 g
Sugars	10 g
Protein	19 g

Chef's Tip: Serve this hearty chowder with warm French bread and a tossed salad.

Teriyaki Chicken

Makes: 4 servings   *Serving Size: 1 chicken breast and 1/2 cup brown rice*   *Prep Time: 10 minutes*

Cooking spray

1/4 cup bottled teriyaki sauce

1/4 cup pineapple juice

1/2 teaspoon hot pepper sauce (optional)

4 4-ounce boneless, skinless chicken breasts

1 tablespoon sesame seeds

1 1-pound bag frozen stir-fry vegetables (broccoli, carrots, and peapods)

2 cups cooked brown rice

1. Preheat oven to 375 degrees. Coat a shallow baking dish with cooking spray.

2. In a small bowl, whisk together teriyaki sauce, pineapple juice, and hot pepper sauce. Reserve 3 tablespoons of the sauce and set aside.

3. Coat a large sauté pan with cooking spray over high heat. Sear chicken breasts about 2 minutes on each side. Transfer chicken to the prepared baking dish. Brush sauce on both sides of chicken, coating well. Sprinkle all of the chicken breasts with sesame seeds and bake for 20 minutes or until done.

4. Meanwhile, add the vegetables and remaining sauce to the pan. Stir-fry vegetables for 2 minutes or until vegetables are tender-crisp.

5. Serve vegetables over 1/2 cup of rice and place chicken on top.

Exchanges

2 Starch	1 Vegetable
3 Very Lean Meat	1/2 Fat

Calories 319
  Calories from Fat 44
Total Fat . . . . 5 g
  Saturated Fat . . . . 1 g
Cholesterol . . . . 68 mg
Sodium . . . . 708 mg
Total Carbohydrate . . . . . . 35 g
  Dietary Fiber . . . . 5 g
  Sugars . . . . 10 g
Protein . . . . 31 g

Chef's Tip: Teriyaki sauce is right next to the soy sauce in your market.

Green Beans Amandine

1 tablespoon margarine
   Cooking spray
1 1-pound bag frozen green
   beans, thawed
1/4 cup slivered almonds, toasted
1/2 teaspoon salt

1. Add margarine and a generous amount of cooking spray to a medium nonstick skillet over medium-high heat.

2. After margarine melts, add in remaining ingredients and sauté for 4–5 minutes.

Exchanges

1 Vegetable	1 Fat

Calories 67	
Calories from Fat 50	
Total Fat . . . . 6 g	
Saturated Fat . . . . 0 g	
Cholesterol . . . . 0 mg	
Sodium . . . . 263 mg	
Total Carbohydrate . . . . 4 g	
Dietary Fiber . . . . 2 g	
Sugars . . . . 1 g	
Protein . . . . 2 g	

Dietitian's Tip: Almonds provide taste and texture to this recipe, along with vitamin E.

Beef and Cheese Skillet Casserole

Makes: 7 servings   *Serving Size: 1 cup*   *Prep Time: 2 minutes*

2 cups rotini pasta, uncooked

1 pound 90% lean ground beef

1 14.5-ounce can crushed
  tomatoes

1 8-ounce can tomato sauce

2 teaspoons chili powder

1/8 teaspoon cayenne pepper

1 teaspoon garlic powder

1 teaspoon sugar

2/3 cup shredded, reduced-fat
  cheddar cheese

1. Cook pasta according to package directions, omitting salt. Drain.

2. In a large nonstick skillet, cook ground beef until beginning to brown, about 8–9 minutes. Drain any excess fat.

3. Add remaining ingredients except cheese and pasta and bring to a boil. Reduce heat and simmer for 6–7 minutes or until beginning to thicken. Fold in cheese and toss with pasta.

Exchanges

1 Starch	2 Vegetable
2 Lean Meat	

Calories 243
  Calories from Fat 74
Total Fat . . . . 8 g
  Saturated Fat . . . . 4 g
Cholesterol . . . . 47 mg
Sodium . . . . 504 mg
Total Carbohydrate . . . . . . 25 g
  Dietary Fiber . . . . 2 g
  Sugars . . . . 6 g
Protein . . . . 19 g

Chef's Tip: This is a quick and easy recipe the whole family will enjoy.

Ham Sandwich with Mushrooms

Makes: 4 servings   *Serving Size: 1 sandwich*   *Prep Time: 5 minutes*

2 tablespoons light mayonnaise

1 tablespoon Dijon mustard

2 teaspoons finely chopped fresh
dill
Cooking spray

1 pint mushrooms, thinly sliced

8 slices whole-wheat bread

8 ounces extra lean, thinly sliced
deli ham

4 1-ounce slices reduced-fat
Swiss cheese

1. Preheat broiler.

2. In a small bowl, whisk together mayonnaise, mustard, and dill.

3. Coat a medium nonstick skillet with cooking spray. Add mushrooms and cook over medium-high heat for 5 minutes, or until the liquid is evaporated. Remove from heat.

4. Place 4 whole-wheat bread slices on a baking sheet. Spread 1 1/2 teaspoons mayonnaise mixture on each slice. Top each with 2 ounces ham, 1 slice cheese, and 1/4 of the mushroom mixture. Top each with another slice of bread.

5. Broil the sandwiches about 4 inches from the heat for 1–2 minutes on each side.

Exchanges

2 Starch	3 Lean Meat

Calories	306
Calories from Fat	87
Total Fat	10 g
Saturated Fat	3 g
Cholesterol	39 mg
Sodium	1037 mg
Total Carbohydrate	31 g
Dietary Fiber	4 g
Sugars	5 g
Protein	25 g

Dietitian's Tip: Just because bread is brown doesn't mean it's whole-wheat bread. Check the label carefully to make sure your brand is made with whole-wheat flour and has plenty of fiber per slice.

Fruit Salad with Yogurt Dressing

Makes: 5 servings   *Serving Size: 1 cup*   *Prep Time: 15 minutes*

FRUIT SALAD

2 cups strawberries, sliced

1 cup blueberries

2 cups green grapes

DRESSING

1/2 cup plain, fat-free yogurt

1 tablespoon honey

1 tablespoon lemon juice

1/4 teaspoon vanilla extract

1. In a medium bowl, toss together strawberries, blueberries, and grapes.

2. In a small bowl, whisk together dressing ingredients. Pour dressing over fruit and gently toss.

 World Diabetes Day is November 14. Celebrate by enjoying healthy food today!

Exchanges

2 Fruit

Calories 107
   Calories from Fat 6
Total Fat . . . . 1 g
   Saturated Fat . . . . 0 g
Cholesterol . . . . 1 mg
Sodium . . . . 26 mg
Total Carbohydrate . . . . . . 26 g
   Dietary Fiber . . . . 3 g
   Sugars . . . . 20 g
Protein . . . . 2 g

Chef's Tip: This quick dressing really jazzes up plain fruit. Try it on more exotic fruits, too.

Tuna Spinach Bake

Makes: 6 servings   *Serving Size: 1 cup*   *Prep Time: 10 minutes*

Cooking spray

4 cups farfalle pasta, uncooked

1 6-ounce bag fresh spinach (about 4 cups)

1/2 teaspoon salt

1/4 teaspoon ground black pepper

2 6-ounce cans tuna packed in spring water, drained

1 10 3/4-ounce can low-fat cream of mushroom condensed soup

1/2 cup shredded, reduced-fat cheddar cheese

1. Preheat oven to 375 degrees. Coat a 9 × 9-inch baking dish with cooking spray. Set aside.

2. Cook pasta according to package directions, omitting salt. Drain.

3. Coat a medium nonstick skillet with cooking spray. Sauté spinach leaves over medium-high heat for 4 minutes.

4. In a medium bowl, mix salt, pepper, tuna, soup, and cooked spinach. Pour pasta in bottom of baking dish. Pour tuna/spinach mixture over the pasta and spread evenly to coat.

5. Sprinkle cheese over the top and bake for 15 minutes.

Exchanges

2 Starch   2 Lean Meat

Calories	259
Calories from Fat	40
Total Fat	4 g
Saturated Fat	1 g
Cholesterol	23 mg
Sodium	653 mg
Total Carbohydrate	33 g
Dietary Fiber	3 g
Sugars	3 g
Protein	21 g

Chef's Tip: If you don't love tuna, try cooked, shredded chicken in this recipe.

November ❖ Week 3

GROCERY LIST

Fresh Produce
Garlic – 1 head
Onions – 3
Celery – small bag
Carrots – small bag
Mushrooms – 1/2 pint
Russet potatoes –
2 pounds
Fresh chives – 1 bunch
Fresh cranberries –
1 pound bag
Navel orange –
1 medium

Meat/Poultry/Fish
Turkey bacon –
1 package

Halibut filets – 4
(4-ounce) filets
Whole turkey –
12–16 pounds

Grains/Bread/Pasta
Small shell pasta – 1 box
Orzo pasta – 1 box

Dairy and Cheese
Fat-free milk
Eggs
Grated Parmesan cheese
Fat-free half-and-half –
1 1/2 pints
Margarine

Canned Goods and Sauces
15-ounce can pumpkin –
1 can
14.5-ounce can fat-free,
reduced-sodium
chicken broth – 5 cans
14.5-ounce can no-salt-
added diced
tomatoes – 2 cans
16-ounce can cannellini
(white kidney)
beans – 3 cans

Staples/Seasonings/ Baking Needs
Salt/ground black pepper
Cooking spray
Olive oil
Canola oil
All-purpose flour
Baking powder
Ground cinnamon
Ground nutmeg
Brown sugar
Dried parsley
Dried basil
Dried oregano
Paprika
Garlic powder
SPLENDA® Granular
sweetener

Pumpkin Pancakes

Makes: 7 servings   *Serving Size: 2 pancakes*   *Prep Time: 5 minutes*

1 1/2 cups all-purpose flour
2 1/4 teaspoons baking powder
1 teaspoon ground cinnamon
1/4 teaspoon ground nutmeg
1/4 teaspoon salt
2 cups fat-free milk
2 tablespoons brown sugar
1 tablespoon canola oil
2 eggs, lightly beaten
1 15-ounce can pumpkin
Cooking spray

1. In a large bowl, sift together flour, baking powder, cinnamon, nutmeg, and salt.

2. In a medium bowl, whisk together milk, brown sugar, canola oil, eggs, and pumpkin. Make a well in the dry ingredients and pour in the wet ingredients. Stir mixture until liquid is incorporated and batter is smooth.

3. Coat a large nonstick skillet with cooking spray over medium heat. Once pan heats up, pour 1/3 cup batter to form pancakes. Cook pancakes until brown on bottom and some bubbles begin to break around edges. Turn pancake over. Cook until brown on bottom and firm to touch in center.

4. Repeat procedure until all batter is gone.

Exchanges

2 Starch	1 Fat

Calories	198
Calories from Fat	36
Total Fat	4 g
Saturated Fat	1 g
Cholesterol	62 mg
Sodium	259 mg
Total Carbohydrate	33 g
Dietary Fiber	3 g
Sugars	10 g
Protein	8 g

Chef's Tip: Serve these pancakes spread with reduced-fat margarine and sprinkled with a mixture of sugar substitute, cinnamon, and nutmeg . . . or just top with a dusting of powdered sugar.

Pasta Fagioli

Makes: 6 servings　　　　*Serving Size: 1 cup*　　　　*Prep Time: 15 minutes*

Cooking spray
4 slices turkey bacon, chopped
1 medium onion, minced
2 garlic cloves, minced
2 medium celery stalks, finely diced
2 medium carrots, finely diced
2 14.5-ounce cans fat-free, reduced-sodium chicken broth
2 16-ounce cans cannellini (white kidney) beans
1 15-ounce can no-salt-added diced tomatoes, drained
1 teaspoon dried parsley
1 teaspoon dried basil
1/2 teaspoon salt (optional)
1/4 teaspoon ground black pepper
1 cup small shell pasta, uncooked
1/4 cup grated Parmesan cheese

1. Coat a large soup pot with cooking spray over high heat. Add bacon and sauté until crisp.

2. Reduce heat to medium and add onion, garlic, celery, and carrots. Sauté about 5–7 minutes or until vegetables begin to brown. Add broth and simmer for 5 minutes.

3. Stir in beans, tomatoes, parsley, basil, salt, and pepper and simmer for 10 minutes. Add the pasta and continue to simmer for 10–15 minutes or until pasta is al dente.

4. Serve soup in a bowl sprinkled with Parmesan cheese.

Exchanges

2 Starch	1/2 Fat
2 Vegetable	

Calories 240	
Calories from Fat 36	
Total Fat . . . . 4 g	
Saturated Fat . . . . 2 g	
Cholesterol . . . . 12 mg	
Sodium . . . . : 1016 mg	
Total Carbohydrate . . . . . . 38 g	
Dietary Fiber . . . . 8 g	
Sugars . . . . 8 g	
Protein . . . . 13 g	

Chef's Tip: Al dente literally means "to the tooth" in Italian, meaning that the pasta should be soft but still have a little bit of a bite to it.

Mushroom Alfredo Halibut

Makes: 4 servings   *Serving Size: 1 filet*   *Prep Time: 15 minutes*

1 teaspoon olive oil
Cooking spray
1/2 pint mushrooms, sliced
1/2 cup fat-free half-and-half
1/4 cup grated Parmesan cheese
2 teaspoons garlic powder
4 4-ounce halibut filets

1. Preheat oven to 350 degrees.

2. Add oil and a generous amount of cooking spray to a medium nonstick skillet over medium heat. Add sliced mushrooms and sauté for 5–7 minutes or until liquid is evaporated.

3. Heat half-and-half in the microwave for 1 minute. Turn off flame under mushrooms. Pour half-and-half over mushrooms. Add cheese and garlic powder and stir well.

4. Place each halibut filet in an aluminum foil piece. Pour 1/4 of mushroom sauce over fish and seal. Repeat procedure for remaining 3 filets. Place foil packets on baking sheet and bake for 15 minutes or until fish flakes with a fork.

Exchanges

4 Very Lean Meat   1/2 Fat
1/2 Carbohydrate

Calories	203
Calories from Fat	58
Total Fat	6 g
Saturated Fat	2 g
Cholesterol	46 mg
Sodium	233 mg
Total Carbohydrate	7 g
Dietary Fiber	1 g
Sugars	3 g
Protein	29 g

Dietitian's Tip: Alfredo sauce is typically very high in fat, but the fat-free half-and-half solves that problem in this recipe.

Garlic Mashed Potatoes

Makes: 8 servings   *Serving Size: 1/2 cup*   *Prep Time: 15 minutes*

2 pounds russet potatoes, peeled and cut into chunks
8 garlic cloves, peeled
1 1/2 cups fat free half-and-half, heated
2 tablespoons margarine
1/4 cup fresh chives, chopped
1 teaspoon salt
1/4 teaspoon ground black pepper

1. Add potatoes and garlic cloves to a large soup pot and cover with cold water. Place on stove over high heat and bring to a boil. Boil for 20 minutes or until potatoes are softened. Drain and return to pot.

2. Add remaining ingredients and beat with an electric mixture until smooth.

✔ *National Family Health Month is in October . . . serve delicious, nutritious meals every day to your family!*

Exchanges

1 1/2 Starch   1/2 Fat

Calories 135
Calories from Fat 32
Total Fat . . . . 4 g
Saturated Fat . . . . 1 g
Cholesterol . . . . 3 mg
Sodium . . . . 394 mg
Total Carbohydrate . . . . . . 23 g
Dietary Fiber . . . . 2 g
Sugars . . . . 5 g
Protein . . . . 3 g

Chef's Tip: This dish is a classic favorite and easy too! Serve these potatoes with a wide variety of entrées.

Roasted Turkey

Makes: 20 servings   Serving Size: 4–5 ounces turkey   Prep Time: 15 minutes with skin

1 12-pound whole turkey
1 tablespoon salt
2 tablespoons margarine, melted

1. Preheat oven to 325 degrees.

2. Remove giblets from turkey. Rinse cavity. Rub cavity of bird lightly with salt.

3. Place turkey breast side up on rack in shallow roasting pan. Brush with melted margarine. Prick skin with fork.

4. When turkey begins to turn golden, place a tent of aluminum foil loosely over it.

5. Turkey will cook for approximately 3 1/2–4 1/2 hours until internal temperature reaches 180 degrees. Place a meat thermometer in thigh muscle so thermometer does not touch bone to ensure proper cooking temperature.

6. Remove from oven and let stand about 15 minutes before slicing.

Exchanges

5 Lean Meat	1/2 Fat

Calories 310
  Calories from Fat 138
Total Fat . . . . 15 g
  Saturated Fat . . . . 5 g
Cholesterol . . . . 117 mg
Sodium . . . . 284 mg
Total Carbohydrate . . . . 0 g
  Dietary Fiber . . . . 0 g
  Sugars . . . . 0 g
Protein . . . . 41 g

Chef's Tip: When roasting a bird this large, be sure to take the temperature in the thigh muscle to ensure the entire thing is cooked to 180 degrees. The thigh meat takes longer to cook than the breast meat, so you'll know the whole bird is done when the thigh meat is done.

Cranberry Salad

Makes: 8 servings   *Serving Size: 1/8 recipe*   *Prep Time: 10 minutes*

1 1-pound bag fresh cranberries

1 medium navel orange, peeled and cut into chunks

3/4 cup SPLENDA® Granular sweetener

1. In a blender or food processor, pulse cranberries and orange chunks until finely ground. Pour into a medium bowl and stir in SPLENDA® Granular until incorporated.

2. Cover and refrigerate overnight.

Exchanges

1 Fruit

Calories 44
  Calories from Fat 1
Total Fat . . . . 0 g
  Saturated Fat . . . . 0 g
Cholesterol . . . . 0 mg
Sodium . . . . 1 mg
Total Carbohydrate . . . . . . 11 g
  Dietary Fiber . . . . 3 g
  Sugars . . . . 8 g
Protein . . . . 0 g

Dietitian's Tip: Cranberries contain several antioxidants that may help fight against heart disease and some cancers.

Turkey Soup with White Beans

Makes: 10 servings   *Serving Size: 1 cup*   *Prep Time: 15 minutes*

1 tablespoon olive oil
2 small onions, finely diced
2 medium carrots, finely diced
2 medium celery stalks, finely diced
3 garlic cloves, minced
3 14.5-ounce cans fat-free, reduced-sodium chicken broth
1 1/2 teaspoons dried oregano
1/2 teaspoon paprika
2 1/2 cups cooked turkey meat, shredded (from Roasted Turkey recipe, page 384)
1 15-ounce can no-salt-added diced tomatoes with juice
1 cup orzo pasta, uncooked
1 16-ounce can cannellini (white kidney) beans, drained and rinsed
1/4 teaspoon salt
1/4 teaspoon ground black pepper

1. Add oil to a large soup pot over medium-high heat. Add onions, carrots, and celery and sauté for 5–7 minutes or until vegetables begin to soften. Stir in garlic and sauté an additional 30 seconds.

2. Add remaining ingredients and bring to a boil. Reduce heat and simmer for 20 minutes.

Exchanges

1 1/2 Starch	1 Vegetable
1 Lean Meat	

Calories 207
  Calories from Fat 33
Total Fat . . . . 4 g
  Saturated Fat . . . . 1 g
Cholesterol . . . . 27 mg
Sodium . . . . 442 mg
Total Carbohydrate . . . . . . 26 g
  Dietary Fiber . . . . 4 g
  Sugars . . . . 5 g
Protein . . . . 17 g

Chef's Tip: Make use of that leftover turkey from Thanksgiving in this tasty soup.

November ❖ Week 4

RECIPE LIST

DAY 1: Unstuffed Cabbage   **388**

DAY 2: Italian Sausage with Pepper Medley   **389**

DAY 3: Cobb Salad   **390**
French Onion Soup   **391**

DAY 4: Angel Hair with Turkey Bacon and Peas   **392**

DAY 5: Roasted Chicken   **393**
Potato Casserole   **394**

DESSERT OF THE MONTH: Sweet Potato Pie   **395**

GROCERY LIST

Fresh Produce
Garlic – 1 head
Cabbage – 1 large head
Onions – 7
Green bell peppers – 2
Red bell pepper – 1
Romaine lettuce –
  1 large head
Endive – 1 head
Tomato – 1 large
Lemons – 2
Sweet potatoes –
  1 1/4 pounds

Meat/Poultry/Fish
Lean ground beef –
  1 pound
Lean turkey Italian
  sausage links – 5
  (3-ounce) sausages
Turkey bacon – 1 package
Boneless, skinless
  chicken breasts –
  1/2 pound

3-pound fryer chicken,
  cut up into 8 pieces –
  1 chicken

Grains/Bread/Pasta
Brown rice
Croutons – small box
Angel hair pasta – 1 box

Dairy and Cheese
Eggs
Egg substitute – 1/2 pint
Shredded, reduced-fat
  Swiss cheese –
  1 package
Shredded, reduced-fat
  cheddar cheese –
  1 package
Grated Parmesan cheese
Margarine
Fat-free sour cream –
  1 container
Fat-free half-and-half –
  1/2 pint
Fat-free milk

Canned Goods and Sauces
14.5-ounce can fat-free,
  reduced-sodium beef
  broth – 4 cans
14.5-ounce can no-salt-
  added diced
  tomatoes – 2 cans
Dijon mustard – small
  bottle
10 3/4-ounce can low-fat
  cream of chicken con-
  densed soup – 1 can

Frozen Foods
Peas – small package
Hash browns – 2 pounds

Staples/Seasonings/Baking Needs
Salt/ground black pepper
Cooking spray
Olive oil
Canola oil
Dried basil
Dried oregano
Crushed red pepper
  flakes
Paprika
White wine vinegar
Red wine vinegar
Brown sugar
9-inch unbaked pie crust
10-ounce can evaporated
  fat-free milk – 1 can
Sugar
Vanilla extract
Ground cinnamon
Ground nutmeg

Unstuffed Cabbage

Makes: 5 servings *Serving Size: 1/5 recipe* *Prep Time: 20 minutes*

1 pound lean ground beef

1 cup fat-free, reduced-sodium beef broth

8 cups cabbage, shredded

1 cup diced onion

2 14.5-ounce cans no-salt-added diced tomatoes with juice

4 tablespoons white wine vinegar

2 tablespoons brown sugar

1 teaspoon salt

1/2 teaspoon ground black pepper

3 1/2 cups white or brown rice, cooked

1. Sauté ground beef in a large, deep skillet until completely cooked. Drain off any excess fat.

2. Add beef broth and shredded cabbage and cook until cabbage begins to soften.

3. Add remaining ingredients except rice and simmer for 20 minutes or until cabbage is completely cooked.

4. Serve over rice.

Exchanges

2 1/2 Starch	3 Vegetable
2 Lean Meat	

Calories 382
  Calories from Fat 75
Total Fat . . . . 8 g
  Saturated Fat . . . . 3 g
Cholesterol . . . . 55 mg
Sodium . . . . 694 mg
Total Carbohydrate . . . . . . 54 g
  Dietary Fiber . . . . 6 g
  Sugars . . . . 16 g
Protein . . . . 24 g

Chef's Tip: This recipe tastes great and is a lot less time-intensive than your grand-mother's stuffed cabbage. It's a one-skillet sensation that's sure to make you want seconds!

Italian Sausage with Pepper Medley

Makes: 5 servings   *Serving Size: 1/5 recipe*   *Prep Time: 10 minutes*

5 lean Italian turkey sausage links (14–15 ounces total)

1 teaspoon olive oil

2 green bell peppers, sliced into 1/2-inch strips

1 red bell pepper, sliced into 1/2-inch strips

1/2 teaspoon salt (optional)

1/8 teaspoon ground black pepper

1/2 teaspoon dried basil

1/2 teaspoon dried oregano

1/4 teaspoon crushed red pepper flakes

2 garlic cloves, minced

1 tablespoon water

1. Cook sausage in a large nonstick skillet over medium-high heat for 8–10 minutes or until done. Remove from pan and set aside.

2. Add oil to skillet. Add remaining ingredients and sauté for 4–5 minutes or until tender-crisp.

3. Serve peppers over sausage links.

Exchanges
2 Medium-Fat Meat   1 Vegetable

Calories 185
  Calories from Fat 91
Total Fat . . . . 10 g
  Saturated Fat . . . . 3 g
Cholesterol . . . . 60 mg
Sodium . . . . 492 mg
Total Carbohydrate . . . . 7 g
  Dietary Fiber . . . . 2 g
  Sugars . . . . 3 g
Protein . . . . 17 g

See photo insert.

Dietitian's Tip: This entrée is a terrific blend of flavors.

Cobb Salad

Makes: 8 servings   *Serving Size: 1/8 recipe*   *Prep Time: 15 minutes*

8 cups chopped romaine lettuce
2 cups chopped endive
6 slices turkey bacon, chopped
1/2 pound boneless, skinless chicken breasts, cooked and cubed
1 large tomato, seeded and diced
2 hard-boiled egg whites, sliced
1/4 cup red wine vinegar
2 tablespoons olive oil
2 teaspoons Dijon mustard

1. In a large salad bowl, toss together romaine and endive. Set aside.

2. Cook bacon in a large nonstick skillet until crisp. Arrange the chicken, tomato, egg whites, and cooled bacon over top of lettuce.

3. In a small bowl, whisk together remaining ingredients. Drizzle dressing over salad and toss to coat.

✔ *National Home Care Month is in November . . . take over a meal to someone who's taking care of a loved one.*

Exchanges

1 Very Lean Meat	1 Fat
1 Vegetable	

Calories 108
Calories from Fat 56
Total Fat . . . . 6 g
Saturated Fat . . . . 1 g
Cholesterol . . . . 25 mg
Sodium . . . . 195 mg
Total Carbohydrate . . . . 3 g
Dietary Fiber . . . . 1 g
Sugars . . . . 2 g
Protein . . . . 10 g

Chef's Tip: You can add almost anything to a Cobb salad—try cucumbers, avocado, bell peppers, or chopped ham.

French Onion Soup

Makes: 4 servings   *Serving Size: 1 cup*   *Prep Time: 10 minutes*

2 teaspoons canola oil
  Cooking spray
5 small or 3 large onions, thinly
  sliced
3 14.5-ounce cans fat-free,
  reduced-sodium beef broth
1/4 teaspoon salt (optional)
1/4 teaspoon ground black pepper
1/2 cup croutons
1/2 cup shredded, reduced-fat
  Swiss cheese

1. Add oil and a generous amount of cooking spray to a medium soup pot over medium-high heat. Add onion and cook for 15–20 minutes until onion is deeply caramelized; stirring occasionally.

2. Add broth, salt, and pepper. Bring to a boil; then reduce heat and simmer for 25 minutes.

3. Pour soup into 4 soup bowls and top each with 2 tablespoons croutons and 2 tablespoons cheese.

Exchanges

1 Fat   1 Carbohydrate

Calories 132
  Calories from Fat 40
Total Fat . . . . 4 g
  Saturated Fat . . . . 1 g
Cholesterol . . . . 5 mg
Sodium . . . . 661 mg
Total Carbohydrate . . . . . . 14 g
  Dietary Fiber . . . . 3 g
  Sugars . . . . 8 g
Protein . . . . 9 g

Chef's Tip: Caramelize means to cook until chocolate brown, but not burned.

Angel Hair with Turkey Bacon and Peas

Makes: 4 servings　　　*Serving Size: 1 cup*　　　*Prep Time: 5 minutes*

8 ounces angel hair pasta, uncooked

1 cup fat-free half-and-half

1 teaspoon grated lemon peel

1 cup frozen peas

6 strips turkey bacon, cooked and chopped

2 teaspoons fresh lemon juice

1/4 cup grated Parmesan cheese

1. Cook pasta according to package directions, omitting salt. Drain. Reserve 1/2 cup pasta cooking liquid.

2. In a large nonstick skillet, simmer half-and-half, pasta liquid, and lemon peel until slightly reduced, about 1 minute. Stir in peas, turkey bacon, and lemon juice. Simmer 2 minutes.

3. Add cooked pasta and cheese to skillet; toss to coat.

Exchanges

3 1/2 Starch　　1 Medium-Fat Meat

Calories 358
Calories from Fat 70
Total Fat . . . . 8 g
Saturated Fat . . . . 4 g
Cholesterol . . . . 27 mg
Sodium . . . . 504 mg
Total Carbohydrate . . . . . . 54 g
Dietary Fiber . . . . 4 g
Sugars . . . . 8 g
Protein . . . . 17 g

Chef's Tip: You'll love the flavor combination of sweet peas, tart lemon, and salty bacon in this dish.

Roasted Chicken

Makes: 6 servings   *Serving Size: 1 breast or 1 thigh*   *Prep Time: 5 minutes*
or 1 leg and wing

Cooking spray
1 3-pound fryer chicken, cut
into 8 pieces
1 tablespoon paprika
1/2 teaspoon salt
1/4 teaspoon ground black pepper

1. Preheat oven to 375 degrees.

2. Coat a 13 × 9-inch roasting pan with cooking spray. Arrange chicken pieces skin side up and spray generously with cooking spray. Season chicken with paprika, salt, and pepper.

3. Bake for 35 minutes or until juices run clear.

Exchanges (without skin)

3 Lean Meat   1 Fat

Calories 140
Calories from Fat 49
Total Fat . . . . 5 g
Saturated Fat . . . . 1 g
Cholesterol . . . . 65 mg
Sodium . . . . 160 mg
Total Carbohydrate . . . . . . 0 g
Dietary Fiber . . . . 0 g
Sugars . . . . 0 g
Protein . . . . 21 g

Dietitian's Tip: Taking the skin off poultry after cooking it is a good way to decrease the fat and extra calories.

Potato Casserole

Makes: 16 servings   *Serving Size: 1/2 cup*   *Prep Time: 10 minutes*

Cooking spray

2 pounds frozen hash browns

1 teaspoon margarine

1/2 cup chopped onion

1/2 teaspoon ground black pepper

1 10 3/4-ounce can low-fat cream of chicken condensed soup

1 cup fat-free sour cream

1 1/4 cups shredded, reduced-fat cheddar cheese

1 cup fat-free milk

1. Preheat oven to 375 degrees.

2. Coat a 13 × 9-inch pan with cooking spray. Spread hash browns on bottom of pan.

3. In a large nonstick skillet, melt margarine over medium-high heat. Add onion and sauté until clear. Add remaining ingredients and mix well. Cook about 5 minutes, stirring occasionally.

4. Pour soup mixture over hash browns. Bake for 50–60 minutes.

Exchanges

1 Starch	1/2 Fat

Calories 105	
Calories from Fat 25	
Total Fat . . . . 3 g	
Saturated Fat . . . . 1 g	
Cholesterol . . . . 9 mg	
Sodium . . . . 189 mg	
Total Carbohydrate . . . . . . 17 g	
Dietary Fiber . . . . 1 g	
Sugars . . . . 3 g	
Protein . . . . 5 g	

Dietitian's Tip: This healthy version of a traditional high-fat recipe takes advantage of great-tasting low-fat and fat-free products. Most recipes still need a little fat to help enhance flavor, but not nearly as much as we used to use.

Sweet Potato Pie

Makes: 10 servings   *Serving Size: 1 slice*   *Prep Time: 10 minutes*

1 9-inch unbaked pie crust

2 cups mashed cooked sweet potatoes

1 cup evaporated fat-free milk

3/4 cup sugar

1 teaspoon vanilla extract

1 teaspoon ground cinnamon

1/4 teaspoon salt

1/2 teaspoon ground nutmeg

1/2 cup egg substitute

1 tablespoon margarine

1 teaspoon lemon juice

1. Preheat oven to 350 degrees.

2. In a medium bowl, combine all ingredients except pie crust and beat with an electric mixer on low-medium speed until smooth.

3. Spoon sweet potato mixture into pie crust. Bake for 45 minutes or until set.

4. Cool completely on wire rack. Serve with light whipped topping if desired.

The ADA recommends eating only a small amount of saturated fat every day. This recipe is higher in saturated fat, so try to balance it by eating foods low in saturated fat at your other meals today.

Exchanges

1 Fat   2 1/2 Carbohydrate

Calories. 227
 Calories from Fat. 50
Total Fat . . . . 6 g
 Saturated Fat . . . . 2 g
Cholesterol . . . . 0 mg
Sodium . . . . 216 mg
Total Carbohydrate. . . . . . 40 g
 Dietary Fiber . . . . 2 g
 Sugars. . . . . 21 g
Protein. . . . . 5 g

Chef's Tip: We recommend roasting the sweet potatoes in the oven at 400 degrees for 1 hour. Remove the sweet potatoes from the oven and peel off the skin. Roasting is a great way to bring out the sweetness in the potato.

December

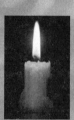

As you relax and enjoy
your friends and family
over the holidays, try some
of this month's recipes—
healthier versions of
old holiday favorites!

Healthy Holiday Eating

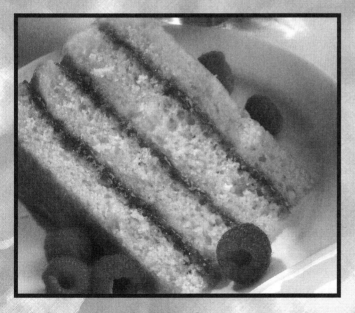

Raspberry Almond Layer Cake (page 431)
Make your holiday festivities extra special with this month's
beautiful and tasty dessert. Your guests will love these fresh
raspberries layered with almond cake and sprinkled with
powdered sugar.

December ❖ Recipes

RECIPE LIST

DAY 1: Pepper Steak over Rice **400**

DAY 2: Spicy Chicken Chili **401**

DAY 3: Shrimp Marsala **402**

DAY 4: Chicken Drumsticks **403**
Mashed Sweet Potatoes **404**

DAY 5: Roast with Vegetables **405**
Sage Stuffing **406**

GROCERY LIST

Fresh Produce
Garlic – 1 head
Green bell peppers –
   2 large
Sliced mushrooms –
   1 pint
Onions – 3 medium
Sweet potatoes – 3 large
Russet potatoes – 4 large
Carrots – small bag

Meat/Poultry/Fish
Boneless top round
   steak – 1 pound
Boneless, skinless
   chicken breasts –
   1 pound
Shrimp – 1 pound
Chicken drumsticks – 12

Beef bottom round
   roast – 3 pounds

Grains/Bread/Pasta
Brown rice
Bread crumbs
Cubed bread stuffing –
   1 bag

Dairy and Cheese
Margarine

Canned Goods
and Sauces
15-ounce can Great
   Northern beans –
   1 can
16-ounce can red kidney
   beans – 1 can
15-ounce can no-salt-
   added diced
   tomatoes – 2 cans

14.5-ounce can fat-free,
   reduced-sodium
   chicken broth – 2 cans
4-ounce can chopped
   green chilies – 1 can
15-ounce can corn –
   1 can
Dijon mustard – small
   bottle

Staples/Seasonings/
Baking Needs
Salt/ground black pepper
Cooking spray
Olive oil
Chili powder
Cumin
Cayenne pepper
Ground cinnamon
Ground nutmeg
Garlic powder
Dried sage
Red wine vinegar
Vanilla extract

Miscellaneous
Marsala wine – small
   bottle
Reduced-sodium beef
   bouillon cubes – small
   jar
Pitted prunes –
   1 package

Pepper Steak over Rice

Makes: 4 servings　　　*Serving Size: 3/4 cup beef*　　　*Prep Time: 10 minutes*
and 1/2 cup rice

1 cup brown rice, uncooked
　Cooking spray
1 pound boneless top round
　steak, cut into thin 1-inch
　slices
2 large green bell peppers,
　sliced into 1/2-inch-thick
　strips
1/4 teaspoon salt
1/4 teaspoon ground black pepper
1/4 cup water

1. Cook rice according to package directions, omitting salt.

2. Coat a large nonstick skillet with cooking spray over high heat. Add steak and sauté for about 4 minutes. Remove from pan and set aside.

3. Reduce heat to medium; add peppers to pan and sauté another 5 minutes. Add steak and any juices back to pan. Add salt, pepper, and water to pan. Sauté for 2 more minutes. Serve over rice.

✔ *World AIDS Day is December 1 every year. This dreadful disease kills many innocent people all over the world—please contribute to relief efforts.*

Exchanges

2 1/2 Starch	1 Vegetable
2 Lean Meat	

Calories 324
　Calories from Fat 59
Total Fat . . . . 7 g
　Saturated Fat . . . . 2 g
Cholesterol . . . . 58 mg
Sodium . . . . 181 mg
Total Carbohydrate . . . . . . 42 g
　Dietary Fiber . . . . 3 g
　Sugars . . . . 3 g
Protein . . . . 24 g

Chef's Tip: Be sure not to overcook the meat in this recipe, or it will be too tough.

Spicy Chicken Chili

Makes: 7 servings   *Serving Size: 1 cup*   *Prep Time: 5 minutes*

Cooking spray

1 pound boneless, skinless chicken breasts, cubed

1 tablespoon chili powder

1 teaspoon cumin

1/4 teaspoon cayenne pepper

1 15-ounce can Great Northern beans, rinsed and drained

1 16-ounce can red kidney beans, rinsed and drained

1 15-ounce can no-salt-added diced tomatoes

1 14.5-ounce can fat-free, reduced-sodium chicken broth

1/2 teaspoon salt (optional)

1/4 teaspoon ground black pepper

1 4-ounce can chopped green chilies

1 15-ounce can corn, drained (or 1 1/2 cups frozen corn, thawed)

1. Coat a large soup pot generously with cooking spray over high heat. Add chicken and sauté for 5 minutes.

2. Add remaining ingredients and bring to a boil. Reduce heat and simmer for 15 minutes.

Exchanges

2 Starch	2 Very Lean Meat

Calories 231
Calories from Fat 24
Total Fat . . . . 3 g
Saturated Fat . . . . 1 g
Cholesterol . . . . 38 mg
Sodium . . . . 501 mg
Total Carbohydrate . . . . . . 29 g
Dietary Fiber . . . . 8 g
Sugars. . . . . 5 g
Protein. . . . . 24 g

Chef's Tip: This is a hearty winter dish that is so easy to make.

Shrimp Marsala

Makes: 5 servings   *Serving Size: 1/5 recipe*   *Prep Time: 5 minutes*

2 teaspoons olive oil

1 pint sliced mushrooms

1 15-ounce can no-salt-added diced tomatoes, drained

1 cup Marsala wine

1 pound uncooked shrimp, peeled and deveined

1/2 teaspoon salt

1/4 teaspoon ground black pepper

1. Add oil to a large nonstick skillet over medium heat. Add mushrooms and sauté for 7–9 minutes. Add tomatoes and wine and simmer for 10 minutes.

2. Add shrimp, salt, and pepper. Sauté 4 more minutes or until shrimp are done.

Exchanges

2 Very Lean Meat   1/2 Fat
1 Vegetable

Calories 121
  Calories from Fat 24
Total Fat . . . . 3 g
  Saturated Fat . . . . 0 g
Cholesterol . . . . 116 mg
Sodium . . . . 400 mg
Total Carbohydrate . . . . 5 g
  Dietary Fiber . . . . 2 g
  Sugars . . . . 3 g
Protein . . . . 14 g

Chef's Tip: This is great over brown rice or linguine.

Chicken Drumsticks

Makes: 6 servings   *Serving Size: 2 drumsticks*   *Prep Time: 25 minutes*

1 small onion, chopped
2 garlic cloves, sliced
1/4 cup red wine vinegar
2 tablespoons Dijon mustard
1 tablespoon olive oil
1/2 teaspoon salt (optional)
1/4 teaspoon ground black pepper
12 chicken drumsticks, skins removed
2 cups bread crumbs

1. Preheat oven to 350 degrees.

2. In a blender or food processor, purée onion, garlic, vinegar, mustard, olive oil, salt, and pepper.

3. In a large bowl, add drumsticks and cover with marinade, turning to coat. Cover and refrigerate for 15 minutes.

4. Remove drumsticks from marinade and roll in bread crumbs, coating well.

5. Arrange drumsticks in the bottom of a shallow baking dish. Bake for 25–30 minutes or until done.

Exchanges

1 1/2 Starch   3 Lean Meat

Calories 280
  Calories from Fat 75
Total Fat . . . . 8 g
  Saturated Fat . . . . 1 g
Cholesterol . . . . 77 mg
Sodium . . . . 391 mg
Total Carbohydrate . . . . . . 21 g
  Dietary Fiber . . . . 1 g
  Sugars . . . . 3 g
Protein . . . . 28 g

Dietitian's Tip: The dark meat in chicken drumsticks has more fat than white breast meat, but removing the skins helps, and they're delicious marinated.

Mashed Sweet Potatoes

Makes: 5 servings   *Serving Size: 1/5 recipe*   *Prep Time: 20 minutes*

3 large sweet potatoes
1 1/2 teaspoons vanilla extract
1/8 teaspoon ground cinnamon
1/8 teaspoon ground nutmeg
1 tablespoon margarine

1. Wash and dry sweet potatoes and pierce on all sides with a fork. Microwave on high for approximately 15 minutes or until soft.

2. Cut potatoes in half lengthwise and scoop the meat out into a medium mixing bowl. Discard skins.

3. Mash the potato pulp with a potato masher or fork until smooth. Add remaining ingredients and mix well.

Look for an ADA Diabetes EXPO® near you. It's an interactive health fair—one-stop shopping for every diabetes-related product you need. Go to www.diabetes.org to find the EXPO® now!

Exchanges
2 Starch

Calories 135
   Calories from Fat 22
Total Fat . . . . 2 g
   Saturated Fat . . . . 0 g
Cholesterol . . . . 0 mg
Sodium . . . . 37 mg
Total Carbohydrate . . . . . . 26 g
   Dietary Fiber . . . . 3 g
   Sugars. . . . . 12 g
Protein . . . . 2 g

Dietitian's Tip: This is a much healthier version of a holiday favorite. Serve this dish any time of the year!

Roast with Vegetables

Makes: 8 servings *Serving Size: 1/8 recipe* *Prep Time: 15 minutes*

Cooking spray
1 3-pound beef bottom round roast
4 large russet potatoes, cut in long wedges (with skins)
1 medium onion, chopped
3 carrots, sliced
1 teaspoon ground black pepper
1 teaspoon garlic powder
1 cup water
2 reduced-sodium beef bouillon cubes

1. Preheat oven to 325 degrees. Place roast in a roasting pan coated with cooking spray.

2. Place potatoes, onion, and carrots around the roast in the pan. Sprinkle roast with pepper and garlic powder.

3. Add water and bouillon cubes to bottom of pan.

4. Bake for 1 1/2 to 2 hours, or until the meat is tender.

5. Slice and serve with vegetables and juice from pan.

Exchanges

1 Starch   1 Vegetable
4 Lean Meat

Calories 328
  Calories from Fat 86
Total Fat . . . . 10 g
  Saturated Fat . . . . 3 g
Cholesterol . . . . 100 mg
Sodium . . . . 230 mg
Total Carbohydrate . . . . . . 20 g
  Dietary Fiber . . . . 3 g
  Sugars . . . . 4 g
Protein . . . . 39 g

Chef's Tip: This roast makes great leftover sandwiches the next day.

Sage Stuffing

Makes: 7 servings   *Serving Size: 1/2 cup*   *Prep Time: 10 minutes*

Cooking spray
1 14.5-ounce can fat-free, reduced-sodium chicken broth
1/4 cup water
6 cups prepackaged cubed bread stuffing
1 teaspoon dried sage
1/2 cup chopped, pitted prunes
1/8 teaspoon salt (optional)
1/8 teaspoon ground black pepper

1. Preheat oven to 350 degrees.

2. Coat an 8-inch casserole dish with cooking spray. In a small saucepan, bring broth and water to a low boil.

3. In a medium bowl, toss stuffing, sage, prunes, salt, and pepper. Pour heated broth over stuffing and let sit, covered, for 5 minutes.

4. Spread stuffing evenly in casserole dish and bake for 20–25 minutes or until golden brown on top.

Exchanges

2 Starch	1/2 Fruit

Calories 193	
Calories from Fat 16	
Total Fat . . . . 2 g	
Saturated Fat . . . . 0 g	
Cholesterol . . . . 0 mg	
Sodium . . . . 575 mg	
Total Carbohydrate . . . . . . 39 g	
Dietary Fiber . . . . 3 g	
Sugars . . . . 8 g	
Protein . . . . 7 g	

Dietitian's Tip: You can buy prepackaged whole-wheat stuffing mix at the market.

December ❖ Week 2

RECIPE LIST

DAY 1: 20-Minute Chicken **408**
        Italian Veggies **409**

DAY 2: Polish Sausage and Sauerkraut **410**

DAY 3: Baked Ham with Mango
        Chutney **411**

DAY 4: Split Pea Soup **412**

DAY 5: Roasted Red Pepper and Goat
        Cheese-Stuffed Chicken **413**
        Mushroom Rice Pilaf **414**

GROCERY LIST

Fresh Produce
Garlic – 1 head
Lemon – 1
Carrots – small bag
Celery – small bag
Shallot – 1
Broccoli – 1 medium
    head
Zucchini – 2 small
Mangoes – 2 medium
Red onion – 1 medium
Mushrooms – 1 pint
Onion – 1

Meat/Poultry/Fish
Boneless, skinless
    chicken breasts –
    8 (4-ounce) breasts
Lean turkey or low-fat
    kielbasa – 1 pound
1 fully cooked boneless
    ham – 2–3 pounds

Grains/Bread/Pasta
Bread crumbs
White rice

Dairy and Cheese
Margarine
Goat cheese – small
    package

Canned Goods and Sauces
14.5-ounce can fat-free,
    reduced-sodium
    chicken broth – 5 cans
15-ounce can no-salt-
    added diced
    tomatoes – 1 can
2-pound jar sauerkraut
    – 1 jar
Roasted red peppers
    (pimientos) – 1 jar

Staples/Seasonings/Baking Needs
Salt/ground black pepper
Cooking spray
Olive oil
Dried basil
Dried sage
Cayenne pepper
Paprika
Brown sugar
Cider vinegar
Bay leaf
Honey

Miscellaneous
16-ounce package green
    split peas – 1 package

20-Minute Chicken

Makes: 4 servings   *Serving Size: 1 chicken breast*   *Prep Time: 5 minutes*

1/4 cup bread crumbs
1 teaspoon dried basil
1/8 teaspoon ground black pepper
2 garlic cloves, minced
4 4-ounce boneless, skinless
chicken breasts
Cooking spray
1 teaspoon margarine
2 tablespoons lemon juice
1/2 cup fat-free, reduced-sodium
chicken broth
1 tablespoon lemon zest

1. In a shallow dish, combine bread crumbs, basil, pepper, and garlic. Set aside.

2. Place each chicken breast between 2 sheets of plastic wrap; flatten to 1/4 inch thick using a meat tenderizer or rolling pin. Spray both sides of chicken with cooking spray. Dredge chicken in bread crumb mixture.

3. Coat a large nonstick skillet with cooking spray and melt margarine over medium-high heat. Add chicken and cook 4 minutes each side or until done. Remove chicken from pan and set aside.

4. Add lemon juice, broth, and lemon zest to skillet and cook 1 minute. Spoon sauce over chicken breasts.

Exchanges

3 Very Lean Meat	1/2 Fat
1/2 Carbohydrate	

Calories 169
Calories from Fat 37
Total Fat . . . . 4 g
Saturated Fat . . . . 1 g
Cholesterol . . . . 68 mg
Sodium . . . . 178 mg
Total Carbohydrate . . . . 5 g
Dietary Fiber . . . . 0 g
Sugars . . . . 1 g
Protein . . . . 26 g

Chef's Tip: Pounding the chicken breasts flat makes them cook more quickly, so they're more tender. If your chicken is too dry, it's overcooked!

Italian Veggies

Makes: 8 servings   *Serving Size: 1/2 cup*   *Prep Time: 10 minutes*

Cooking spray
1 tablespoon olive oil
3 garlic cloves, minced
2 cups carrots, sliced (about
  2 medium or 1 large carrot)
2 cups broccoli florets (one
  medium head)
2 cups zucchini, thinly sliced
  (2 small zucchini)
1/2 teaspoon salt
1 tablespoon water

1. Add oil and a generous amount of cooking spray to a large nonstick skillet over medium-high heat. Add remaining ingredients except water and sauté for 5–6 minutes.

2. Turn heat to high, add water, and cover vegetables. Steam for 3–4 minutes or until tender-crisp.

Exchanges

1 Vegetable	1/2 Fat

Calories 39	
Calories from Fat 17	
Total Fat . . . . 2 g	
Saturated Fat . . . . 0 g	
Cholesterol . . . . 0 mg	
Sodium . . . . 162 mg	
Total Carbohydrate . . . . . . 5 g	
Dietary Fiber . . . . 2 g	
Sugars . . . . 3 g	
Protein . . . . 1 g	

Chef's Tip: Sautéing these veggies with garlic before steaming them adds great flavor.

Polish Sausage and Sauerkraut

Makes: 6 servings   *Serving Size: 1 cup*   *Prep Time: 5 minutes*

Cooking spray

1 pound lean turkey or low-fat kielbasa, cut into 1-inch chunks

1 15-ounce can no-salt-added diced tomatoes with juice

1 2-pound jar sauerkraut, drained

1 tablespoon brown sugar

1. Coat a large, deep nonstick skillet with cooking spray and sauté sausage over medium-high heat until beginning to brown, about 5 minutes. Add tomatoes and increase heat to high; simmer for 5 minutes.

2. Add sauerkraut and brown sugar and simmer 10 more minutes.

Exchanges

1 Medium-Fat Meat   3 Vegetable

Calories 168
  Calories from Fat 63
Total Fat . . . . 7 g
  Saturated Fat . . . . 3 g
Cholesterol . . . . 43 mg
Sodium . . . . 1087 mg
Total Carbohydrate . . . . . . 15 g
  Dietary Fiber . . . . 5 g
  Sugars . . . . 10 g
Protein . . . . 12 g

Dietitian's Tip: This lean Polish turkey sausage means you can enjoy Polish sausage again!

Baked Ham with Mango Chutney

Makes: 6 servings   *Serving Size: 1/6 recipe*   *Prep Time: 10 minutes*
                           (see Chef's Tip)

1 2 1/2-pound fully cooked boneless ham

1 tablespoon olive oil

2 10-ounce mangoes, peeled and cut into cubes

1 medium red onion, thinly sliced

1/2 cup water

1/4 cup cider vinegar

2 tablespoons honey

1/4 teaspoon cayenne pepper

1. Preheat oven to 325 degrees. Place ham on a rack in a shallow roasting pan. Bake for 40 minutes.

2. Add oil to a medium saucepan over high heat. Add mangoes and red onion and sauté for 5 minutes. Add remaining ingredients and bring to a boil, stirring occasionally. Reduce heat and simmer for 15 minutes or until thickened.

3. Spoon chutney over sliced ham.

Exchanges

4 Lean Meat   1/2 Carbohydrate
1 Fruit

Calories 301	
Calories from Fat 108	
Total Fat . . . . 12 g	
Saturated Fat . . . . 4 g	
Cholesterol . . . . 70 mg	
Sodium . . . . 1711 mg	
Total Carbohydrate . . . . . . 21 g	
Dietary Fiber . . . . 2 g	
Sugars . . . . 18 g	
Protein . . . . 28 g	

Chef's Tip: Reserve 1 cup chopped ham without chutney for tomorrow's Split Pea Soup recipe.

Split Pea Soup

Makes: 8 servings   *Serving Size: 1/8 recipe*   *Prep Time: 15 minutes*

1 tablespoon olive oil
1 large carrot, finely diced
2 celery stalks, finely diced
1 shallot, minced
1 garlic clove, minced
1 teaspoon salt
1/4 teaspoon ground black pepper
1 16-ounce package green split peas
3 14.5-ounce cans fat-free, reduced-sodium chicken broth
1 cup chopped ham

1. Add oil to a large soup pot over medium-high heat. Sauté carrots, celery, and shallots for 3–4 minutes or until shallots begin to turn clear. Add garlic and sauté 1 more minute.

2. Add remaining ingredients except ham and bring to a boil. Simmer uncovered for 25–30 minutes.

3. Purée soup in a blender or with an immersion blender until smooth. Stir in ham and bring back to a simmer over medium heat for 2–3 minutes.

✔ *Did you know you can organize a School Walk for Diabetes®? Earn money, raise school spirit, and help the community at the same time! Go to www.diabetes.org to find out how.*

Exchanges

2 Starch   2 Very Lean Meat

Calories	232
Calories from Fat	33
Total Fat	4 g
Saturated Fat	1 g
Cholesterol	10 mg
Sodium	634 mg
Total Carbohydrate	33 g
Dietary Fiber	12 g
Sugars	6 g
Protein	18 g

Chef's Tip: This soup freezes well and tastes great reheated.

Roasted Red Pepper and Goat Cheese-Stuffed Chicken

Makes: 4 servings   *Serving Size: 1 chicken breast   Prep Time: 15 minutes*

4 4-ounce boneless, skinless chicken breasts
1 cup jarred roasted red peppers, finely chopped
1/4 cup goat cheese
2 garlic cloves, minced
1/2 teaspoon salt
1/2 teaspoon ground black pepper
1 teaspoon paprika
   Cooking spray

1. Preheat oven to 350 degrees.

2. Place each chicken breast between 2 sheets of plastic wrap; flatten to 1/4 inch thick using a meat tenderizer or rolling pin. Set aside.

3. In a medium bowl combine roasted red peppers, goat cheese, and garlic. Spread 3 tablespoons of this mixture on one side of the pounded chicken breast. Roll breast and secure the seam with a toothpick. Repeat procedure for remaining 3 chicken breasts.

4. Sprinkle all sides of rolled chicken breasts with salt, pepper, and paprika.

5. Coat a medium glass or metal baking dish with cooking spray and place chicken in dish seam side down. Spray chicken breasts generously with cooking spray. Bake for 30 minutes or until chicken is done.

6. To serve, remove toothpicks and slice each piece into 5 rounds. Serve over Mushroom Rice Pilaf (see recipe, page 414).

Exchanges

3 Very Lean Meat	1/2 Fat

Calories. 135
  Calories from Fat. 36
Total Fat . . . . 4 g
  Saturated Fat . . . . 2 g
Cholesterol . . . . 59 mg
Sodium . . . . 501 mg
Total Carbohydrate. . . . . . . 3 g
  Dietary Fiber . . . . 1 g
  Sugars. . . . . 3 g
Protein. . . . . 21 g

Chef's Tip: Impress your gourmet friends with this easy and healthy meal!

Mushroom Rice Pilaf

Makes: 5 servings   *Serving Size: 2/3 cup*   *Prep Time: 10 minutes*

1 teaspoon olive oil

1 pint mushrooms, finely chopped

1 medium onion, finely diced

1 cup white rice, uncooked

3 cups fat-free, reduced-sodium chicken broth

1/4 teaspoon dried sage

1 bay leaf

1/2 teaspoon salt (optional)

1/4 teaspoon ground black pepper

1. Add oil to a medium saucepan over medium-high heat. Sauté mushrooms and onion for 6–7 minutes or until liquid is evaporated.

2. Add rice and stir constantly over heat for 2 minutes. Pour chicken broth, sage, and bay leaf over mixture and stir. Bring to a boil.

3. Reduce heat and simmer, covered, for 20 minutes.

4. Remove bay leaf. Season with salt and pepper and fluff rice with a fork.

Exchanges

2 Starch	1 Vegetable

Calories 171
Calories from Fat 12
Total Fat . . . . 1 g
Saturated Fat . . . . 0 g
Cholesterol . . . . 0 mg
Sodium . . . . 304 mg
Total Carbohydrate . . . . . . 34 g
Dietary Fiber . . . . 1 g
Sugars . . . . 3 g
Protein . . . . 5 g

Chef's Tip: It's important to brown the rice after cooking the mushrooms and before adding the liquid. This imparts great toasted flavor to the rice and elevates this dish from the ordinary to the extraordinary.

December ❖ Week 3

GROCERY LIST

Fresh Produce
Garlic – 1 head
Fresh parsley – 1 bunch
Lemons – 2
Tomato – 1 medium
Onions – 2 small
Red new potatoes –
1 pound
Celery – small bag
Green bell pepper –
1 small

Meat/Poultry/Fish
Salmon filets – 4
(4-ounce) filets
Cornish game hens – 4
Pork tenderloin –
1 pound
Lean smoked turkey
sausage – 1 pound
Boneless, skinless
chicken breasts –
1 pound

Grains/Bread/Pasta
Manicotti pasta – 1 box

Dairy and Cheese
Eggs
Fat-free ricotta cheese –
30 ounces
Shredded, reduced-fat
mozzarella cheese –
1 package
Fresh Parmesan cheese –
1 wedge

Canned Goods and Sauces
26-ounce jar marinara
pasta sauce – 2 jars
Lite soy sauce – small
jar
14-ounce can artichoke
hearts – 2 cans
2-ounce can sliced black
olives – 1 can
Light sugar-free apricot
preserves – small jar
8-ounce can no-salt-
added tomato sauce –
1 can
14.5-ounce can fat-free,
reduced-sodium
chicken broth – 2 cans

Frozen Foods
10-ounce package sliced
okra – 1 package

Staples/Seasonings/ Baking Needs
Salt/ground black pepper
Cooking spray
Olive oil
Canola oil
Rice wine vinegar
Red wine vinegar
Balsamic vinegar
Sesame oil
Crushed red pepper
flakes
Dried oregano
Dried thyme
Cayenne pepper
All-purpose flour
Hot pepper sauce
Honey

Miscellaneous
Orange juice – small
carton
Sesame seeds
Pitted prunes (dried
plums) – 1 package

415

Manicotti

Makes: 6 servings   Serving Size: 2–3 manicotti shells   Prep Time: 25 minutes

1 8-ounce package manicotti noodles

2 eggs

30 ounces fat-free ricotta cheese

1 1/4 cups shredded, reduced-fat mozzarella cheese, divided

1/4 cup grated fresh Parmesan cheese

1/4 cup chopped fresh parsley
    Cooking spray

2 26-ounce jars marinara pasta sauce

1. Preheat oven to 350 degrees.

2. Cook manicotti according to package directions, omitting salt; drain.

3. In a large bowl, beat eggs, then stir in ricotta cheese, 1 cup mozzarella cheese, Parmesan cheese, and parsley. Mix well.

4. Coat the bottom of a 15 × 10 × 2-inch glass baking dish with cooking spray.

5. Spread 1 jar pasta sauce on bottom of baking dish. Fill each cooked manicotti with ricotta mixture. Arrange filled manicotti in baking dish. Top with other jar pasta sauce and 1 cup mozzarella cheese.

6. Cover with foil and bake until bubbly, about 45 minutes. Uncover and continue cooking until cheese begins to brown, about 10–15 minutes.

Exchanges

2 1/2 Starch	4 Vegetable
4 Lean Meat	

Calories 440
  Calories from Fat 62
Total Fat . . . . 7 g
  Saturated Fat . . . . 4 g
Cholesterol . . . . 133 mg
Sodium . . . . 1064 mg
Total Carbohydrate . . . . . . 58 g
  Dietary Fiber . . . . 8 g
  Sugars . . . . 23 g
Protein . . . . 39 g

Chef's Tip: Try adding a small box of frozen chopped spinach to this dish—thaw and drain it, and mix it into the ricotta cheese mixture.

Salmon with Citrus Sauce

Makes: 4 servings   *Serving Size: 1 salmon filet*   *Prep Time: 10 minutes*

Cooking spray
4   4-ounce salmon filets
1/4   teaspoon ground black pepper
1   cup orange juice
1/4   cup lemon juice
3   tablespoons lite soy sauce
1   tablespoon rice wine vinegar
2   teaspoons sesame oil
1/4   teaspoon crushed red pepper flakes

1. Preheat oven to 350 degrees. Coat a shallow baking dish with cooking spray.

2. Season both sides of salmon filets with pepper and arrange in bottom of the baking dish. Bake for 18–20 minutes or until done.

3. While salmon is baking, add remaining ingredients to a medium saucepan over high heat. Bring to a boil, stirring constantly. Reduce heat and simmer for 15 minutes.

4. Remove salmon from pan and serve with sauce.

Exchanges

3 Lean Meat	1 Fat
1/2 Fruit	

Calories 248
Calories from Fat 109
Total Fat . . . . 12 g
Saturated Fat . . . . 2 g
Cholesterol . . . . 77 mg
Sodium . . . . 516 mg
Total Carbohydrate . . . . 9 g
Dietary Fiber . . . . 0 g
Sugars . . . . 8 g
Protein . . . . 25 g

Chef's Tip: This is an easy way to cook salmon steaks.

Artichoke Salad

DRESSING

1/2 teaspoon dried oregano

1/4 cup red wine vinegar

2 tablespoons olive oil

1/8 teaspoon salt

1/8 teaspoon ground black pepper

SALAD

2 14-ounce cans artichoke hearts, drained and quartered

1 2-ounce can sliced black olives, drained

1 medium tomato, seeded and finely diced

1 small onion, thinly sliced

1. In a small bowl, whisk together all dressing ingredients; set aside.

2. In a large bowl, combine all salad ingredients. Pour dressing over salad and toss to coat.

Exchanges

1 Vegetable	1 Fat

Calories	73
Calories from Fat	45
Total Fat	5 g
Saturated Fat	1 g
Cholesterol	0 mg
Sodium	270 mg
Total Carbohydrate	7 g
Dietary Fiber	1 g
Sugars	2 g
Protein	2 g

Dietitian's Tip: This is another great luncheon salad—so easy and elegant!

Asian Sesame Cornish Game Hens

Makes: 8 servings   *Serving Size: 1/2 Cornish hen*   *Prep Time: 5 minutes*

Cooking spray
1/4 cup light sugar-free apricot preserves
1 teaspoon lite soy sauce
1 teaspoon rice wine vinegar
1 teaspoon sesame oil
1/4 teaspoon hot pepper sauce
2 tablespoons sesame seeds
4 Cornish game hens

1. Preheat oven to 350 degrees. Coat a large glass or metal baking dish with cooking spray.

2. In a small saucepan, combine preserves, soy sauce, vinegar, sesame oil, and hot pepper sauce over medium heat. Bring to a simmer, stirring occasionally. Simmer about 10 minutes or until the sauce becomes glaze-like.

3. Wash and pat dry Cornish game hens. Arrange hens breast side up in the baking dish. Brush each hen generously with glaze. Sprinkle with sesame seeds and bake for 30–35 minutes or until done.

Exchanges (without skin)
3 Lean Meat

Calories	143
Calories from Fat	46
Total Fat	5 g
Saturated Fat	1 g
Cholesterol	85 mg
Sodium	81 mg
Total Carbohydrate	2 g
Dietary Fiber	0 g
Sugars	0 g
Protein	21 g

Dietitian's Tip: Be sure to remove the skins of these moist hens before eating them, to reduce saturated fat and calories!

Pork Loin with Dried Plums

Makes: 4 servings   *Serving Size: 1/4 recipe*   *Prep Time: 15 minutes*

PORK

 1 pound pork tenderloin
15 pitted prunes (dried plums)
1/2 teaspoon salt
1/4 teaspoon ground black pepper
      Cooking spray

GLAZE

 1 cup balsamic vinegar
1/4 cup pitted prunes
 1 tablespoon honey

Exchanges

3 Very Lean Meat	2 Fruit
1 Carbohydrate	

Calories 292	
Calories from Fat 39	
Total Fat . . . . 4 g	
Saturated Fat . . . . 1 g	
Cholesterol . . . . 65 mg	
Sodium . . . . 340 mg	
Total Carbohydrate . . . . . . 43 g	
Dietary Fiber . . . . 3 g	
Sugars . . . . 31 g	
Protein . . . . 25 g	

1. Preheat oven to 375 degrees.

2. Using a small sharp knife, make 6–8 slits in the side of the tenderloin to form several small pockets in a row. Do not cut all the way through. Stuff 1-2 dried plums into each pocket. Season the tenderloin well with salt and pepper.

3. Coat a large sauté pan with cooking spray and heat over high heat. Add whole pork tenderloin and sear on each side for 3 minutes. Remove from pan and set aside.

4. Add vinegar, prunes, and honey to pan over high heat. Bring to a boil for 5 minutes. Purée mixture in blender and set aside.

5. Spread 2 tablespoons glaze on all sides of the tenderloin and transfer to a baking sheet. Bake for 25–30 minutes or until done.

6. Reheat the glaze, if necessary, and pour over cooked tenderloin. Slice thinly and serve.

Dietitian's Tip: Prunes (dried plums) are a good source of fiber and potassium.

Garlic Olive Oil Potatoes

1 pound red new potatoes, quartered

1 1/2 teaspoons olive oil

1/2 teaspoon salt

1/2 teaspoon ground black pepper

2 garlic cloves, minced

1. Preheat oven to 400 degrees.

2. In a large bowl, toss all ingredients together and spread evenly on a baking sheet. Bake 30 minutes or until golden brown.

Exchanges

1 1/2 Starch

Calories	103
Calories from Fat	16
Total Fat	2 g
Saturated Fat	0 g
Cholesterol	0 mg
Sodium	300 mg
Total Carbohydrate	20 g
Dietary Fiber	2 g
Sugars	2 g
Protein	2 g

Chef's Tip: Another classic recipe with wonderful flavor—this can be a side dish for any meat or poultry entrée.

Chicken Sausage Gumbo

Makes: 7 servings   *Serving Size: 1 cup*   *Prep Time: 15 minutes*

Cooking spray

1 small onion, finely diced (about 1/2 cup)

2 stalks celery, finely diced (about 1/2 cup)

1 small green bell pepper, finely diced (about 1 cup)

1 pound lean smoked turkey sausage, diced

1 8-ounce can no-salt-added tomato sauce

1 10-ounce package frozen sliced okra

1/2 teaspoon dried thyme

1/4 teaspoon cayenne pepper

1/4 teaspoon dried oregano

2 14.5-ounce cans fat-free, reduced-sodium chicken broth

1 tablespoon canola oil

2 tablespoons all-purpose flour

1 pound boneless, skinless chicken breasts, cubed

1. Coat a large soup pot with cooking spray over high heat. Add onion, celery, and green pepper and sauté for 6–7 minutes or until beginning to brown. Add sausage and sauté another 5 minutes.

2. Add tomato sauce, okra, thyme, cayenne pepper, oregano, and chicken broth and bring to a boil. Reduce heat and simmer for 15 minutes.

3. In a small nonstick skillet, heat oil over medium heat. Stir in flour and, stirring occasionally, cook until beginning to brown, creating a roux. Stir roux into gumbo and bring back to a boil.

4. Reduce heat to a simmer and add chicken. Simmer for 10–12 minutes or until chicken is done.

Exchanges

3 Lean Meat   1 Carbohydrate

Calories 247
  Calories from Fat 85
Total Fat . . . . 9 g
  Saturated Fat . . . . 2 g
Cholesterol . . . . 80 mg
Sodium . . . . 1308 mg
Total Carbohydrate . . . . . . 12 g
  Dietary Fiber . . . . 2 g
  Sugars . . . . 7 g
Protein . . . . 26 g

Chef's Tip: Serve this hearty gumbo over brown rice.

December ❖ Week 4

GROCERY LIST

Fresh Produce
Garlic – 1 head
Red onion – 1 large
Onion – 1 small
Fresh parsley – 1 bunch
Raspberries – 1 1/2 pints
Mixed baby field
greens – 4 cups
Asparagus – 1 pound
Fresh basil – 1 bunch

Meat/Poultry/Fish
Lean ground beef –
1 pound
Center-cut boneless pork
chops – 4 (4-ounce)
chops
3-pound fryer chicken,
cut into 8 pieces –
1 chicken

Grains/Bread/Pasta
6-inch corn tortillas – 10
Bread crumbs
Penne pasta – 1 box
Kluski-style noodles –
1 bag or box

Dairy and Cheese
Shredded, reduced-fat
Mexican-style cheese
– 1 package
Egg substitute – 1/2 pint
Eggs

Canned Goods and Sauces
16-ounce can fat-free
refried beans – 1 can
8-ounce can no-salt-
added tomato sauce –
2 cans
14.5-ounce can fat-free,
reduced-sodium
chicken broth – 6 cans
4-ounce can no-salt-
added tomato paste –
1 can
Unsweetened apple-
sauce – small jar
10-ounce jar light sugar-
free seedless rasp-
berry preserves – 1 jar

Staples/Seasonings/Baking Needs
Salt/ground black pepper
Cooking spray
Olive oil
Canola oil
Red wine vinegar
White wine vinegar
Crushed red pepper
flakes
Chili powder
Cumin
Cayenne pepper
Dried oregano
Dried parsley
All-purpose flour
18.25-ounce package
yellow cake mix
(3 grams of fat per
serving) – 1 box
Almond extract
Powdered sugar – small
box

Miscellaneous
Honey
2.5-ounce package
Matzo ball mix –
1 package
Pine nuts – small package
Sun-dried tomatoes –
small package (not
packed in oil)

Enchiladas

Makes: 5 servings   *Serving Size: 2 enchiladas*   *Prep Time: 15 minutes*

Cooking spray
3/4 pound 90% lean ground beef
1 16-ounce can fat-free refried beans
1/3 cup shredded, reduced-fat Mexican-style cheese, divided
1/4 teaspoon crushed red pepper flakes
1/2 teaspoon salt (optional)
1/4 teaspoon ground black pepper
10 6-inch corn tortillas, steamed
2 8-ounce cans no-salt-added tomato sauce
2 teaspoons chili powder
1 teaspoon cumin
1/4 teaspoon cayenne pepper

1. Preheat oven to 375 degrees. Coat a large glass or metal baking dish with cooking spray.

2. In a large nonstick skillet, cook ground beef for 7–9 minutes or until beginning to brown; drain excess fat. Stir in refried beans, half the cheese, red pepper flakes, salt, and pepper. Reduce heat and cook for 3 minutes.

3. Fill one tortilla with about 1/4 cup of meat and bean mixture and roll tortilla. Repeat for remaining tortillas.

4. Line baking dish with enchiladas, seam side down.

5. In a small bowl, combine remaining ingredients except the cheese. Pour tomato sauce over enchiladas and sprinkle with remaining cheese. Bake for 20–25 minutes or until cheese is bubbly.

Exchanges

2 1/2 Starch	1 Vegetable
2 Lean Meat	1/2 Fat

Calories 351
  Calories from Fat 84
Total Fat . . . . 9 g
  Saturated Fat . . . . 4 g
Cholesterol . . . . 51 mg
Sodium . . . . 562 mg
Total Carbohydrate . . . . . . 42 g
  Dietary Fiber . . . . 8 g
  Sugars . . . . 6 g
Protein . . . . 24 g

Chef's Tip: To steam tortillas, layer them in between sheets of damp paper towels and microwave on high for 1 minute.

Breaded Pork Cutlets

Makes: 4 servings   *Serving Size: 1 cutlet*   *Prep Time: 15 minutes*

1/3 cup all-purpose flour
1/2 cup egg substitute
1/2 teaspoon salt
1/4 teaspoon ground black pepper
1/2 cup bread crumbs
4 4-ounce boneless, center-cut
  pork chops
  Cooking spray

1. Preheat oven to 350 degrees.

2. Place flour in a shallow dish. Place egg substitute in a shallow dish. Add salt and pepper to bread crumbs and place in a shallow dish.

3. Place 1 pork chop between two sheets of plastic wrap. Using a meat tenderizer or rolling pin, pound chops to 1/4 inch thickness. Repeat for remaining 3 chops.

4. Dredge each chop in flour, coating all sides, then dip into egg substitute and roll in bread crumb mixture, coating well.

5. Coat a baking dish with cooking spray and line the bottom of the pan with chops. Spray each chop with more cooking spray. Bake for 20–25 minutes.

Exchanges

1 Starch	3 Lean Meat

Calories	229
Calories from Fat	63
Total Fat	7 g
Saturated Fat	2 g
Cholesterol	54 mg
Sodium	382 mg
Total Carbohydrate	14 g
Dietary Fiber	0 g
Sugars	1 g
Protein	26 g

Chef's Tip: Add herbs to the bread crumbs for an extra kick. Try one teaspoon each of dried oregano, thyme, and basil.

Red Onion Marmalade

Makes: 4 servings   *Serving Size: 1/4 recipe*   *Prep Time: 10 minutes*

1 tablespoon olive oil

1 large red onion, thinly sliced
(about 1 1/2 cups)

1/3 cup red wine vinegar

1 1/2 tablespoons honey

1/4 teaspoon salt

Dash ground black pepper

1. Add oil to a medium saucepan over high heat. Add onion and sauté for 7–10 minutes or until beginning to caramelize.

2. Add remaining ingredients and bring to a boil. Reduce heat and simmer for 15–20 minutes or until thickened.

Exchanges

1/2 Fat   1/2 Carbohydrate

Calories 72
Calories from Fat 31
Total Fat . . . . 3 g
Saturated Fat . . . . 0 g
Cholesterol . . . . 0 mg
Sodium . . . . 147 mg
Total Carbohydrate . . . . . . 11 g
Dietary Fiber . . . . 1 g
Sugars . . . . 9 g
Protein . . . . 1 g

Chef's Tip: Be sure to cook this tasty meat accompaniment until the onions are nice and soft.

Matzo Ball Soup

Makes: 4 servings   *Serving Size: 1/4 cup soup with 3 matzo balls*   *Prep Time: 20 minutes*

2 eggs
1 tablespoon canola oil
1 2.5-ounce package Matzo ball mix
  Cooking spray
1 small onion, thinly sliced
3 14.5-ounce cans fat-free, reduced-sodium chicken broth
2 tablespoons finely chopped fresh parsley
1/2 teaspoon salt

1. In a small bowl, whisk eggs and oil together. Using a fork, stir in Matzo ball mix until blended. Refrigerate for 15 minutes.

2. Coat a large soup pot with cooking spray. Cook onions over medium heat for 5–6 minutes or until just beginning to caramelize. Add broth and turn heat to high. Bring to a boil.

3. Wet hands and form Matzo ball batter into 1-inch balls, making 12–13 balls. Drop balls into boiling water. Reduce heat and simmer, covered, for 15 minutes.

4. Add parsley and salt, cover, and simmer 5 more minutes.

Exchanges

1 Starch   1 Medium-Fat Meat

Calories 156
  Calories from Fat 53
Total Fat . . . . 6 g
  Saturated Fat . . . . 1 g
Cholesterol . . . . 107 mg
Sodium . . . . 1560 mg
Total Carbohydrate . . . . . . 16 g
  Dietary Fiber . . . . 2 g
  Sugars . . . . 3 g
Protein . . . . 8 g

Chef's Tip: If you want to use dried parsley in this recipe, reduce the amount to 1 tablespoon and add at the same time as the broth.

Green Salad with Raspberry Vinaigrette

Makes: 5 servings   *Serving Size: 1 cup*   *Prep Time: 5 minutes*

DRESSING

- **1/4** cup white wine vinegar
- **1/2** cup fresh raspberries, puréed
- **1 1/2** tablespoons olive oil
- **1/4** teaspoon salt
- Pinch ground black pepper

SALAD

- **4** cups mixed baby field greens
- **1** cup fresh raspberries
- **1** tablespoon pine nuts

1. In a small bowl, whisk dressing ingredients.

2. In a medium salad bowl, toss together salad ingredients. Drizzle dressing over salad and toss gently to coat.

Exchanges

1 Vegetable	1 Fat

Calories 72	
Calories from Fat 48	
Total Fat . . . . 5 g	
Saturated Fat . . . . 1 g	
Cholesterol . . . . 0 mg	
Sodium . . . . 122 mg	
Total Carbohydrate . . . . 6 g	
Dietary Fiber . . . . 3 g	
Sugars . . . . 3 g	
Protein . . . . 1 g	

See photo insert.

Chef's Tip: Serve this beautiful, tasty salad to your holiday party guests.

Pasta with Asparagus and Sun-Dried Tomatoes

Makes: 4 servings   *Serving Size: 1/4 recipe*   *Prep Time: 5 minutes*

8 ounces penne pasta, uncooked
1 tablespoon olive oil, divided
1 pound asparagus, trimmed, cut into 1/2-inch pieces
1/2 cup chopped sun-dried tomatoes
1/2 cup chopped fresh basil
2 large garlic cloves, minced
1/2 teaspoon dried oregano
1/4 teaspoon crushed red pepper flakes
1 14.5-ounce can fat-free, reduced-sodium chicken broth
2 tablespoons tomato paste

1. Cook pasta according to package directions, omitting salt; drain.

2. Heat 2 teaspoons oil in a large nonstick skillet over medium-high heat. Add asparagus and sauté about 5 minutes. Remove asparagus from pan and set aside.

3. Add 1 teaspoon oil to skillet over medium-high heat. Add sun-dried tomatoes, basil, garlic, oregano, and crushed red pepper flakes and sauté about 3 minutes.

4. Add broth and tomato paste to skillet and bring to a low boil. Stir occasionally and cook for 5–7 minutes or until sauce thickens.

5. Add sauce and cooked asparagus to cooked pasta and toss to coat.

Exchanges

3 Starch	1/2 Fat
1 Vegetable	

Calories 290
  Calories from Fat 44
Total Fat . . . . 5 g
  Saturated Fat . . . . 1 g
Cholesterol . . . . 0 mg
Sodium . . . . 267 mg
Total Carbohydrate . . . . . . 51 g
  Dietary Fiber . . . . 4 g
  Sugars . . . . 6 g
Protein . . . . 11 g

Chef's Tip: Sprinkle this pasta with Parmesan cheese before serving.

Chicken and Noodles

Makes: 6 servings   *Serving Size: 1 cup*   *Prep Time: 5 minutes*

Cooking spray
1 3-pound fryer chicken, cut up into 8 pieces
2 14.5-ounce cans reduced sodium, fat-free chicken broth
2 cups water
3 cups kluski-style noodles, uncooked
1 tablespoon dried parsley
4 tablespoons cold water
2 tablespoons all-purpose flour
1/2 teaspoon salt

1. Preheat oven to 350 degrees. Coat a shallow baking dish with cooking spray. Remove skin from chicken pieces and trim any excess fat.

2. Lay chicken pieces in bottom of baking dish and spray generously with cooking spray. Bake for 25 minutes or until done. Set aside to cool. Once cool enough to handle, shred chicken meat from bone and set aside.

3. In a large saucepan, bring chicken broth and water to a boil. Add noodles and parsley and cook for 15 minutes or until noodles are softened.

4. In a small bowl, whisk together water and flour. Stir into broth and boil for 2–3 minutes. Reduce heat to simmer. Add salt and shredded chicken until heated through.

Exchanges

1 1/2 Starch	3 Lean Meat

Calories 281
  Calories from Fat 69
Total Fat . . . . 8 g
  Saturated Fat . . . . 2 g
Cholesterol . . . . 129 mg
Sodium . . . . 596 mg
Total Carbohydrate . . . . . . 24 g
  Dietary Fiber . . . . 1 g
  Sugars . . . . 2 g
Protein . . . . 27 g

Chef's Tip: Kluski-style noodles are a dense, egg-style noodle that looks like really fat pasta.

Raspberry Almond Layer Cake

Makes: 14 servings   *Serving Size: 1 slice*   *Prep Time: 15 minutes*

CAKE

Cooking spray
1   18.25-ounce package yellow cake mix (3 grams of fat per serving)
1 1/4   cups water
1   egg
3   egg whites
1/4   cup canola oil
3   tablespoons unsweetened applesauce
1   teaspoon almond extract

FILLING

1   10-ounce jar light sugar-free seedless raspberry preserves

TOPPING

1/4   cup powdered sugar
1   cup fresh raspberries

1. Preheat oven to 350 degrees. Coat two 8-inch cake pans with cooking spray.

2. In a large bowl, mix together cake ingredients and beat with an electric mixer on low speed for 30 seconds. Increase speed to medium and beat for 2 minutes.

3. Divide batter evenly between cake pans and bake for 30–35 minutes or until a toothpick inserted in the center comes out clean. Cool 10 minutes in pan. Run knife around side of pan before removing. Cool completely.

4. To prepare filling, heat preserves in a small saucepan over low heat for 3–4 minutes or until they just begin to thin. Do not simmer or boil.

5. To assemble cake, using a long, sharp knife, slice cakes in half lengthwise to create 4 cake halves. Place one of the bottom cake halves on a large plate or cake plate, cut side up. Spoon 1/3 of the raspberry preserves on top and spread evenly over entire cake within 1/4 inch of the sides. Top with one of the top cake halves, cut side up. Spoon another 1/3 of the raspberry preserves on top and spread over entire cake within 1/4 inch of the sides. Top with the other bottom half, cut side up. Spoon the remaining raspberry preserves on top and spread over entire cake within 1/4 inch of the sides. Top with the last top cake half, cut side down.

6. To top cake, sift 1/4 cup powdered sugar over entire cake, letting some sprinkle down onto the plate. Line the fresh raspberries along the bottom edge of the cake and pile 3 of them on the top middle of the cake to garnish.

See photo insert.

Chef's Tip: Use mint leaves in your garnish for added color.

Exchanges

1 Fat	2 1/2 Carbohydrate

Calories	225
Calories from Fat	69
Total Fat	8 g
Saturated Fat	2 g
Cholesterol	15 mg
Sodium	248 mg
Total Carbohydrate	38 g
Dietary Fiber	1 g
Sugars	22 g
Protein	3 g

Index

Alphabetical List of Recipes

Subject Index

Appetizers

Beans

Beef

Breads and Muffins

Breakfast

Broccoli

Chicken

Chicken Breasts with Raspberry
   Balsamic Glaze, 23
Chicken Cacciatore, 102
Chicken Caesar Salad, 292
Chicken Caesar Wrap, 245
Chicken Couscous Salad, 298
Chicken Drumsticks, 403
Chicken Fajita Pizza, 150
Chicken Fajitas, 138
Chicken Fingers, 301
Chicken Guacamole Salad, 212
Chicken Gyros, 86
Chicken Hash, 172
Chicken Kabobs, 241
Chicken Marsala, 256
Chicken Parmesan, 283
Chicken Pasta Salad with Fresh
   Mozzarella, 320
Chicken Sausage Gumbo, 422
Chicken Tacos, 170
Chicken Tostadas, 159
Chicken Vesuvio, 69
Chicken with Portabello Tofu Sauce,
   130
Greek Lemon Chicken and Rice, 280
Honey Lime Chicken, 220
Jerk Chicken, 62
Kung Pao Chicken, 268
Lemon Chicken with Bell Peppers,
   201
Mandarin Orange Chicken Salad, 308
Mango Salsa Chicken over Rice, 190
Marinated Grilled Chicken, 192
Mediterranean Chicken, 277
Orange Chicken, 113
Pecan Chicken, 15
Pecan Chicken Salad, 246
Penne with Chicken and Vegetables,
   44
Pesto Chicken Pita, 366
Roasted Chicken, 393

Roasted Red Pepper and Goat
   Cheese-Stuffed Chicken, 413
Spinach and Pine Nut-Stuffed
   Chicken, 97
Tasty "Fried" Chicken, 265
Teriyaki Chicken, 373
Thai-Spiced Roasted Chicken with
   Potatoes, 314
Toasted Almond Chicken Salad
   Sandwich, 333

Couscous

Chicken Couscous Salad, 298
Curried Eggplant Couscous, 260
Mediterranean Couscous, 234

Desserts

Apple Crisp, 359
Banana Chocolate Chip Bread, 35
Banana Split Cake, 215
Caramel Brownie Sundae, 143
Cherry Tarts, 251
Chocolate Mousse Pie, 71
Cookie Ice Cream Pie, 323
Lemon Poppy Seed Bundt Cake,
   107
Pretzel and Strawberry Delight, 179
Raspberry Almond Layer Cake, 431
Sweet Potato Pie, 395
Tiramisu, 287

Fruit

Fruit Salad, 87
Fruit Salad with Yogurt Dressing, 377
Fruit Smoothies, 132
Fruit with Dip, 203
Grilled Fruit, 221
Melon Salad, 161
Pear Pecan Salad, 242
Pear Salad with Almonds, 70

About the
American Diabetes Association

The American Diabetes Association is the nation's leading voluntary health organization supporting diabetes research, information, and advocacy. Its mission is to prevent and cure diabetes and to improve the lives of all people affected by diabetes. The American Diabetes Association is the leading publisher of comprehensive diabetes information. Its huge library of practical and authoritative books for people with diabetes covers every aspect of self-care—cooking and nutrition, fitness, weight control, medications, complications, emotional issues, and general self-care.

To order American Diabetes Association books: Call 1-800-232-6733. Or log on to http://store.diabetes.org

To join the American Diabetes Association: Call 1-800-806-7801. www.diabetes.org/membership

For more information about diabetes or ADA programs and services: Call 1-800-342-2383. E-mail: AskADA@diabetes.org or log on to www.diabetes.org

To locate an ADA/NCQA Recognized Provider of quality diabetes care in your area: www.ncqa.org/dprp

To find an ADA Recognized Education Program in your area: Call 1-888-232-0822. www.diabetes.org/recognition/education.asp

To join the fight to increase funding for diabetes research, end discrimination, and improve insurance coverage: Call 1-800-342-2383. www.diabetes.org/advocacy

To find out how you can get involved with the programs in your community: Call 1-800-342-2383. See below for program Web addresses.

- *American Diabetes Month:* educational activities aimed at those diagnosed with diabetes—month of November. www.diabetes.org/ADM
- *American Diabetes Alert:* annual public awareness campaign to find the undiagnosed—held the fourth Tuesday in March. www.diabetes.org/alert
- *The Diabetes Assistance & Resources Program (DAR):* diabetes awareness program targeted to the Latino community. www.diabetes.org/DAR
- *African American Program:* diabetes awareness program targeted to the African American community. www.diabetes.org/africanamerican
- *Awakening the Spirit: Pathways to Diabetes Prevention & Control:* diabetes awareness program targeted to the Native American community. www.diabetes.org/awakening

To find out about an important research project regarding type 2 diabetes: www.diabetes.org/ada/research.asp

To obtain information on making a planned gift or charitable bequest: Call 1-888-700-7029. www.diabetes.org/ada/plan.asp

To make a donation or memorial contribution: Call 1-800-342-2383. www.diabetes.org/ada/cont.asp